Handbook of Juvenile Idiopathic Arthritis

Handbook of Juvenile Idiopathic Arthritis

Editor: Dave Santiago

AMERICAN
MEDICAL PUBLISHERS
www.americanmedicalpublishers.com

AMERICAN
MEDICAL PUBLISHERS
www.americanmedicalpublishers.com

Cataloging-in-Publication Data

Handbook of juvenile idiopathic arthritis / edited by Dave Santiago.
p. cm.
Includes bibliographical references and index.
ISBN 978-1-63927-421-5
1. Rheumatoid arthritis in children. 2. Rheumatism in children. 3. Pediatric rheumatology.
I. Santiago, Dave.
RJ482.A77 H36 2022
618.927 227--dc23

American Medical Publishers,
41 Flatbush Avenue,
1st Floor, New York,
NY 11217, USA

ISBN 978-1-63927-421-5 (Hardback)

Contents

Preface

Juvenile idiopathic arthritis (JIA) is an arthritis which occurs in children and adolescents. It is a noninfective, autoimmune, inflammatory disease of the joints, commonly occurring in children between the ages of 1 and 6. JIA often presents nonspecific symptoms initially such as reduced physical activity, lethargy and poor appetite. Its first noticeable manifestation may be limping. Children may become quite ill with flu-like symptoms. Persistent swelling around the knee, wrist, ankle and the joints of the hands and feet is a clinical manifestation of the condition. The diagnosis of JIA is difficult to establish as the symptoms can indicate other causes. Therefore, often times, a combination of blood tests, X-rays, analysis of the fluid from the joint and clinical presentation are done for making a correct diagnosis. The goal of therapy in JIA is to enable the child to regain a normal level of physical and social activity. This is done with physical therapy, social support and pain management strategies. Children may also be treated with intra-articular corticosteroid injections and nonsteroidal anti-inflammatory drugs. This book elucidates the causes, symptoms and pathophysiology of juvenile idiopathic arthritis in a comprehensive manner. It strives to provide a fair idea about the modern practices in the management of JIA. A number of latest researches have been included to keep the readers up-to-date with the global concepts in this medical condition.

All of the data presented henceforth, was collaborated in the wake of recent advancements in the field. The aim of this book is to present the diversified developments from across the globe in a comprehensible manner. The opinions expressed in each chapter belong solely to the contributing authors. Their interpretations of the topics are the integral part of this book, which I have carefully compiled for a better understanding of the readers.

At the end, I would like to thank all those who dedicated their time and efforts for the successful completion of this book. I also wish to convey my gratitude towards my friends and family who supported me at every step.

Editor

1

Radiographic damage in hands and wrists of patients with juvenile idiopathic arthritis after 29 years of disease duration

Anne M. Selvaag[1*], Eva Kirkhus[2,3], Lena Törnqvist[2,4], Vibke Lilleby[1], Hanne A. Aulie[1,5] and Berit Flatø[1,3]

Abstract

Background: There are few studies on radiographic outcome after long-term disease duration in juvenile idiopathic arthritis (JIA). We wanted to evaluate 29-year radiographic outcome in hands/wrists and predictors of damage in patients with long-term active JIA.

Methods: Patients diagnosed from 1980 to 1985, who had active disease at 15-, 23- or 29-year follow-up and arthritis in the wrists during the disease course, were reexamined with radiographs of hands/wrists. We used the adapted version of the Sharp van der Heijde (aSvdH) score and Carpal Height Ratio (CHR) to evaluate radiographic outcome.

Results: Sixty patients, mean age 38 years, were reexamined at median 29-year follow-up. 33 patients (55%) had an aSvdH score >0, median score was 4.0 (range 0–313), and 25% of the scores were high (≥53). Most patients with radiographic damage (88%) had both erosions and JSN. 52% of the patients had damage in the wrists, 43% in the MCP joints and 40% in the PIP joints.
The CHR correlated strongly with the aSvdH. Both scores had high correlations with the Juvenile Arthritis Damage Index and the number of joints with limited range of motion (LROM) (r_s = -0.688 to 0.743, $p \leq 0.001$). The aSvdH correlated weakly with measures of disease activity.
The number of joints with LROM, ESR and the HAQ disability score at 15 years and HLAB27 positivity predicted the aSvdH score and the CHR at 29-year follow-up.

Conclusions: The majority of patients with long-term active JIA had modest radiographic damage, but more frequently in wrists than in fingers. The radiographic scores correlated well with measures of disease damage. Restricted mobility in joints at 15 years was the most important predictor of radiographic damage at 29 years.

Keywords: Radiography, Juvenile idiopathic arthritis, Follow-up studies, Disease progression, Prognosis, Risk factors, Longitudinal studies

Background

Juvenile idiopathic arthritis (JIA) is a chronic inflammatory autoimmune disease which affects the joints of a child. This chronic inflammation can cause growth disturbances, joint space narrowing (JSN) and erosions in the joints. Patients with a polyarticular disease course have the highest probability of attaining joint destructions [1].

Until recently a standard for radiographic assessment in JIA did not exist. Several methods have been suggested and evaluated [2–6]. One has looked for an index joint which could represent the radiographic status of a child with JIA, and found that the joints most often affected in polyarticular disease are the hands and wrists [1, 7–9].

Recently an adapted version of the Sharp/van der Heijde (aSvdH) score has been developed for radiographic scoring of patients with JIA [10]. It has proved to be reliable, has shown good construct validity and is capable of detecting radiographic progression [10]. In most late studies on radiographic outcome in patients with adult rheumatoid arthritis (RA), the method of Sharp and van der Heijde is frequently applied with a

* Correspondence: anselv@ous-hf.no
[1]Department of Rheumatology, Oslo University Hospital, Rikshospitalet, Post-box 4950 Nydalen, 0424 Oslo, Norway

focus on hands and feet. We therefore chose to use the aSvdH method to score radiographs of hands/wrists in our adult JIA group.

The Poznanski score, an expression of damage in the carpal area, has been used in several studies of radiological damage of hands/wrists in JIA [5, 6, 11, 12]. The Poznanski score is dependent on a growth plate in the distal radius and thus not suitable for adults. However, the Carpal Height Ratio (CHR) has some similarities with the Poznanski score, assesses carpal damage and is applicable in adults [13, 14].

Nutritional factors which influence mineral homeostasis, differentiation of the osteoblasts and the immune system, such as vitamin D and vitamin A, have not previously been included in long-term studies of radiographic outcome in JIA [15, 16].

There is a lack of long-term radiographic outcome studies of adult patients with JIA. The aim of our study was to describe radiographic damage in hands/wrists of patients with long-term active JIA after 29 years of disease duration, by applying the aSvdH score and the CHR in these patients. We also wanted to assess correlations between radiographic outcome and disease variables after 29 years and evaluate possible predictors of radiographic outcome.

Methods

Patients

A total of 260 patients with juvenile idiopathic arthritis (JIA), first time referred to Oslo University Hospital, Rikshospitalet from 1980 to 1985, were reexamined clinically after median 15 years of disease duration and by mailed questionnaires after median 23 years [17, 18]. A total of 176 of these patients were assessed with questionnaires after median 29.6 years [19]. Those who had signs of active disease either at 15, 23 or 29.6 years came to an additional clinical examination. Long-term active disease was defined as having active disease at 15-year follow-up or later. Of the 90 patients examined with long-term active disease, 60 patients (67%) had a history of previous or present arthritis in the wrists and underwent radiographs of hands/wrists.

The patients were classified according to the International League of Associations for Rheumatology (ILAR) criteria for JIA after 15 years of disease duration [18, 20]. Data from baseline was available to fulfil the criteria. Disease onset was defined as the day the physician diagnosed the arthritis.

The study was approved by the Regional Committee for Medical and Health Research Ethics. Written informed consent was obtained from all the participants according to the Declaration of Helsinki.

Clinical examination

The patients were examined by one of three pediatric rheumatologists at follow-up (BF, VL, AMS). The clinical examination included registration of number of joints with swelling, tenderness and limited range of motion (LROM), number of active joints (swelling or both tenderness and LROM), and physician's global assessment of disease activity [on a 10 cm Visual Analogue Scale (VAS), where 0 means no disease activity and 10 means very severe disease activity].

We used the Juvenile Arthritis Damage Index (JADI) to assess clinical damage, the Health Assessment Questionnaire (HAQ) and the Juvenile Arthritis Disease Activity Score (JADAS-71) to evaluate physical disability and disease activity and the Medical Outcome Study 36-item Short Form Health Survey (SF-36) to assess quality of life [21–24]. The preliminary criteria for remission in select categories of JIA was applied as described in a previous study on the same cohort [19].

Blood samples were drawn after an overnight fast. Erythrocyte sedimentation rate (ESR), C-reactive protein (CRP), rheumatoid factor (RF) IgM, anti-cyclic citrullinated peptides (anti-CCP) and antinuclear antibody (ANA) were analysed by standard methods. Vitamin A was measured by ultra high-performance liquid chromatography with UV detection and 25-hydroxy vitamin D was measured by liquid chromatography–tandem mass spectrometry.

Radiographic examinations

Conventional radiographs of the hand/wrist in the posteroanterior view, digital technique, were assessed in consensus by two musculoskeletal radiologists experienced in radiology of children with rheumatic diseases (EK, LT). The aSvdH method was used to score the radiographs of the hands/wrists [10]. The score is based on the assessment of joint space narrowing in 15 areas and bone erosions or deformity in 21 areas, on a 0–4 and a 0–5 point severity scale, respectively. Bone erosions and deformity were considered as equivalent. The total aSvdH score is calculated as the sum of the scores for JSN (range 0–120) and erosion (range 0–210) and ranges from 0 to 330. We defined a score above the 75-percentile as a high score/severe damage.

The CHR was calculated as the ratio between the carpal height (measured between the base of metacarpal III and the distal radial articular surface, measured along the axis of metacarpal III) and the length of metacarpal III [13]. The average CHR in normal controls (Belgian volunteers) has been found to be 0.52 ± 0.07 [14].

Six patients had signs of previous operations (prosthesis and/or arthrodesis) in joints scored by the aSvdH method and these joints were given the highest erosion and JSN sores.

Thus we obtained complete aSvdH scores for all the patients. CHR could not be scored in 7 patients due to joint fusion or prosthesis in the third carpometacarpal joint or in the third metacarpophalangeal (MCP) joint.

Statistical analyses

The differences between 2 patient groups were analyzed by t tests for continuous normality distributed data, Mann–Whitney U test for non-normality distributed data and χ^2 for frequencies. Because of non-normality distribution, we used the Kruskal-Wallis test to analyze differences in the aSvdH scores across the JIA categories. We used a one way analysis of variance with Bonferroni correction to look for differences in CHR between JIA categories. Spearman's correlation coefficient (r_s) was used for non-normality distributed variables.

Missing data was observed in up to 7% of all variables except for JADAS-71 (10%) and CHR scores (12%). Missing data was replaced by median substitution except for CHR scores which were replaced by the worst recorded CHR as missing scores were due to bone damage in the wrists which made it impossible to score.

Initial univariate linear regression analyses tested the relation between patient characteristics, HLA alleles, disease variables at baseline, core set variables at 15-year follow-up and aSvdH or CHR scores at 29 years [25]. Subsequent multivariate linear regression analyses were used to identify a set of statistically significant predictors, where variables with a p value <0.05 in the univariate tests were analyzed as possible predictors. Highly intercorrelated independent variables (r >0.7) were avoided. Backward and forward regression models were used.

For all analyses, p values <0.05 (2 tailed tests) were considered statistically significant. All analyses were performed on the SPSS software program (SPSS Inc., Chicago, IL, USA) version 21.0.

Results

Patients

Out of the original cohort of 260 patients, 60 patients with long-term active JIA and a history of previous or present arthritis in the wrists underwent radiographs of the hands and wrist joints after median 29.4 years (range 26–38) of disease duration (Fig. 1). We missed one patient, who had swelling in the wrist and two proximal interphalangeal (PIP) joints at 29 years, but underwent no radiographs of the hands, thus not included in the study. The 60 patients had significantly more affected wrists both at 6 months and 15-year follow-up compared to those 200 not examined ($p \leq 0.001$). Physician's global, number of active joints, number of joints with LROM, HAQ, SF-36 PCS and patient's global were all significantly worse at 15-year follow-up in the study group than in the 200 patients not examined ($p \leq 0.05$, data not shown).

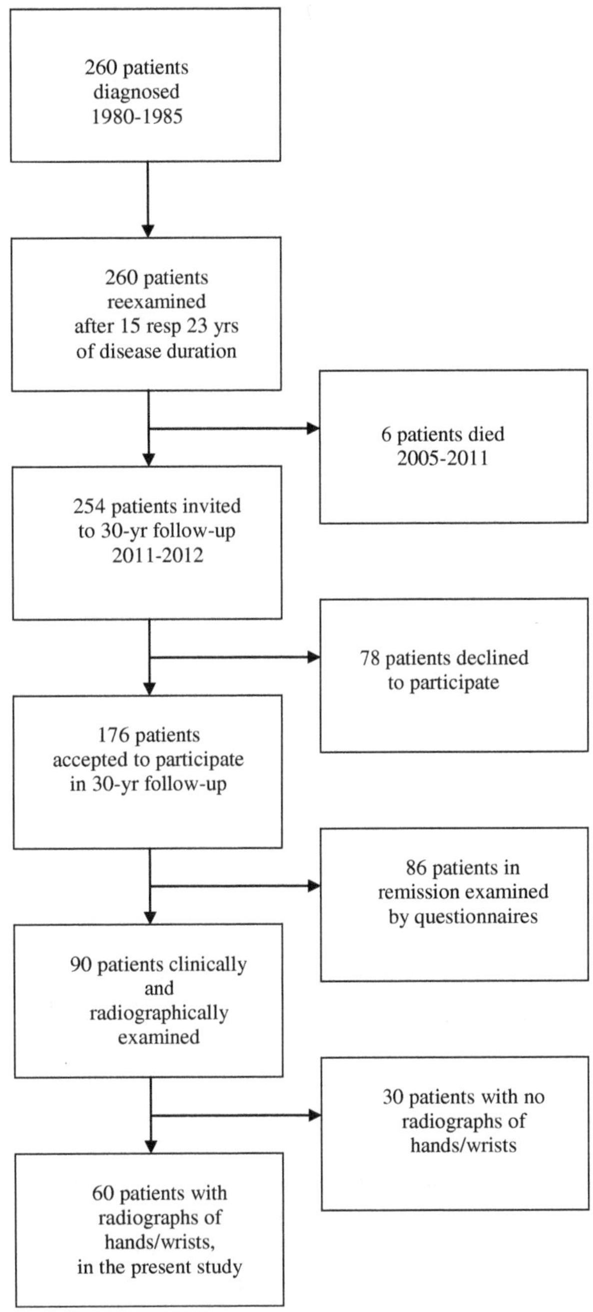

Fig. 1 Flow chart of how the 60 patients were selected from the original cohort of 260 patients

Table 1 shows a description of the patient group. The patients had a median age of 38.2 years (range 30–45) and 70% were female. In general patients had modest disease activity (median 0 swollen joints, 4 joints with LROM, 0 active joints), but 48 patients (80%) had active disease and only 12 patients (20%) were in remission off medication at 29-year follow-up. Four patients (7%) were

Table 1 Demographic and clinical characteristics of 60 patients with JIA after 29 years of disease duration

Characteristics	Value
Age, years	38.2 (30–45)
Female	42 (70)
Disease duration, years	29.4 (26–38)
Number of swollen joints	0 (0–12)
Number of tender joints	1 (0–16)
Number of joints with LROM	4 (0–56)
Number of active joints	0 (0–13)
PGA, VAS cm	1.5 (1–7.6)
Patient's global well-being, VAS cm	2.0 (1–5.9)
HAQ	0.5 (0–1.6)
JADAS	4.8 (0.2–27.1)
JADI total	6 (0–73)
CRP, mg/l	2.0 (0–38)
ESR, mm/h	6.0 (2–60)
Vitamin A µmol/L	1.6 (0.9–2.4)
Vitamin D nmol/L	64 (26–100)
Patients in remission off medication	12 (20)
Patients with inactive disease on medication	8 (13)
Patients with persistently active disease	40 (67)
Patients on sDMARDs	19 (32)
Patients on biological immunosuppressants	21 (35)
Patients on glucocorticosteroids	6 (10)
Employed[a]	46 (77)

Numbers are median (range) or number (%). [a]Employed is full or part time
LROM limited range of motion, *PGA* physician's global assessment of disease activity, *JADAS* juvenile arthritis disease activity score, *JADI* juvenile arthritis damage index, *sDMARDs* synthetic disease-modifying anti-rheumatic drugs

RF IgM-positive, 6 patients (10%) were anti-CCP-positive and 19 (32%) were ANA positive.

Radiographic scores of the hand and wrist after 29 years

Thirty three patients (55%) had radiographic damage (aSvdH > 0), 9 patients (15%) had aSvdH scores between 1 and 20, 9 patients (15%) had aSvdH scores between 21 and 52, and 15 (25%) had aSvdH scores ≥53 (range 53–313).

The aSvdH scores of the radiographs of hands/wrists were median 4 (range 0–313), and the scores of erosions and JSN were 1 (range 0–205) and 3 (range 0–110), respectively (Table 2). Patients with systemic or polyarticular RF-positive JIA had the highest frequency of damage. Patients with polyarticular RF-positive JIA also showed the highest aSvdH scores (median 222, range 0–313) (Table 2 and Fig. 2). Their scores were significantly higher than the scores from patients with polyarticular RF-negative JIA (median 22, $p = 0.038$), extended oligoarticular JIA (median 3, $p = 0.028$), enthesitis related arthritis (ERA) (median 0, $p = 0.019$) and psoriatic arthritis (PsA) (median 1, $p = 0.028$). Likewise, patients with polyarticular RF-positive JIA had significantly worse erosion and JSN scores (median 127 and 95, respectively) than those with polyarticular RF-negative JIA, extended oligoarticular JIA, ERA and PsA ($p \leq 0.05$). The aSvdH scores were also significantly worse in anti-CCP-positive patients compared to anti-CCP-negative (mean 238 vs 2, $p = 0.001$).th=tlb=

We found that 2 patients (3%) had only erosions, 2 patients (3%) had only JSN, 29 patients (48%) had both erosions and JSN (scores > 0) and 27 patients (45%) had no radiographic damage. The total erosion score correlated with the total JSN score ($r_s = 0.945$, $p < 0.001$) and the erosion scores in right and left hand correlated with the respective JSN scores ($r_s = 0.950$ and $r_s = 0.897$, respectively, $p < 0.001$).

When dividing radiographic damage into carpal area, MCP and PIP joints, we found that 31 patients (52%) had damage in the carpal area, 26 (43%) had in MCP joints and 24 (40%) had damage in PIP joints ($p < 0.001$).

The mean CHR was 0.49 ± 0.08 (Table 3). The patients with polyarticular RF-positive JIA had significantly lower CHR than patients with polyarticular RF-negative JIA, persistent oligoarticular JIA, extended oligoarticular JIA, ERA and PsA ($p \leq 0.005$ for all). Patients with systemic JIA had significantly lower CHR than patients with persistent oligoarticular JIA, ERA and PsA ($p < 0.05$). Eight patients had a mean score ≤0.38. The mean CHR correlated significantly with aSvdH scores ($r_s = -0{,}779$ $p < 0.001$).

The relation between radiographic scores and measures of disease activity and damage

After 29 years, the total aSvdH, erosion and JSN scores correlated strongly with JADI scores and the number of joints with LROM ($r_s = 0.659$ to 0.721, $p < 0.001$, Table 4). The CHR had also a high correlation with JADI scores and joints with LROM ($r_s = -0.660$ to-0.645, $p < 0.001$). The aSvdH score had weak correlations with JADAS-71 and CRP ($r_s = 0.266$ to 0.268, $p < 0.05$). The erosion and JSN scores correlated with HAQ ($r_s = 0.278$ and $r_s = 0.259$, respectively, $p < 0.05$). All the radiographic scores of the hands/wrists had a weak to moderate correlation with vitamin A levels ($r_s = -0.299$ to 0.430, $p < 0.05$). Vitamin D levels did not correlate consistently with any of the scores, nor did the number of swollen, tender or active joins, pain, ESR, well-being or variables on smoking habits.

The aSvdH score for those in remission at 29 years was significantly lower than the score for those with active disease [median 0 (range 0–45) vs median 11.5 (range 0–313), $p = 0.038$]. When analysing JSN scores separately, there was a significantly lower JSN score in

Table 2 The aSvdH score in hands and wrists of patients with JIA at 29-year follow-up

JIA categories	No. of patients	No. of patients with a score > 0	Total aSvdH score	Erosion score	JSN score	JADI Articular damage	JADI Extra-articular damage	JADI Total damage
Total	60 (100)	33 (55)	4 (0–313)	1 (0–205)	3 (0–110)	5 (0–68)	1 (0–7)	6 (0–73)
Systemic arthritis	3 (5)	3 (100)	45 (28–121)	25 (10–75)	20 (18–46)	13 (8–24)	1 (0–2)	13 (9–26)
Polyarticular RF-negative	11 (18)	8 (61)	22 (0–131)	5 (0–76)	8 (0–69)	8 (0–36)	1 (0–2)	6 (0–38)
Polyarticular RF-positive	5 (8)	4 (80)	222 (0–313)[a]	127 (0–205)[b]	95 (0–108)[b]	30 (0–68)	1 (0–5)	31 (0–73)
Persistent oligoarticular	5 (8)	1 (20)	0 (0–3)	0 (0–1)	0 (0–2)	0	1 (0–3)	1 (0–3)
Extended oligoarticular	10 (17)	5 (50)	3 (0–95)	0 (0–56)	3 (0–39)	7 (0–24)	1 (0–3)	8 (0–24)
Enthesitis related arthritis	13 (22)	5 (38)	0 (0–117)	0 (0–69)	0 (0–48)	3 (8–28)	1 (0–3)	5 (0–30)
Psoriatic arthritis	10 (17)	5 (50)	1 (0–115)	1 (0–68)	0 (0–47)	3 (0–42)	0 (0–2)	3 (0–42)
Undifferentiated arthritis	3 (5)	2 (67)	31 (0–308)	25 (0–128)	6 (0–110)	7 (2–43)	4 (0–7)	11 (2–50)

Numbers are median (range) or number (%). [a]Significantly different from scores in patients with polyarticular RF-negative JIA, extended oligoarticular JIA, enthesitis related arthritis and psoriatic arthritis (all $p < 0.05$). [b]Significantly different from scores in patients with polyarticular RF-negative JIA, persistent oligoarticular JIA, extended oligoarticular JIA, enthesitis related arthritis and psoriatic arthritis (all $p < 0.05$). *aSvdH* adapted Sharp van der Heijde, *JSN* joint space narrowing, *JADI* juvenile arthritis damage index

those in remission compared to those with active disease [median 0 (range 0–20) vs median 6 (range 0–110), $p = 0.023$]. We found the same tendency for erosions, but the difference was not statistically significant ($p = 0.054$).

At 15-year follow-up, 53 (88%) of the 60 patients had used median 2.5 (range 1–7) different synthetic(s) DMARDs during their disease course (data not shown). At 29 years, 33 (69%) out of total 48 patients with active disease, used sDMARDs, biological immunosuppressants and/or prednisolone. When comparing these patients with those not treated with sDMARDs, biological immunosuppressants and/or prednisolone ($n = 15$), those on treatment had significantly higher aSvdH scores [median 28 (range 0–313) vs median 0 (range 0–113), $p = 0.014$], but there were no significant differences in disease activity measures (ESR, CRP, number of active joints, joints with

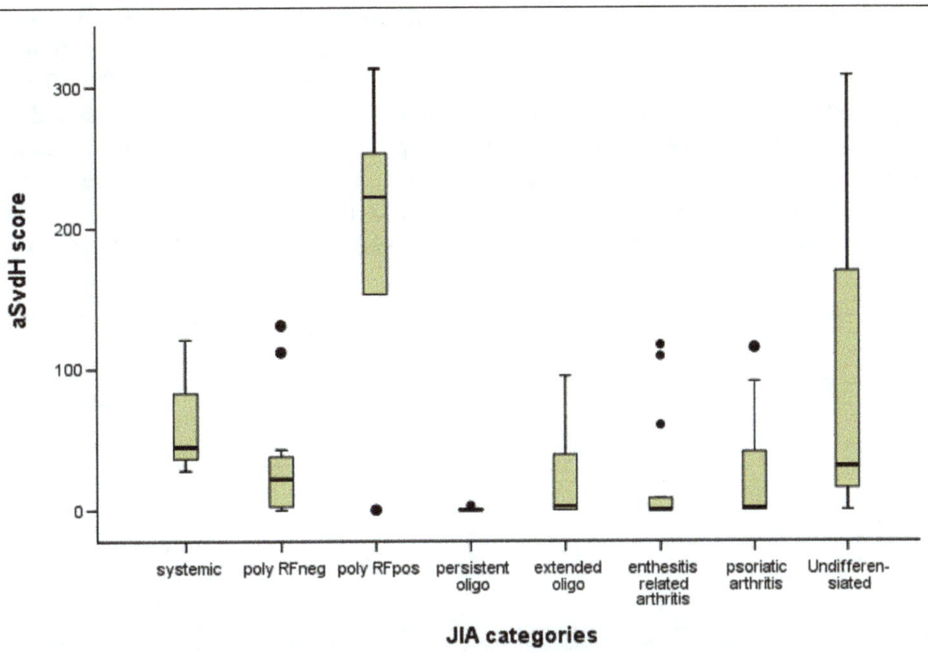

Fig. 2 The distribution of the aSvdH scores according to JIA category. aSvdH = adapted Sharp van der Heijde, RF = rheumatoid factor

Table 3 The CHR of patients with JIA at 29-year follow-up

JIA categories	No. of patients	CHR Right	CHR Left	Mean CHR
Total	60 (100)	0.52 (0.31–.64)	0.52 (0.31–0.63)	0.49 (0.08)
Systemic arthritis	3 (5)	0.32 (0.31–0.48)	0.34 (0.31–0.48)	0.37 (0.09)[a]
Polyarticular RF-negative	11 (18)	0.51 (0.43–0.57)	0.51 (0.31–0.59)	0.50 (0.05)
Polyarticular RF-positive	5 (8)	0.31 (0.31–0.53)	0.31 (0.31–0.53)	0.35 (0.10)[b]
Persistent oligoarticular	5 (8)	0.56 (0.52–0.58)	0.56 (0.52–0.56)	0.55 (0.02)
Extended oligoarticular	10 (17)	0.50 (0.31–0.55)	0.51 (0.47–0.56)	0.50 (0.04)
Enthesitis related arthritis	13 (22)	0.55 (0.42–0.64)	0.54 (0.31–0.62)	0.54 (0.06)
Psoriatic arthritis	10 (17)	0.52 (0.32–0.62)	0.52 (0.45–0.63)	0.52 (0.06)
Undifferentiated arthritis	3 (5)	0.40 (0.31–0.53)	0.40 (0.31–0.58)	0.42 (0.12)

Numbers are median (range), number (%) or mean (SD). [a]Significantly different from scores in patients with persistent oligoarticular arthritis, enthesitis related arthritis and psoriatic arthritis ($p < 0.05$). [b]Significantly different from scores in patients with polyarticular RF-negative JIA, persistent oligoarticular JIA, extended oligoarticular JIA, enthesitis related arthritis and psoriatic arthritis ($p \leq 0.005$). *CHR* carpal height ratio

LROM, patient's and physician's global assessment). There were no significant differences between aSvdH score or CHR in those employed versus those not employed (data not shown).

Predictors of radiographic scores from clinical variables at baseline and 15 years

All the core set variables from 15-year follow-up (except patient's global assessment of well-being), HLA-DR4, HLA-B27, onset and course type were associated with the aSvdH scores and CHR after 29 years (Table 5). In a multivariate linear regression analysis a higher number of joints with LROM and ESR from 15-year follow-up, predicted a higher aSvdH score at 29-year follow-up, $R^2 = 65\%$. The number of joints with LROM and HAQ at 15 years and HLA-B27 positivity were predictors of the mean CHR at 29 years, $R^2 = 51\%$.

Discussion

In the present study of 60 patients with long-term active JIA and clinical arthritis in the wrist during their disease course, more than half of these patients had radiographic damage measured by the aSvdH score in the hands/wrists after 29 years. The damage was modest in most patients, but 25% had severe damage. Patients with polyarticular RF-positive or anti-CCP-positive JIA had the worst damage. The majority of patients with radiographic damage had both erosions and JSN. Most damage occurred in the carpus area compared to the rest of the hand. Both the radiographic scores correlated strongly with other measures of disease damage at 29-year follow-up. The number of joints with LROM at 15 years was the most important predictor of the radiographic scores after 29 years of disease duration.

We found that 55% of the patients with long-term active disease and previous or present arthritis in the wrist had developed radiographic damage in the hands/wrists. There are few studies on radiographic long-term outcome in JIA patients, and reports of radiographic outcome especially in hands/wrists are even more scarce. A study from the sixties reported presence of erosions in hands/wrists of 68% of patients with juvenile rheumatoid arthritis (JRA) after 18 years [26]. The majority of their patients had polyarticular disease and 28% of them were RF-positive. Damage in this study refers to erosions only which is not comparable to the aSvdH score. Another study reported radiographic damage in hands/wrists in 79% of patients with polyarticular JIA (54% RF-positive)

Table 4 Correlations between radiographic scores and measures of disease damage and disease activity at 29-year follow-up

Variables	aSvdH scores 4.0 (0–313)	Erosion scores 1.0 (0–205)	JSN scores 3.0 (0–110)	Mean CHR 0.52 (0.31–0.63)
JADI total	0.706[a]	0.721[a]	0.714[a]	−0.660[a]
Joints with LROM	0.669[a]	0.659[a]	0.665[a]	−0.645[a]
JADAS	0.268[b]	0.255[b]	0.266[b]	NS
HAQ	NS	0.278[b]	0.259[b]	NS
CRP	0.266[b]	NS	0.273[b]	NS
Vitamin A	−0.272[b]	−0.275[b]	−0.299[b]	0.430[a]

Numbers are median scores (range) and Spearman's correlation coefficients. The radiographic scores did not correlate with the number of swollen, tender and active joints, pain, well-being, ESR or vitamin D. [a]$p \leq 0.001$, [b]$p < 0.05$. *aSvdH* adapted Sharp van der Heijde, *JSN* joint space narrowing, *CHR* carpal height ratio, *JADI* juvenile arthritis damage index, *LROM* limited range of motion, *JADAS* juvenile arthritis disease activity score, *NS* not significant

Table 5 Predictors of the aSvdH score and mean CHR at 29-year follow-up

	aSvdH				Mean CHR			
	Univariate analyses		Multivariate analyses		Univariate analyses		Multivariate analyses	
Variables assessed within 15 years:	B (95% CI)	*P* value	B (95% CI)	*P* value	B (95% CI)	*P* value	B (95% CI)	*P* value
Oligoarticular onset[a]	−48.1 (−85.3 to −10.9)	0.012			0.047 (0.005 to 0.090)	0.028		
Polyarticular course[b]	NA	NA			−0.060 (−0.120 to 0.000)	0.048		
HLA-DRB1*04 positive	67.2 (28.8 to 105.5)	0.001			NA	NA		
HLA-B27 positive	NA	NA			0.057 (0.011 to 0.102)	0.016	0.047 (0.013 to 0.082)	0.009
No. joints with LROM at 15 years[c]	5.9 (4.7 to 7.2)	<0.001	4.8 (3.4 to 6.3)	<0.001	−0.005 (−0.007 to−0.004)	<0.001	−0.004 (−0.006 to−0.002)	<0.001
ESR at 15 years, mm/h	2.6 (1.7 to 3.5)	<0.001	1.1 (0.3 to 1.9)	0.010	−0.002 (−0.003 to−0.001)	<0.001		
CRP at 15 years, mg/l	2.3 (1.2 to 3.3)	<0.001			NA	NA		
HAQ at 15 years	53.5 (22.2 to 84.7)	0.001			−0.065 (−0.100 to −0.031)	<0.001	−0.042 (−0.071 to −0.012)	0.007
Total time with active disease at 15-year follow-up, years	5.1 (1.0 to 9.1)	0.015			−0.007 (−0.011 to −0.002)	0.005		

[a]Oligoarticular onset: ≤ 4 active joints first 6 months, from all JIA categories except polyarticular JIA. [b]Polyarticular course: having in total ≥ 5 active joints after 6 months of disease, from all JIA categories except persistent oligoarticular JIA. [c]Number of joints with LROM at 15 years correlated highly ($r > 0.7$) with physician's global assessment and number of active joints at 15 years so only joints with LROM was chosen in the model. *aSvdH* adapted Sharp van der Heijde, *CHR* carpal height ratio, *LROM* limited range of motion, *NA* not applicable

after 13.3 years compared to 86% in patients with RA (79% RF-positive, not significant) after 11 years [27]. Other studies have reported worse radiographic outcome in patients with RA compared to patients with JIA [28].

Patients with polyarticular RF-positive JIA showed the most serious damage in hands/wrists and most of them had been through surgical operations in the wrist. It is well known that patients in this JIA category have the most aggressive disease and thus the most damage [19, 29–32]. Studies have shown that after 10–15 years of disease duration the most severely affected joints in RF-positive polyarticular juvenile arthritis were hands/wrists, and erosions were most commonly seen in these joints [1, 8, 27, 33]. We found that aSvdH scores were significantly worse in anti-CCP-positive patients compared to anti-CCP-negative patients, which is in harmony with other studies [34, 35].

In the present study most patients (29/33) with radiographic damage had both erosions and JSN after 29 years and very few had only erosions or JSN. Erosion and JSN scores correlated highly. There are few studies that have assessed this issue up to now in JIA [36]. One study found that erosions and JSN occurred at almost equal frequencies in patients with polyarticular JRA examined after 8 years of disease [32].

Patients had more often radiographic damage in the carpal area than in MCPs and PIPs in our study. A recent study supports this as they reported more damage in carpus and less in MCPs after up to 10 years of disease duration in patients with JIA and polyarticular course [36]. On the other hand, another study found damage in the MCP joints of all patients with polyarticular JIA after 13 years of disease duration and in 97% of the carpal area [27].

We chose to include the CHR to compare radiographic damage in the carpal area as measured by aSvdH and CHR. Both methods defined patients with polyarticular RF-positive JIA as having the worst damage and patients with systemic JIA as having the second worst damage. A study which applied the Poznanski method also found significant damage in the wrist of these two JIA categories [37]. The aSvdH scores correlated strongly with the CHR, in the same way as other studies have shown moderate to high correlations between the Sharp/aSvdH and the Poznanski score [6, 10]. Thus the aSvdH score performs well in scoring wrist damage in JIA.

We observed high correlations between the radiographic scores aSvdH or CHR and scores for disease damage (JADI and joints with LROM), and lower correlations for the disease activity score (JADAS-71). This is in harmony with other studies on JIA which have reported associations between radiographic measures and JADI and with the number of joints with LROM [6, 10, 11, 21, 32, 38]. Also in adult RA radiographic scores are reported to be associated with other measures of disease damage and disability [39, 40].

Eighty percent of our patients had active disease, but only 69% of them used sDMARDs, biological immunosuppressants and/or prednisolone. This may indicate that some of them are not optimally treated, but on the other hand they may have a mild disease course as the aSvdH scores of those not on advanced treatment were in the lower range.

There were persistent correlations between vitamin A levels and all the radiographic scores. Fifteen percent of the patients had vitamin A levels ≤ 1.2 μmol/L and this subgroup had the highest radiographic scores. Retinoic acid is known to be involved in proliferation and differentiation of osteoblasts and low levels of retinoic acid can have a harmful effect on bone metabolism [41, 42]. However, this correlation needs to be confirmed. There is a lot of research in the field of retinoic acid and its importance in regulation of T cells and other immune cells [43, 44] . Alternatively, our finding of an association with low vitamin A status may be connected to deficiency in immune cells and thus the inflammatory process and not directly on bone metabolism.

We found that the number of joints with LROM and ESR from 15-year follow-up were predictors of aSvdH after 29 years. This is supported by previous studies, which have found ESR as an important predictor for joint destruction [45, 46]. We have in an earlier 3-year follow-up study, revealed the number of joints with LROM as a predictor of radiographic changes [7]. Others have reported that continuing disease activity is a predictor of joint damage [47]. HLA-B27 positivity protected against radiographic damage measured as CHR. This seems to be explained by the fact that 11 out of 18 HLAB27 positive patients had ERA and they had less damage in the wrists as shown in Tables 2 and 3. Alternatively HLA-B27 represents a marker for ERA. When ERA patients were excluded from the analysis, HLA-B27 was no longer a predictor of CHR. On the other hand, a previous study found HLA-B27 positivity associated with worse radiographic outcome in JIA [9].

The strength of the study is the long-term follow-up over 29 years of this cohort that has been described in several publications [17–19, 46, 48]. There are however some limitations of the study. We have examined only patients with long-term active disease who also had current or previous clinical arthritis in the wrist joints, thus a selection of those with severe disease. Optimally we could have taken radiographs of all the patients, including those who went into remission before 15 years. We would have registered the progression of bone damage compared to previous radiographs, but these were unfortunately not available. There were few patients with persistent oligoarticular JIA, therefore their results must be interpreted with caution. The radiographic method we used, the aSvdH score, is evaluated for children with JIA, but we have used it in adults with JIA. However, the Sharp van der Heijde method is widely used in adults with RA and the main difference in this adapted version is the adding of locations in the carpal area in which patients with JIA have more changes than adults with RA [10]. Another limitation is that the JADAS is not validated for adults with JIA. On the other hand, we used the JADAS in a recent study and found that the JADAS correlated strongly with categories of disease activity in adult patients, but JADAS may capture some other aspects of the burden of disease like damage and overall well-being in adults [19].

We did not perform intra- and interrater reliability testing among raters of the radiographs. Our two raters agreed by consensus. The Sharp/Sharp van der Heijde method has previously been evaluated as having good reliability and reproducibility [6, 49], and a good inter- and intraobserver agreement has been demonstrated for the aSvdH in JIA [10].

Conclusions

In the present cohort of patients with prolonged active JIA and wrist involvement during 29 years of disease duration, we found that about half of the patients had radiographic damage in hands/wrists. Changes were modest for most patients, but one out of four had severe damage. Patients with JIA and arthritis in hands/wrist should be examined regularly with radiographs and especially patients who have joints with LROM. Our patients were diagnosed early in the methotrexate era. Patients nowadays receive more aggressive therapy and will most likely have better radiographic outcome in long-term follow-up than patients in the present study. Similar long-term radiographic outcome studies are needed to continually survey the effectiveness of the present medical regimes, and hopefully document improved outcomes compared to the present study in the future.

Abbreviations

ANA: Antinuclear antibody; anti-CCP: Anti-cyclic citrullinated peptides; aSvdH score: The adapted version of the Sharp van der Heijde score; CHR: Carpal height ratio; CRP: C-reactive protein; ERA: Enthesitis related arthritis; ESR: Erythrocyte sedimentation rate; HAQ: Health assessment questionnaire; HLA: Human leukocyte antigen; ILAR: International League of Associations for Rheumatology; JADAS: Juvenile arthritis disease activity score; JADI: Juvenile arthritis damage index; JIA: Juvenile idiopathic arthritis; JSN: Joint space narrowing; LROM: Limited range of motion; MCP: Metacarpophalangeal; PIP: Proximal interphalangeal; PsA: Psoriatic arthritis; RA: Rheumatoid arthritis; RF: Rheumatoid factor; sDMARDs: Synthetic disease-modifying anti-rheumatic drugs; SF-36: Medical outcome study 36-item short form health survey; VAS: Visual analogue scale

Acknowledgements

The authors thank Torhild Garen for assistance in data management, the Hormone Laboratory, Aker, for the analyses of vitamin D and the Department of Medical Biochemistry at Oslo University Hospital for the analyses of vitamin A.

Funding

The study was funded by the Norwegian Women's Public Health Association (H3/2012).

Authors' contributions

BF, EK, HAA and AMS contributed to the design and conception of the study. BF, VL, HAA, and AMS administered and examined the patients clinically. EK and LT scored the radiographs. AMS analyzed the data and drafted the manuscript. All authors revised the manuscript critically. All authors read and approved the final manuscript.

Competing interests

The authors declare that they have no competing interests.

Consent for publication

Not applicable.

Author details

[1]Department of Rheumatology, Oslo University Hospital, Rikshospitalet, Post-box 4950 Nydalen, 0424 Oslo, Norway. [2]Department of Radiology and Nuclear Medicine, Oslo University Hospital, Rikshospitalet, Oslo, Norway. [3]Institute of Clinical Medicine, Faculty of Medicine, University of Oslo, Oslo, Norway. [4]Present address: Department of Radiology, Linköping University, Linköping, Sweden. [5]Present address: Department of Internal Medicine, Diakonhjemmet Hospital, Oslo, Norway.

References

1. Ravelli A. The time has come to include assessment of radiographic progression in juvenile idiopathic arthritis clinical trials. J Rheumatol. 2008; 35:553–7.
2. van Rossum MA, Boers M, Zwinderman AH, van Soesbergen RM, Wieringa H, Fiselier TJ, et al. Development of a standardized method of assessment of radiographs and radiographic change in juvenile idiopathic arthritis: introduction of the Dijkstra composite score. Arthritis Rheum. 2005;52:2865–72.
3. Dale K, Paus AC, Laires K. A radiographic classification system in juvenile rheumatoid arthritis applied to the knee. Eur Radiol. 1994;4:27–32.
4. Poznanski AK, Hernandez RJ, Guire KE, Bereza UL, Garn SM. Carpal length in children–a useful measurement in the diagnosis of rheumatoid arthritis and some concenital malformation syndromes. Radiology. 1978;129:661–8.
5. Magni-Manzoni S, Rossi F, Pistorio A, Temporini F, Viola S, Beluffi G, et al. Prognostic factors for radiographic progression, radiographic damage, and disability in juvenile idiopathic arthritis. Arthritis Rheum. 2003;48:3509–17.
6. Rossi F, Di Dia F, Galipo O, Pistorio A, Valle M, Magni-Manzoni S, et al. Use of the Sharp and Larsen scoring methods in the assessment of radiographic progression in juvenile idiopathic arthritis. Arthritis Rheum. 2006;55:717–23.
7. Selvaag AM, Flato B, Dale K, Lien G, Vinje O, Smerdel-Ramoya A, et al. Radiographic and clinical outcome in early juvenile rheumatoid arthritis and juvenile spondyloarthropathy: a 3-year prospective study. J Rheumatol. 2006;33:1382–91.
8. Mason T, Reed AM, Nelson AM, Thomas KB, Patton A, Hoffman AD, et al. Frequency of abnormal hand and wrist radiographs at time of diagnosis of polyarticular juvenile rheumatoid arthritis. J Rheumatol. 2002;29:2214–8.
9. van Rossum MA, Zwinderman AH, Boers M, Dijkmans BA, van Soesbergen RM, Fiselier TJ, et al. Radiologic features in juvenile idiopathic arthritis: a first step in the development of a standardized assessment method. Arthritis Rheum. 2003;48:507–15.
10. Ravelli A, Ioseliani M, Norambuena X, Sato J, Pistorio A, Rossi F, et al. Adapted versions of the Sharp/van der Heijde score are reliable and valid for assessment of radiographic progression in juvenile idiopathic arthritis. Arthritis Rheum. 2007;56:3087–95.
11. Palmisani E, Solari N, Magni-Manzoni S, Pistorio A, Labo E, Panigada S, et al. Correlation between juvenile idiopathic arthritis activity and damage measures in early, advanced, and longstanding disease. Arthritis Rheum. 2006;55:843–9.

12. Aoki C, Inaba Y, Choe H, Kaneko U, Hara R, Miyamae T, et al. Discrepancy between clinical and radiological responses to tocilizumab treatment in patients with systemic-onset juvenile idiopathic arthritis. J Rheumatol. 2014; 41:1171–7.
13. Youm Y, McMurthy R, Flatt AE, Gillespie TE. Kinematics of the wrist. I. An experimental study of radial-ulnar deviation and flexion-extension. J Bone Joint Surg Am. 1978;60:423–31.
14. Feipel V, Rinnen D, Rooze M. Postero-anterior radiography of the wrist. Normal database of carpal measurements. Surg Radiol Anat. 1998;20:221–6.
15. Jeffery LE, Raza K, Hewison M. Vitamin D in rheumatoid arthritis-towards clinical application. Nat Rev Rheumatol. 2016;12:201–10.
16. Dadon Bar-El S, Reifen R. Vitamin A and the Epigenome. Crit Rev Food Sci Nutr. 2015. doi:10.1080/10408398.2015.1060940.
17. Flato B, Lien G, Smerdel A, Vinje O, Dale K, Johnston V, et al. Prognostic factors in juvenile rheumatoid arthritis: a case–control study revealing early predictors and outcome after 14.9 years. J Rheumatol. 2003;30:386–93.
18. Flato B, Hoffmann-Vold AM, Reiff A, Forre O, Lien G, Vinje O. Long-term outcome and prognostic factors in enthesitis-related arthritis: a case–control study. Arthritis Rheum. 2006;54:3573–82.
19. Selvaag AM, Aulie HA, Lilleby V, Flato B. Disease progression into adulthood and predictors of long-term active disease in juvenile idiopathic arthritis. Ann Rheum Dis. 2016;75:190–5.
20. Petty RE, Southwood TR, Manners P, Baum J, Glass DN, Goldenberg J, et al. International League of Associations for Rheumatology classification of juvenile idiopathic arthritis: second revision, Edmonton, 2001. J Rheumatol. 2004;31:390–2.
21. Viola S, Felici E, Magni-Manzoni S, Pistorio A, Buoncompagni A, Ruperto N, et al. Development and validation of a clinical index for assessment of long-term damage in juvenile idiopathic arthritis. Arthritis Rheum. 2005;52:2092–102.
22. Fries JF, Spitz P, Kraines RG, Holman HR. Measurement of patient outcome in arthritis. Arthritis Rheum. 1980;23:137–45.
23. Consolaro A, Ruperto N, Bazso A, Pistorio A, Magni-Manzoni S, Filocamo G, et al. Development and validation of a composite disease activity score for juvenile idiopathic arthritis. Arthritis Rheum. 2009;61:658–66.
24. Loge JH, Kaasa S, Hjermstad MJ, Kvien TK. Translation and performance of the Norwegian SF-36 Health Survey in patients with rheumatoid arthritis. I. Data quality, scaling assumptions, reliability, and construct validity. J Clin Epidemiol. 1998;51:1069–76.
25. Giannini EH, Ruperto N, Ravelli A, Lovell DJ, Felson DT, Martini A. Preliminary definition of improvement in juvenile arthritis. Arthritis Rheum. 1997;40: 1202–9.
26. Jeremy R, Schaller J, Arkless R, Wedgwood RJ, Healey LA. Juvenile rheumatoid arthritis persisting inot adulthood. Am J Med. 1968;45:419–34.
27. Elhai M, Bazeli R, Freire V, Feydy A, Drape JL, Quartier P, et al. Radiological peripheral involvement in a cohort of patients with polyarticular juvenile idiopathic arthritis at adulthood. J Rheumatol. 2013;40:520–7.
28. Koivuniemi R, Leirisalo-Repo M. Juvenile chronic arthritis in adult life: a study of long-term outcome in patients with juvenile chronic arthritis or adult rheumatoid arthritis. Clin Rheumatol. 1999;18:220–6.
29. Wallace CA, Huang B, Bandeira M, Ravelli A, Giannini EH. Patterns of clinical remission in select categories of juvenile idiopathic arthritis. Arthritis Rheum. 2005;52:3554–62.
30. Ringold S, Seidel KD, Koepsell TD, Wallace CA. Inactive disease in polyarticular juvenile idiopathic arthritis: current patterns and associations. Rheumatology (Oxford). 2009;48:972–7.
31. Guzman J, Oen K, Tucker LB, Huber AM, Shiff N, Boire G, et al. The outcomes of juvenile idiopathic arthritis in children managed with contemporary treatments: results from the ReACCh-Out cohort. Ann Rheum Dis. 2015;74:1854–60.
32. Oen K, Reed M, Malleson PN, Cabral DA, Petty RE, Rosenberg AM, et al. Radiologic outcome and its relationship to functional disability in juvenile rheumatoid arthritis. J Rheumatol. 2003;30:832–40.
33. Williams RA, Ansell BM. Radiological findings in seropositive juvenile chronic arthritis (juvenile rheumatoid arthritis) with particular reference to progression. Ann Rheum Dis. 1985;44:685–93.
34. Lipinska J, Brozik H, Stanczyk J, Smolewska E. Anticitrullinated protein antibodies and radiological progression in juvenile idiopathic arthritis. J Rheumatol. 2012;39:1078–87.
35. Omar A, Abo-Elyoun I, Hussein H, Nabih M, Atwa H, Gad S, et al. Anti-cyclic citrullinated peptide (anti-CCP) antibody in juvenile idiopathic arthritis (JIA): correlations with disease activity and severity of joint damage (a multicenter trial). Joint Bone Spine. 2013;80:38–43.
36. Giancane G, Pederzoli S, Norambuena X, Ioseliani M, Sato J, Gallo MC, et al. Frequency of radiographic damage and progression in individual joints in children with juvenile idiopathic arthritis. Arthritis Care Res (Hoboken). 2014; 66:27–33.
37. Ozawa R, Inaba Y, Mori M, Hara R, Kikuchi M, Higuchi R, et al. Definitive differences in laboratory and radiological characteristics between two subtypes of juvenile idiopathic arthritis: systemic arthritis and polyarthritis. Mod Rheumatol. 2012;22:558–64.
38. Susic GZ, Stojanovic RM, Pejnovic NN, Damjanov NS, Soldatovic II, Jablanovic DB, et al. Analysis of disease activity, functional disability and articular damage in patients with juvenile idiopathic arthritis: a prospective outcome study. Clin Exp Rheumatol. 2011;29:337–44.
39. Bejia I, Braham R, Said M, Salem KB, Touzi M, Bergaoui N. Reliability of the rheumatoid arthritis articular damage score in Tunisian patients. Clin Rheumatol. 2005;24:593–4.
40. Odegard S, Landewe R, van der Heijde D, Kvien TK, Mowinckel P, Uhlig T. Association of early radiographic damage with impaired physical function in rheumatoid arthritis: a ten-year, longitudinal observational study in 238 patients. Arthritis Rheum. 2006;54:68–75.
41. Bosetti M, Sabbatini M, Calarco A, Borrone A, Peluso G, Cannas M. Effect of retinoic acid and vitamin D3 on osteoblast differentiation and activity in aging. J Bone Miner Metab. 2016;34:65–78.
42. Tanaka K, Tanaka S, Sakai A, Ninomiya T, Arai Y, Nakamura T. Deficiency of vitamin A delays bone healing process in association with reduced BMP2 expression after drill-hole injury in mice. Bone. 2010;47:1006–12.
43. Brown CC, Esterhazy D, Sarde A, London M, Pullabhatla V, Osma-Garcia I, et al. Retinoic acid is essential for Th1 cell lineage stability and prevents transition to a Th17 cell program. Immunity. 2015;42:499–511.
44. Chatterjee A, Gogolak P, Blottiere HM, Rajnavolgyi E. The impact of ATRA on shaping human myeloid cell responses to epithelial cell-derived stimuli and on T-lymphocyte polarization. Mediators Inflamm. 2015. doi:10.1155/2015/579830.
45. Guillaume S, Prieur AM, Coste J, Job-Deslandre C. Long-term outcome and prognosis in oligoarticular-onset juvenile idiopathic arthritis. Arthritis Rheum. 2000;43:1858–65.
46. Flato B, Smerdel A, Johnston V, Lien G, Dale K, Vinje O, et al. The influence of patient characteristics, disease variables, and HLA alleles on the development of radiographically evident sacroiliitis in juvenile idiopathic arthritis. Arthritis Rheum. 2002;46:986–94.
47. Gilliam BE, Chauhan AK, Low JM, Moore TL. Measurement of biomarkers in juvenile idiopathic arthritis patients and their significant association with disease severity: a comparative study. Clin Exp Rheumatol. 2008;26:492–7.
48. Aulie HA, Selvaag AM, Gunther A, Lilleby V, Molberg O, Hartmann A, et al. Arterial haemodynamics and coronary artery calcification in adult patients with juvenile idiopathic arthritis. Ann Rheum Dis. 2015;74:1515–21.
49. Boini S, Guillemin F. Radiographic scoring methods as outcome measures in rheumatoid arthritis: properties and advantages. Ann Rheum Dis. 2001;60: 817–27.

2

Predictors of the response to etanercept in patients with juvenile idiopathic arthritis without systemic manifestations within 12 months: results of an open-label, prospective study conducted at the National Scientific and Practical Center of Children's Health, Russia

Ekaterina I. Alexeeva[1,2,3*], Leyla S. Namazova-Baranova[1], Tatyana M. Bzarova[1,2], Saniya I. Valieva[1], Rina V. Denisova[1], Tatyana V. Sleptsova[1], Kseniya B. Isaeva[1], Alexandra M. Chomahidze[1], Nikolay I. Taibulatov[1], Anna N. Fetisova[1], Anna V. Karaseva[1] and Alexandr A. Baranov[1]

Abstract

Background: The aim of this study was to investigate the efficacy of etanercept treatment and to identify predictors of response to therapy within 12 months in patients with juvenile idiopathic arthritis (JIA) without systemic manifestations.

Methods: A total of 197 juvenile patients were enrolled in this study. Response to therapy was assessed using the ACRPedi 30/50/70/90 criteria, the Wallace criteria, and the Juvenile Arthritis Disease Activity Score 71 (JADAS-71). Univariate and multivariate logistic regression analyses were performed to identify potential baseline factors associated with treatment response in different JIA categories.

Results: One year after treatment initiation, 179 (90.9%) patients achieved ACRPedi30; 177 (89.8%) patients achieved ACRPedi50; 168 (85.3%) patients achieved ACRPedi70; and 135 (68.5%) patients achieved ACRPedi90 response. A total of 132 (67.0%) and 92 (46.7%) patients achieved inactive disease according to the Wallace criteria and the JADAS-71 cut-off point, respectively. Excellent response (achieving ACRPedi90 and clinically inactive disease according both to the Wallace criteria and the JADAS71 cut-off point) was associated with persistent oligoarticular JIA category, shorter disease duration before the start of etanercept, a lower number of DMARDs used before the introduction of etanercept, a lower number of joints with limited motion, and lower C-reactive protein at baseline. Poor response (failure to achieve ACR 70 or active disease according to both the Wallace criteria and JADAS71 even when ACR 70 was achieved) was associated with the polyarticular or enthesitis-related JIA categories, higher disease duration before the start of etanercept, and older age at disease onset.

(Continued on next page)

* Correspondence: alekatya@yandex.ru
[1]Federal State Autonomous Institution "National Scientific and Practical Center of Children's Health" Of the Ministry of Health of the Russian Federation, Moscow, Russia
[2]Federal State Autonomous Educational Institution of Higher Education I.M. Sechenov First Moscow State Medical University of the Ministry of Health of the Russian Federation, Moscow, Russia
Full list of author information is available at the end of the article

(Continued from previous page)

Conclusion: Almost half (45.7%) of the patients who initiated etanercept treatment achieved an excellent response (inactive disease and ACRPedi90) after 1 year. What may be novel is our finding that the response to etanercept therapy was strongly associated with the JIA category. The response to etanercept therapy was also associated with the disease duration before the start of etanercept treatment.

Keywords: Juvenile idiopathic arthritis, Anti-TNF treatment, Etanercept, Factors associated with treatment response

Background

Juvenile idiopathic arthritis (JIA) is among the most common autoimmune diseases of the musculoskeletal system in children [1, 2]. Its prevalence in Russia is 53.8 per 100,000 children [3]. For each of the 7 JIA categories, there are appropriate recommendations for initial therapy and guidelines for switching medications if they fail or cause serious adverse effects [4].

Searches for novel therapies and response predictors have been initiated because many patients exhibit disease progression and need subsequent treatment when receiving conventional treatments, including MTX [5].

The efficacy of etanercept, a TNFα inhibitor, in daily practice for JIA was confirmed in controlled clinical trials where at least 70% of patients in all categories except RF-positive polyarthritis achieved ACR Pedi 30 and at least 40% of patients in all categories achieved ACR70 [6–8]; CHAQ scores decreased in approximately 53% of patients after 12 weeks of treatment [9], and 41.8% of patients receiving long-term therapy with etanercept (approximately 2.5 years) achieved inactive disease according to the Wallace criteria [10]. Despite the growing use of biological agents that have made it possible for patients to achieve the ACR70 and ACR90 criteria, minimal disease activity and clinical remission still have not been achieved during etanercept treatment in a substantial proportion of cases [6].

Several observational studies with sample sizes ranging from 61 to 863 patients have been published with the aim of determining the factors associated with children's responses to etanercept treatment [6, 11, 12]. Based on the results of these studies, researchers have identified some factors potentially associated with a better response to etanercept treatment in various combinations: nonsystemic disease onset [13], younger age at disease onset [12, 13], shorter disease duration [6, 13], age at therapy initiation, lower disability scores at therapy initiation (CHAQ and VAS by Physician) [6, 13], higher erythrocyte sedimentation rate (ESR) [13], absence of wrist involvement [12], history of acute anterior uveitis [10], absence of concomitant steroid use [11, 13], and a smaller number of previously used DMARDs [6]. However, no reliable predictors of a good nor poor response to treatment with most drugs have been found because of a lack of consistency in data.

Most of the demographic, clinical, and laboratory characteristics of patients are also associated with the JIA category, defined according to the International League of Associations for Rheumatology (ILAR) classification, that was initially proposed to gather further information on the patterns of clinical presentation [14]. Both certain individual parameters and the comprehensive clinical presentation should be taken into account to create and clarify a reliable model for predicting disease progression and response to etanercept therapy. Further research and analysis of a large body of data are needed to identify the JIA category and clinical characteristics of an "ideal patient" for each modern drug.

Agreement among the conclusions derived from various local data is one of the main criteria for data reliability. There is a clear lack of studies conducted in Russia in the scientific literature. We initiated a prospective study at the Department of Rheumatology of the Scientific Centre for Children's Health (Moscow) in December 2009 to investigate the efficacy and safety of etanercept treatment, identify the predictors of response to therapy and define the optimal time and conditions for the initiation of etanercept therapy in patients with JIA without systemic manifestations.

Methods

Study design and patient enrolment

This open-label, prospective study was conducted at the Department of Rheumatology of the Scientific Centre for Children's Health, Russian Academy of Medical Sciences, Russia. The children enrolled in the study had taken etanercept between December 2009 and August 2014 and met the following eligibility criteria: ILAR criteria for JIA, no systemic symptoms, no signs of tuberculosis, and being naïve to etanercept before treatment. The study was conducted in compliance with the good clinical practice guidelines to ensure that the data design, implementation, and communication were reliable, that patients' rights were protected and that the integrity of subjects was maintained through maintaining the confidentiality of their data.

The study was approved by the local Ethics Committee of the Scientific Centre for Children's Health (protocol no. 36, dated October 16, 2008). All patients and their parents provided written informed consent in accordance with the principles of the Declaration of Helsinki, which included their consent for their data to be used in analyses and to be presented.

Treatment protocol and data collection

Etanercept was administered via subcutaneous injection at a dose of 0.4 mg per kg body weight (maximum single dose, 25 mg) twice a week. The following parameters were measured and collected at each follow-up point: the JIA disease activity score (JADAS71), physician global assessment of disease activity (0- to 100-mm Visual Analogue Scale, with 0 as the best score, phyVAS); the Childhood Health Assessment Questionnaire (CHAQ; range 0 – 3, with 0 being the best score) for patients or parents, including global assessment of well-being using the Visual Analogue Scale (patVAS); the number of active joints, swollen joints, painful joints, and joints with limited range of motion; erythrocyte sedimentation rate (ESR); C-reactive protein (CRP); and duration of morning stiffness in minutes.

Assessment of inactive disease

Response to therapy was assessed using the ACR Pedi criteria [7]. The ACR Pedi 30, 50, 70, and 90 response is defined as at least 30%, 50%, 70%, or 90% improvement in 3 or more variables of the JIA core set compared to the baseline, with no more than one variable worsening by more than 30%. We used the JADAS-71 cut-off point [15] and the modified Wallace criteria [16] (no active arthritis, no systemic manifestations, no uveitis, normal ESR (<20 mm/h), duration of morning stiffness ≤15 min, and the physician's global assessment of disease activity score indicating no disease activity (0 – 10 cm)).

We defined an excellent treatment response as inactive disease after 12 months (the Wallace criteria), achieving the JADAS71 cut-off point, and achieving the ACR 90. A poor treatment response was defined as a failure to achieve ACR 70 or inactive disease according to at least one of the Wallace criteria or the JADAS71 cut-off point, even if ACR 70 was achieved. The intermediate treatment response group comprised all patients not included in the excellent and poor treatment response groups.

Factors associated with treatment response according to JIA categories

The following potential baseline predictors of response to etanercept treatment were selected based on the literature data: demographic indicators (sex, age at disease onset, disease duration before initiation of etanercept therapy), indicators of disease activity (the number of affected joints; the CHAQ, phyVAS, and patVAS scores; duration of morning stiffness), previous therapy (amount of DMARDs and/or biologicals used), background therapy (oral glucocorticoids, NSAIDs, and sulfasalazine), and laboratory tests (ESR, CRP). Potential predictors were analysed for each of four ILAR categories (persistent oligoarthritis, extended oligoarthritis, rheumatoid factor-negative polyarthritis, and enthesitis-related arthritis).

Statistical analysis

The R Statistical Package (http://www.r-project.org) was used for calculations. Descriptive statistics were reported as absolute frequencies or as median values with IQR. Depending on the type of the processed data, we used either the Mann-Whitney U test, the Pearson's chi-squared test, or Fisher's exact test and the non-parametric Kruskal-Wallis analysis of variance by rank and median for multiple comparisons.

Univariate and multivariate logistic regression analyses were used to determine the significance of potential predictors of the response to etanercept treatment among baseline indicators (comparing excellent response to poor and intermediate response combined and comparing poor response to intermediate and excellent responses combined). Independent parameters for modelling were chosen based on statistical and clinical significance and correlations. The results are presented as adjusted odds ratios (OR; the OR for each covariate was adjusted to the effects of the other covariates) with 95% confidence intervals; P values were calculated.

All the reported P values were based on two-tailed significance tests; P values <0.05 were considered statistically significant. We used STATISTICA 7.0 software (StatSoft, Tulsa, USA) and RStudio software version 0.99.484 (Free Software Foundation, Inc., Boston, USA) with R packages version 3.2.2 (The R Foundation for Statistical Computing, Vienna, Austria) for the analyses.

Results

Baseline characteristics of the complete cohort

The study initially included 198 children with JIA who had begun etanercept therapy; 137 (69.2%) were females [Table 1]. One male patient withdrew early from the study because of a severe allergic reaction to etanercept. Hence, 197 children were enrolled in the efficacy analysis. Since there was only one patient (1; 0.51%) in each of the polyarticular RF positive and psoriatic arthritis groups, univariate and multivariate efficacy analyses could not be performed for these categories.

At baseline, the median patient age was 7.25 years (IQR 4 – 12 years), and the disease duration was 2.1 years (IQR 1 – 5 years). The median CHAQ score was 1.25 (IQR 0.5 – 1.875).

At baseline, 136 (69.0%) patients were receiving concomitant treatment with MTX; 10 (5.0%) were receiving concomitant treatment with oral steroids; 6 (3.0%) were receiving concomitant treatment with

Table 1 Characteristics of children with JIA starting treatment with etanercept (N = 197) at baseline

Characteristics	All patients (n = 197)	Persistent oligoarticular (n = 84)	Extended oligoarticular (n = 23)	Polyarticular RF negative (n = 64)	Enthesitis-related (n = 24)
Female, n (%)	137 (69.5)	68 (81.0)	16 (69.6)	46 (71.9)	5(20.8)^{d}
Age at JIA onset, median (IQR), years	3 (2 – 7)	2.3 (1.7 – 3.7)^{a}	2 (1.5 – 4)	3.25 (2 – 7.5)^{a}	9 (5 – 11.8)^{d}
Age at start of etanercept, median (IQR), years	7.25 (4 – 12)	5.1 (2.9 – 8.9)^{a}	7.5 (3.5 – 10)	9 (5.8 – 13)^{a}	13 (10.9 – 15.0)^{d}
Disease duration before start etanercept, median (IQR), years	2.1 (1 – 5)	1.9 (0.9 – 4)^{a}	3 (1.7 – 7)	3.5 (1.8 – 6)^{a}	3 (1.5 – 5)
History of chronic anterior uveitis, n (%)	7 (3.6)	3 (3.6)	1 (4.3)	3 (4.7)	0 (0)
History of at least 1 DMARD use except MTX, n (%)	84 (42.6)	24 (28.6)^{ab}	7 (30.4)^{c}	34 (53.1)^{a}	18 (75.0)^{bc}
History of at least 1 DMARD use, n (%)	170 (86.3)	69 (82.1)	22 (95.7)	57 (89.1)	22 (91.7)
History of ≥2 DMARDs use, n (%)	76 (38.6)	21 (25.0)^{ab}	6 (26.1)	32 (50.0)^{a}	15 (62.5)^{b}
History of at least 1 biologic use, n (%)	44 (22.3)	10 (11.9)^{a}	5 (21.7)	20 (31.3)^{a}	7 (29.2)
History of ≥2 biologics use, n (%)	7 (3.6)	1 (1.2)	0 (0)	5 (7.8)	1 (4.2)
History of oral steroid use, n (%)	55 (27.9)	8 (9.5)^{ab}	7 (30.4)	30 (46.9)^{a}	8 (33.3)^{b}
Concurrent MTX use, n (%)	136 (69.0)	51 (60.7)^{a}	21 (91.3)^{ab}	51 (79.7)	12 (50.0)^{b}
Concurrent sulfasalazin use, n (%)	6 (3.0)	1 (1.2)	0 (0)	2 (3.1)	3 (12.5)
Concurrent oral steroid use, n (%)	10 (5.1)	0 (0)	2 (8.7)	5 (7.8)	3 (12.5)
NSAID use, n (%)	121 (61.4)	44 (52.4)	15 (65.2)	43 (67.2)	18 (75.0)

Paired superscript letters (^{a}, ^{b}, ^{c}) denote the existence of differences between two groups in each line ($p < 0.05$). The superscript letter ^{d} denotes the difference between indicators in one group and those in all other groups. *RF* rheumatoid factor, *IQR* interquartile range, *DMARD* disease-modifying antirheumatic drugs, *MTX* Methotrexate, *NSAID* nonsteroidal anti-inflammatory drugs

sulfasalazine; and 121 (61.4%) were receiving NSAIDs. No patients received any intra-articular steroids during the entire study period. One hundred sixty-three (82.7%) patients had a history of using at least one DMARD, and 17 (8.6%) patients had previously received two or more DMARDs. Etanercept was the first biological agent taken by 153 (77.7%) patients. Seven (3.6%) patients had previously used two or more biologicals.

Baseline characteristics according to JIA categories

An analysis of the data across JIA categories revealed a significant difference in the baseline parameters among different JIA types. In the enthesitis-related group, male patients predominated considerably over females (20.8% females). In the other three groups (persistent oligoarticular, extended oligoarticular, and polyarticular RF-negative), female patients were prevalent (81.0%, 69.6%, and 71.9%, respectively). The median age at JIA onset in the enthesitis-related group differed significantly from that of the other groups: 9 years for the enthesitis-related JIA group (min-max 1-16 years) compared with 2.3 years (min-max 10 months – 15 years) in the persistent oligoarticular group, 2 years (min-max 6 months – 12 years) in the extended oligoarticular group, and 3.25 years (min-max 8 months – 13 years) in the polyarticular RF-negative group. The persistent oligoarticular and polyarticular RF-negative groups differed significantly in terms of treatment duration (1.9 vs 3.5 years, respectively). The patient groups differed significantly in terms of previous treatment. Less than one-third of the patients in the oligoarthritis groups had a history of using at least one DMARD other than MTX (28.6 and 30.4% in the persistent oligoarticular and the extended oligoarticular groups, respectively). Meanwhile, the percentage of these patients in the polyarticular RF-negative and enthesitis-related groups was >50% (53.1 and 75%, respectively). The administration of biologicals (11.9%) and oral steroids (9.5%) was minimal in the persistent oligoarticular group.

Response to therapy within 12 months

Of the 197 patients enrolled in the study, 17 (8.6%) discontinued etanercept within the first year: 5 due to the occurrence of AEs (three patients had acute infusional reactions, and two had drug-induced hepatotoxicity), five due to primary failure, two due to de novo uveitis, and one due to uveitis flare; four additional patients withdrew because of non-adherence to therapy. Of the remaining 180 patients, 36 withdrew during the first year: six discontinued the study due to age (they were transferred to adult care centres), and 30 were transferred to local medical centres for further follow-up.

According to the final measurements taken after 12 months, 179 (90.9%) patients achieved ACR Pedi 30,177(89.8%) patients achieved ACR Pedi 50, 168(85.3%) patients achieved ACR Pedi 70, 135(68.5%) patients achieved ACR Pedi 90; 132(67.0%) patients achieved inactive disease according to the Wallace criteria; and 92 (46.7%) patients achieved inactive disease according to the JADAS cut-off point [Tables 2 and 3].

Of 197 patients, 90 (45.7%) achieved an excellent response to etanercept therapy after 1 year, while 48 (24.4%) were considered poor responders. The remaining 59 (29.9%) were considered intermediate responders.

We found a significant relationship between diagnosis according to JIA category and the response level. In the patients with persistent oligoarticular JIA, the percentage of excellent responders (65.5%) after 1 year of etanercept treatment was significantly higher than that in polyarticular RF-negative patients (23.4%) and in enthesitis-related arthritis patients (37.5%) [Fig. 1]. More than-one third of the patients in the polyarticular RF-negative and enthesitis-related groups were poor responders (39.1% and 33.3%, respectively). The highest percentage of patients who achieved inactive disease was observed in the group with persistent oligoarticular JIA (86.9%), whereas the lowest percentage was observed among the polyarticular RF-negative patients (45.3%).

All 7 patients with a history of uveitis before starting etanercept treatment had no active uveitis at the time of etanercept initiation. Uveitis flare occurred in one patient (0.5%) during the first year of treatment, resulting in the discontinuation of etanercept. The patient was subsequently switched to abatacept. Two cases of de novo uveitis (1%) developed 6 months after the initiation of etanercept therapy among all patients without a history of uveitis: one patient started etanercept monotherapy at the age of 10.7 years, and the second patient started receiving etanercept in combination with MTX at the age of 3.9 years. After the discontinuation of etanercept, both patients were switched to adalimumab.

Analysis of predictors of response to etanercept within 12 months

For each JIA category, we analysed the factors that initially differed in the patients with different response levels. Univariate analysis of all baseline characteristics was performed for each diagnosis. For the multivariate analysis in each group of patients, we selected independent factors associated with response to therapy based on the univariate analysis data and literature data. We used logistic regression to determine the significance of the variables in the univariate and multivariate analyses [Tables 4 and 5].

For the persistent oligoarthritis group, no factor was significant for poor response according to the multivariate analysis. In the group of excellent responders, a lower number of DMARDs was associated with better response.

In the extended oligoarticular group, none of the factors was significant for poor response according to the multivariate analysis. Excellent response was associated with a shorter disease duration.

In the polyarticular RF-negative group, poor response to treatment was associated with longer disease duration and older age. Excellent response was associated with a smaller number of joints with limited functions, a lower CRP level at the initiation of etanercept therapy, and younger age at disease onset.

In the enthesitis-related group, poor response to therapy was associated with longer disease duration. No significant factors were associated with excellent response.

Discussion

This open-label study of children with JIA without active systemic manifestations provides evidence supporting the efficacy and safety of the first course of etanercept treatment in the largest cohort of JIA patients in Russia. According to an intention-to-treat analysis after 12 months of etanercept treatment, only 18 (9.1%) patients failed to achieve ACR Pedi 30, while 135 (68.5%) patients achieved ACR Pedi 90 and 132 (67.0%) patients achieved inactive disease according to the Wallace criteria. The JIA categories differed in terms of the level of response to ETA. Hence, to determine the optimal time and conditions for initiating etanercept treatment in JIA patients without systemic manifestations, we identified baseline predictors associated with excellent and poor responses to treatment in the studied JIA categories.

Previous research on the efficacy of anti-TNF drugs, and etanercept in particular, demonstrated different responses to treatment in JIA patients with systemic manifestations [17]. However, differences in other diagnoses have not been examined in many studies. In one study [18], the authors attempted to determine the contribution of diagnosis to the response to treatment but did not find any significant differences. This may be explained by the relatively small sample size (24 patients in two oligoarticular categories and 13 patients in the polyarticular category). We enrolled only patients without systemic manifestations because the Scientific Centre for Children's Health uses different treatment strategies for these categories of patients, as published previously [19]. Since the literature indicates that many demographic and clinical characteristics (onset; further characteristics of the arthritis; disease course; the presence of ANA, chronic or acute anterior uveitis, HLA allelic associations, etc.) are actually determined by the JIA category [14], we decided to analyse the response individually for each category. Because we found that the patients within the diagnostic groups differed in

Table 2 Dynamic of basic clinical and laboratory parameters among children with JIA starting treatment with etanercept (*N* = 197) at baseline and at the final measurement during 1 year follow-up

Characteristics	Baseline, median (IQR)	1 year follow-up, median (IQR)
Active joint count	4 (2-10)	0 (0-3)
Persistent oligoarticular	2 (2-4)	0 (0-0)
Extended oligoarticular	6 (5-10)	0 (0-0)
Polyarticular RF-	14 (6-23.5)	0 (0-2)
Enthesitis-related	5 (2.5-9)	0 (0-1.5)
Limited joint count	4 (2-11)	0 (0-2)
Persistent oligoarticular	2 (2-3.5)	0 (0-0)
Extended oligoarticular	6 (3-10)	0 (0-1)
Polyarticular RF-	15 (6.5-25.5)	0 (0-6)
Enthesitis-related	4.5 (4-9)	0 (0-1.5)
Swollen joint count	4 (2-8)	0 (0-0)
Persistent oligoarticular	2 (2-4)	0 (0-0)
Extended oligoarticular	6 (4-6)	0 (0-0)
Polyarticular RF-	9 (5-12.5)	0 (0-2)
Enthesitis-related	4 (2-7)	0 (0-0)
Pained joint count	4 (2-10)	0 (0-0)
Persistent oligoarticular	2 (1.5-3)	0 (0-0)
Extended oligoarticular	6 (3-9)	0 (0-0)
Polyarticular RF-	12 (4-23)	0 (0-0)
Enthesitis-related	4.5 (3-9)	0 (0-1)
Morning stiffness, min	30 (0-60)	0 (0-15)
Persistent oligoarticular	30 (0-60)	0 (0-0)
Extended oligoarticular	35 (0-60)	0 (0-3)
Polyarticular RF-	60 (20-120)	0 (0-0)
Enthesitis-related	60 (15-120)	0 (0-1)
Physician global of disease (0-100 mm)	60 (45-80)	5 (0-15)
Persistent oligoarticular	50 (42-70)	0 (0-4)
Extended oligoarticular	65 (46-80)	3 (0-14)
Polyarticular RF-	70 (56-86)	6 (2-19)
Enthesitis-related	68.5 (54.5-82.5)	4.5 (0.5-11)
Parent/patient global of well-being (0-100 mm)	68 (50-82.5)	6.5 (2.8-14.3)
Persistent oligoarticular	60 (49-70)	2 (0-7)
Extended oligoarticular	68 (50-81)	5 (3-10)
Polyarticular RF-	73.5 (60-87)	9 (2-15.5)
Enthesitis-related	70 (50-90)	4.5 (0-12)
Childhood health assessment questionnaire (0-3)	1.3 (0.5-1.9)	0 (0-0.2)
Persistent oligoarticular	0.78 (0.5-1.5)	0 (0-0)
Extended oligoarticular	1.5 (1-1.9)	0 (0-0.25)
Polyarticular RF-	1.75 (13-2.25)	0 (0-0.75)
Enthesitis-related	1.5 (0.75-2.5)	0 (0-0.25)
Juvenile arthritis disease activity score-71	19.2 (13.8-28.5)	1.1 (0.3-3.9)
Persistent oligoarticular	14.9 (11.7-18.9)	0.5 (0-1.1)
Extended oligoarticular	21.8 (16.3-28.5)	1 (0-2.5)
Polyarticular RF-	29.6 (20.6-39.8)	1.45 (0.65-6.4)
Enthesitis-related	20.6 (15.6-30.7)	1.1 (0.1-3.6)
Erythrocyte sedimentation rate, mm/h	21 (12-35)	5 (3-11)
Persistent oligoarticular	19.5 (10-28)	5 (2-7)
Extended oligoarticular	20 (15-35)	4 (2-12)
Polyarticular RF-	25.5 (16-41.5)	5 (3-15.5)
Enthesitis-related	30 (8.5-59.5)	5 (4-13.5)
C-reactive protein, mg/l	6.6 (1.9-19.7)	1 (0-4.6)
Persistent oligoarticular	2.6 (1-10)	0 (0-1)
Extended oligoarticular	6.4 (2.4-15)	1 (0-3)
Polyarticular RF-	9.8 (4-27)	1 (0-6.5)
Enthesitis-related	16.7 (7.6-52.3)	3.7 (0.9-12.6)

RF rheumatoid factor, *IQR* interquartile range

their response to therapy, we analysed the predictors for each JIA category.

We used the clustering method for the response to therapy to single out three levels (poor, intermediate, and excellent response) according to the results of 1 year of etanercept treatment. Other researchers have focused on analyses using a similar approach [6, 11, 12] since it is promising for building predictive models and elaborating the algorithms for treatment selection. The results of the analysis enabled us to identify the consistency and inconsistency of our results with real-world data on the efficacy of etanercept treatment.

The results of various studies show that some baseline demographic characteristics can predict treatment response. The factors identified among the literature data are as follows: female sex [6], age at initiation of treatment [7, 13], age of JIA onset [6, 12], and disease duration [6, 12, 20]. We found that sex was not a significant predictor of response, regardless of diagnosis. However, because polyarthritis and oligoarthritis are characterized by female predominance, while male predominance is typical of only enthesitis-related arthritis, the associations between sex and response level that some researchers have found may be due to the relationship between sex and diagnosis.

Table 3 Final disease activity parameters achieved in different ILAR categories during one year etanercept treatment

JIA subtype	ACR Pedi, %				Inactive disease, %
	ACR Pedi 30	ACR Pedi 50	ACR Pedi 70	ACR Pedi 90	
All patients (*n* = 197)	90,9	89,8	85,3	68,5	67
Persistent oligoarticular (*n* = 84)	90,5	90,5	88,1	77,4	86,9
Extended oligoarticular (*n* = 23)	95,7	95,7	95,7	73,9	65,2
Polyarticular RF negative (*n* = 64)	90,6	87,5	85,4	57,8	45,3
Polyarticular RF positive (*n* = 1)	100	100	0	0	0
Psoriatic (*n* = 1)	100	100	100	100	100
Enthesitis-related (*n* = 24)	87,5	87,5	83,3	62,5	58,3

n number, *RF* rheumatoid factor, *JADAS-71* juvenile arthritis disease activity score 71; inactive disease defined by Wallace criteria

In our study, the cohorts of patients in different JIA categories had different age characteristics. Shorter disease duration was associated with excellent response in the extended oligoarthritis group, while longer disease duration was associated with poor response in the polyarthritis and enthesitis arthritis groups. The higher efficacy of etanercept in patients in the early disease stage (up to 1.4 – 2 years of disease) may indicate a "window of opportunity" when the use of etanercept appears to be more effective if there are no irreversible changes in the joints.

The patient's past medical history is very important when prescribing treatment for JIA. Studies have separately assessed the effect of previous use of different classes of medications [6]. In our study, only the number of previously used DMARDs was a significant predictor of response in the persistent oligoarthritis group.

Among all the laboratory parameters analysed in our study, only lower CRP was a significant predictor of excellent response in polyarticular patients.

Indicators of joint involvement are very important characteristics of the clinical presentation in JIA patients. In our study, the small number of joints with limitation of motion in children with arthritis correlated with an excellent response to etanercept treatment. This is related to the fact that a large number of joints with LOM are observed in children who experienced the onset of arthritis at an older age (median, 6 years) and who have been suffering for a long time and therefore experienced irreversible changes in joints and tendons.

At the beginning of the study, only 7 patients had a history of JIA-associated uveitis, but none of them had active uveitis when etanercept therapy was initiated. A history of this disease was insignificant in the multivariate analysis because of the small sample size. However, it should be mentioned that etanercept was discontinued within the first year of treatment in 2 of these7 patients: one because of uveitis flare (the patient administered a combination of etanercept and methotrexate) and the other because of treatment nonadherence. In addition,

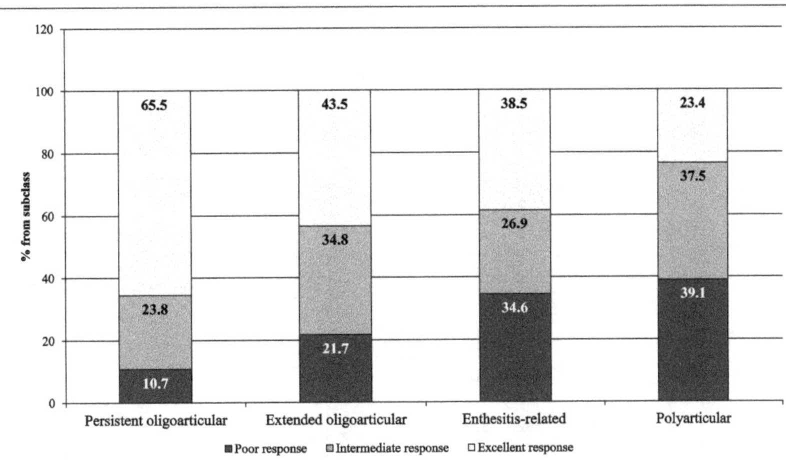

Fig. 1 Distribution of responses to etanercept in different JIA categories within 12 months after beginning treatment

Table 4 Univariable and multivariable analysis of factors associated with response to etanercept for polyarticular RF-negative and enthesitis-related JIA

Baseline characteristics	Poor vs Intermediate and Excellent Responders				Excellent vs Intermediate and Poor Responders			
	Univariable analysis		Multivariable analysis		Univariable analysis		Multivariable analysis	
	Odds ratio (95% CI)	*p* value	Odds ratio (95% CI)	*p* value	Odds ratio (95% CI)	*p* value	Odds ratio (95% CI)	*p* value
Polyarticular RF-negative JIA								
Demographic								
Gender	0.886 (0.519-1.461)	0.642			1.334 (0.765-2.283)	0.295		
Disease duration before start of etanercept	0.55 (0.312-0.917)	0.027	*0.313 (0.116-0.730)*	*0.012*	0.995 (0.573-1.818)	0.985		
Age of disease onset	0.659 (0.391-1.087)	0.106	*0.418 (0.176-0.866)*	*0.028*	1.535 (0.84-3.14)	0.193	*0.518 (0.267-0.945)*	*0.039*
Disease activity								
CHAQ score at start of etanercept	0.58 (0.321-0.984)	0.053	0.801 (0.300-2.108)	0.649	1.745 (0.982-3.255)	0.065	1.089 (0.469-2.543)	0.841
VAS disease activity by patient/parent at start of etanercept	0.946 (0.565-1.562)	0.828			1.1 (0.617-1.934)	0.741		
VAS disease activity by physician at start of etanercept	0.76 (0.436-1.266)	0.308			1.375 (0.785-2.444)	0.261		
No. of joints with LOM	0.575 (0.328-0.96)	0.041	0.438 (0.150-1.129)	0.103	2.081 (1.069-4.712)	0.049	*0.430 (0.185-0.900)*	*0.033*
Morning stiffness, min	0.505 (0.259-0.876)	0.026	0.524 (0.214-1.130)	0.121	4.592 (1.54-20.62)	0.021	0.680 (0.326-1.312)	0.267
Previous therapy								
No. of DMARDs used before start of etanercept	0.638 (0.366-1.065)	0.095	1.272 (0.558-3.069)	0.573	0.707 (0.386-1.253)	0.243		
Fact of biologics using before start of etanercept	0.696 (0.42-1.146)	0.155	0.604 (0.283-1.224)	0.170	0.891 (0.513-1.589)	0.685		
Laboratory tests								
CRP at start of etanercept	0.712 (0.41-1.171)	0.189	0.658 (0.304-1.333)	0.252	3.361 (1.166-19.326)	0.088	*0.539 (0.271-0.959)*	*0.046*
Enthesitis-related JIA								
Demographic								
Gender	-	-			0.6 (0.242-1.365)	0.226		
Disease duration before start of etanercept	0.17 (0.021-0.59)	0.029	*3.980 (1.294-23.095)*	*0.048*	3.219 (0.995-19.183)	0.12	0.385 (0.051-1.531)	0.263
Age of disease onset	2.286 (0.885-7.397)	0.114			0.404 (0.13-1.002)	0.073	1.200 (0.308-5.023	0.789
Previous therapy								
No. of DMARDs used before start of etanercept	0.737 (0.275-1.816)	0.51			3.587 (1.261-15.132)	0.039	0.351 (0.047-1.416)	0.205
Fact of biologics using before start of etanercept	0.419 (0.161-0.997)	0.056	2.030 (0.714-6.369)	0.185	2.052 (0.81-8.276)	0.184	1.046 (0.220-4.252)	0.948

All entries in italic are statistically significant

Table 5 Univariable and multivariable analysis of factors associated with response to etanercept for extended and persistant oligoarticular JIA

Baseline characteristics	Poor vs Intermediate and Excellent Responders				Excellent vs Intermediate and Poor Responders			
	Univariable analysis		Multivariable analysis		Univariable analysis		Multivariable analysis	
	Odds ratio (95% CI)	*p* value	Odds ratio (95% CI)	*p* value	Odds ratio (95% CI)	*p* value	Odds ratio (95% CI)	*p* value
Extended oligoarticular JIA								
Demographic								
Disease duration before start of etanercept	0.449 (0.146-1.144)	0.114	1.066 (0.184-7.261)	0.942	1.729 (0.723-4.87)	0.245	*6.808 (1.520-63.332)*	*0.036*
Age of disease onset	0.561 (0.195-1.363)	0.213			2.091 (0.788-9.563)	0.218	3.447 (1.106-15.630)	0.053
Disease activity								
VAS disease activity by physician at start of etanercept	0.361 (0.1-0.98)	0.07	0.841 (0.173-3.997)	0.816	1.271 (0.543-3.149)	0.582		
Pain joint count	0.838 (0.333-2.186)	0.695			0.668 (0.242-1.577)	0.373	0.340 (0.070-1.097)	0.104
Previous therapy								
No. of DMARDs used before start of etanercept	0.533 (0.19-1.343)	0.198	0.518 (0.087-2.841)	0.431	1.064 (0.449-2.613)	0.885		
Fact of biologics using before start of etanercept	0.497 (0.188-1.193)	0.123	0.440 (0.138-1.337)	0.136	1.794 (0.729-6.57)	0.253		
Persistant oligoarticular JIA								
Demographic								
Disease duration before start of etanercept	0.671 (0.385-1.216)	0.157	1.118 (0.522-2.736)	0.785	1.154 (0.731-1.807)	0.527		
Disease activity								
Morning stiffness, min	0.746 (0.429-1.391)	0.302			1.386 (0.886-2.25)	0.16	1.448 (0.902-2.413)	0.129
Previous therapy								
Oral corticosteroids before start of etanercept	0.681 (0.389-1.095)	0.093	0.927 (0.482-5.718)	0.858	0.768 (0.149-1.297)	0.487		
No. of DMARDs used before start of etanercept	0.633 (0.343-1.171)	0.131	0.562 (0.250-1.232)	0.145	1.629 (1.025-2.748)	0.049	*1.691 (1.04-2.958)*	*0.046*
Background therapy								
Concomitant NSAID at start of etanercept	0.838 (0.408-1.637)	0.609			0.711 (0.445-1.12)	0.145	0.649 (0.388-1.058)	0.089
Laboratory tests								
CRP at start of etanercept	0.869 (0.515-1.791)	0.635			1.3 (0.833-2.099)	0.247	1.385 (0.874:2.274)	0.164

CHAQ **child health assessment questionnaire,** ***CI*** **confidence interval,** ***DMARD*** **disease-modifying antirheumatic drug,** ***ESR*** **erythrocyte sedimentation rate,** ***JIA*** **juvenile idiopathic arthritis,** ***VAS*** **visual analog scale**
All entries in italic are statistically significant

two children without a history of uveitis developed it after 6 months of etanercept use. Hence, the total rate of uveitis or uveitis flares was 3 cases (1.5%) within the first year of treatment: one case using monotherapy and two cases using combination therapy with methotrexate. This rate is somewhat lower than the data reported by other authors, particularly the large cohort of children from the Italian Registry) [10, 21], which could be due to both population features and differences in the total cohort of patients with respect to age and JIA category. Nevertheless, meticulous long-term monitoring of children receiving etanercept therapy is needed to reveal the development of risks and associations.

In our study, the VAS scores for disease activity as assessed by physician and patients were insignificant in the univariate analysis regardless of diagnostic category. The CHAQ score was significant in the univariate analysis for the polyarticular RF-negative group in the poor response model but was insignificant in the multivariate analysis.

However, the current study had some limitations. Despite its prospective design, the study lacked a control group. Hence, we could not assess the identified predictors as prognostic markers and could not evaluate whether a different treatment would be more effective than etanercept therapy for the poor responders. We did not consider immunological and genetic parameters as predictors of treatment response. Researchers are currently extensively investigating these parameters, so their value as predictors of treatment response may be determined in the future.

Conclusion

Our findings demonstrated that the response to etanercept therapy was strongly associated with the JIA category. While our results confirm earlier findings that etanercept is an effective and safe medication that resulted in ACR 90 and inactive disease in 45% of children with JIA after 1 year of treatment, few clinical, laboratory, and historical parameters can predict treatment success. The revealed predictors of treatment efficacy included persistent oligoarticular JIA, a shorter disease duration before the initiation of etanercept therapy, a smaller number of DMARDs used before the initiation of etanercept therapy, and a smaller number of joints with LOM. Lower C-reactive protein levels at baseline were a laboratory predictor. Polyarticular and enthesitis-related arthritis with a longer disease duration before the initiation of etanercept were predictors of poor response to etanercept treatment. These factors may help physicians to identify patients who might benefit from earlier treatment with etanercept.

Key messages

Almost half of children with JIA achieved an excellent response to etanercept treatment after 1 year.

Children with persistent oligoarthritis and a shorter disease duration were more likely to achieve an excellent response to etanercept treatment.

Abbreviations

CRP: C-reactive protein; DMARD: Disease-modifying antirheumatic drug; JADAS71: JIA disease activity score; JIA: Juvenile idiopathic arthritis;; MTX: Methotrexate; NSAID: Nonsteroidal anti-inflammatory drug

Acknowledgements

This study would not have been possible without the collaboration of numerous Russian paediatric rheumatologists, patients and patients' parents.

Funding

This research received no specific grants from any funding agency in the public, commercial or not-for-profit sectors.

Authors' contributions

All the authors contributed to all aspects of the work leading to the production of this paper. All authors read and approved the final manuscript.

Competing interests

The authors declare that they have no competing interests.

Consent for publication

All patients and their parents provided written informed consent for their data to be used in analyses and reported.

Author details

[1]Federal State Autonomous Institution "National Scientific and Practical Center of Children's Health" Of the Ministry of Health of the Russian Federation, Moscow, Russia. [2]Federal State Autonomous Educational Institution of Higher Education I.M. Sechenov First Moscow State Medical University of the Ministry of Health of the Russian Federation, Moscow, Russia. [3]Rheumatology Department, Federal State Autonomous Institution "National Scientific and Practical Center of Children's Health" Of the Ministry of Health of the Russian Federation, Moscow, Russia.

References

1. Prahalad S, Glass DN. A comprehensive review of the genetics of juvenile idiopathic arthritis. Pediatr Rheumatol Online J. 2008;6:11.
2. Kahn P. Juvenile idiopathic arthritis - an update on pharmacotherapy. Bull NYU Hosp Jt Dis. 2011;69:264–76.
3. Overall incidence in children in Russia (under age of 14 years) in 2011. Report of the Russian Federation Ministry of Health; 2015. https://static-3.rosminzdrav.ru/system/attachments/attaches/000/015/822/original/ZD6.DOC?1389768574.
4. Ringold S, Weiss PF, Beukelman T, DeWitt EM, Ilowite NT, Kimura Y, et al. 2013 update of the 2011 American College of Rheumatology recommendations for the treatment of juvenile idiopathic arthritis: recommendations for the medical therapy of children with systemic juvenile idiopathic arthritis and tuberculosis screening among children receiving biologic medications. Arthritis Rheum. 2013;65:2499–512.

5. Beukelman T, Patkar NM, Saag KG, Tolleson-Rinehart S, Cron RQ, DeWitt EM, et al. 2011 American College of Rheumatology recommendations for the treatment of juvenile idiopathic arthritis: initiation and safety monitoring of therapeutic agents for the treatment of arthritis and systemic features. Arthritis Care Res (Hoboken). 2011;63(4):465–82. doi:10.1002/acr.20460.
6. Otten MH, Prince FH, Armbrust W, ten Cate R, Hoppenreijs EP, Twilt M, et al. Factors associated with treatment response to etanercept in juvenile idiopathic arthritis. JAMA. 2011;306:2340–7.
7. Giannini EH, Ilowite NT, Lovell DJ, Wallace CA, Rabinovich CE, Reiff A, et al. Pediatric Rheumatology Collaborative Study Group. Long-term safety and effectiveness of etanercept in children with selected categories of juvenile idiopathic arthritis. Arthritis Rheum. 2009;60(9):2794–804.
8. Windschall D, Müller T, Becker I, Horneff G. Safety and efficacy of etanercept in children with the JIA categories extended oligoarthritis, enthesitis-related arthritis and psoriasis arthritis. Clin Rheumatol. 2015;34(1):61–9.
9. Horneff G, Burgos-Vargas R, Constantin T, Foeldvari I, Vojinovic J, Chasnyk VG, et al. Paediatric Rheumatology International Trials Organisation (PRINTO). Efficacy and safety of open-label etanercept on extended oligoarticular juvenile idiopathic arthritis, enthesitis-related arthritis and psoriatic arthritis: part 1 (week 12) of the CLIPPER study. Ann Rheum Dis. 2014;73(6):1114–22.
10. Verazza S, Davì S, Consolaro A, Bovis F, Insalaco A, Magni-Manzoni S, et al. Italian Pediatric Rheumatology Study Group.. Disease status, reasons for discontinuation and adverse events in 1038 Italian children with juvenile idiopathic arthritis treated with etanercept. Pediatr Rheumatol Online J. 2016;14(1):68.
11. Kearsley-Fleet L, Davies R, Lunt M, Southwood TR, Hyrich KL. Factors associated with improvement in disease activity following initiation of etanercept in children and young people with Juvenile Idiopathic Arthritis: results from the British Society for Paediatric and Adolescent Rheumatology Etanercept Cohort Study. Rheumatology (Oxford). 2016;55:840–7.
12. Solari N, Palmisani E, Consolaro A, Pistorio A, Viola S, Buoncompagni A, et al. Factors associated with achievement of inactive disease in children with juvenile idiopathic arthritis treated with etanercept. J Rheumatol. 2013;40: 192–200.
13. Geikowski T, Becker I, Horneff G, German BIKER Registry Collaborative Study Group. Predictors of response to etanercept in polyarticular-course juvenile idiopathic arthritis. Rheumatology (Oxford). 2014;53:1245–9.
14. Petty RE, Southwood TR, Manners P, Baum J, Glass DN, Goldenberg J, et al. International League of Associations for Rheumatology. International League of Associations for Rheumatology classification of juvenile idiopathic arthritis: second revision, Edmonton, 2001. J Rheumatol. 2004;31:390–2.
15. Consolaro A, Bracciolini G, Ruperto N, Pistorio A, Magni-Manzoni S, Malattia C, et al. Paediatric Rheumatology International Trials Organization. Remission, minimal disease activity, and acceptable symptom state in juvenile idiopathic arthritis: defining criteria based on the juvenile arthritis disease activity score. Arthritis Rheum. 2012;64:2366–74.
16. Wallace CA, Giannini EH, Huang B, Itert L, Ruperto N, Childhood Arthritis Rheumatology Research Alliance, et al. American College of Rheumatology provisional criteria for defining clinical inactive disease in select categories of juvenile idiopathic arthritis. Arthritis Care Res (Hoboken). 2011;63:929–36.
17. van Dijkhuizen EH, Wulffraat NM. Early predictors of prognosis in juvenile idiopathic arthritis: a systematic literature review. Ann Rheum Dis. 2015;74: 1996–2005.
18. Quartier P, Taupin P, Bourdeaut F, Lemelle I, Pillet P, Bost M, et al. Efficacy of etanercept for the treatment of juvenile idiopathic arthritis according to the onset type. Arthritis Rheum. 2003;48:1093–101.
19. Alexeeva EI, Valieva SI, Bzarova TM, Semikina EL, Isaeva KB, Lisitsyn AO, et al. Efficacy and safety of repeat courses of rituximab treatment in patients with severe refractory juvenile idiopathic arthritis. Clin Rheumatol. 2011;30:1163–72.
20. Papsdorf V, Horneff G. Complete control of disease activity and remission induced by treatment with etanercept in juvenile idiopathic arthritis. Rheumatology (Oxford). 2011;50:214–21.
21. Foeldvari I, Becker I, Horneff G. Uveitis Events During Adalimumab, Etanercept, and Methotrexate Therapy in Juvenile Idiopathic Arthritis: Data From the Biologics in Pediatric Rheumatology Registry. Arthritis Care Res (Hoboken). 2015;67(11):1529–35.

3

Methotrexate-induced nausea in the treatment of juvenile idiopathic arthritis

Sonja Falvey[1], Lauren Shipman[2], Norman Ilowite[3] and Timothy Beukelman[2*]

Abstract

Background: Methotrexate is the most commonly used disease modifying antirheumatic drug in the treatment of juvenile idiopathic arthritis and can be effective in controlling disease in many patients.

Main body: A significant proportion of patients experience nausea and vomiting induced by methotrexate therapy, which can lead to decreased quality of life and discontinuation of treatment with methotrexate. Many strategies have been employed in attempts to reduce methotrexate-induced nausea, including folate supplementation, switching from oral to subcutaneous methotrexate, anti-emetic therapy, behavioral therapy, and others. Anticipatory nausea can be difficult to treat, making primary prevention of nausea with anti-emetics an attractive approach.

Conclusion: Understanding the prevalence and impact of methotrexate-induced nausea, as well as potentially effective interventions, may help maximize the therapeutic benefits of methotrexate.

Keywords: Methotrexate, MTX, Nausea, Vomiting, Juvenile idiopathic arthritis, JIA

Background

Juvenile idiopathic arthritis (JIA) is defined by the International League of Associations for Rheumatology as arthritis of an unknown etiology that persists for at least 6 weeks in children under the age of sixteen [1] and is the most common rheumatic disease in childhood [2]. Effective and timely treatment is necessary to ensure present and future quality of life for children with JIA [2].

After initially serving in the 1950's as a treatment for acute leukemia and other malignancies, methotrexate (MTX) was shown to be efficacious in the treatment of children with chronic arthritis. This was first published in 1992 in the breakthrough US-USSR controlled study [3], with subsequent controlled trials and observational studies supporting its findings [4–6]. MTX became the most commonly used disease modifying antirheumatic drug (DMARD) to treat JIA and remains the most common to the present day [7–9]. Treatment with MTX has the infrequent but serious potential to cause significant hepatotoxicity or bone marrow suppression; however, the frequency and consequences of MTX-induced nausea likely have a greater clinical impact in practice [10, 11].

* Correspondence: tbeukelman@peds.uab.edu
[2]Division of Pediatric Rheumatology, University of Alabama Birmingham, Birmingham, USA
Full list of author information is available at the end of the article

The gastrointestinal (GI) adverse effects of MTX, most commonly MTX-induced nausea, frequently lead to non-adherence or discontinuation of this otherwise effective and low-cost drug. Different strategies have been employed to diminish the adverse GI effects of MTX, and these have met with variable success. In this paper, we aim to review the published data about MTX-induced nausea in the treatment of JIA, as well as possible management approaches including the use of newer anti-nausea medications.

Frequency and significance of MTX-induced nausea

Although nausea is one of the most frequent adverse effects of MTX, its prevalence and epidemiology in children with JIA has not been completely characterized. One cross-sectional descriptive study performed in the Netherlands reported the prevalence of MTX intolerance owing to GI effects as determined by the Methotrexate Intolerance Severity Score (MISS) to be 50.5% in a cohort of 297 children with JIA. In the same study, 191 (64%) patients experienced MTX-induced nausea, and 81 (27%) reported MTX-associated vomiting [11]. A cohort study of new MTX initiators in the Netherlands reported a 1 year incidence of 42% for MTX intolerance owing to GI effects [12]. An international randomized clinical trial of two doses of methotrexate involving 80 patients with polyarticular JIA reported nausea in 21% and vomiting in 11% of patients [6]. In a survey of 49 adolescents in England with inflammatory arthritis who were receiving MTX, 73% reported nausea and 43% reported vomiting [10]. In a multicenter, double blind, placebo-controlled crossover clinical trial that analyzed the use of low-dose oral methotrexate in 88 children with JIA, nausea was reported in 28% [4]. One survey of 171 mothers of children with JIA reported that almost a third of the JIA patients felt sick every week and 15% vomited every week after taking MTX [13]. A recent survey regarding MTX related nausea and vomiting in patients with JIA was completed by 84 pediatric rheumatology care providers in the United Kingdom (UK). Approximately one-half of the respondents reported the development of nausea and vomiting associated with MTX in greater than 25% of their patients during the first year of treatment with MTX [14].

In summary, there is a wide range of reported rates of MTX-induced nausea in the treatment of JIA (Table 1). The minimum estimate appears that at least 1 out of 5 patients, and perhaps as many as 3 out of 4 patients, suffer from MTX-induced nausea, depending on the definition of nausea used and the method of ascertainment. Importantly, MTX-induced nausea has been associated with significantly decreased quality of life in children with JIA [13] and the presence of significant GI symptoms in general has been associated with worse quality of life in children with JIA [15].

MTX-induced nausea often results in discontinuation of MTX and consequent initiation of other medications. In the open label screening phase of a randomized study of MTX dosing, 9 of the 25 (36%) children who discontinued low-dose MTX did so owing to GI complaints [6]. In a retrospective review of 58 children with JIA who received leflunomide, 39 (67%) of them had discontinued MTX because of nausea [16]. In the recent survey of pediatric rheumatology care providers in the UK, it was estimated that greater than 10% of patients who initiated treatment with biologic agents did so because of intolerance of MTX-induced nausea [14].

Clinical factors associated with MTX-induced nausea

A few clinical factors have been reported to be associated with an increased incidence of MTX-induced nausea. A survey of patients with inflammatory arthritis demonstrated an inverse relationship between age and MTX-induced nausea and vomiting; adolescent patients had over six times higher odds of reporting nausea when compared to adult patients (odds ratio (OR) 6.31 [95% confidence interval (CI) 2.38-16.75]). This study also found that patients who were taking MTX for more than 1 year had almost four times higher odds of developing nausea compared to patients on MTX for only 3–11 months (OR 3.86 [95% CI 1.71-11.79]) [10].

Anticipatory nausea associated with MTX

Anticipatory nausea is a known psychological adverse effect of MTX that develops through classical conditioning. Nausea may be triggered by cues such as seeing MTX or simply hearing the word spoken [17]. Although anticipatory nausea is well-studied in cancer patients receiving chemotherapy treatment and has a reported frequency of 30% [11], it has only been assessed in a few studies of children with JIA (Table 1). In the aforementioned survey of adolescents who receive MTX, anticipatory nausea was reported in 41% of the participants [10]. In the aforementioned survey of mothers of children with JIA receiving MTX, nearly 25% reported anticipatory nausea with every weekly dose of MTX and more than 35% reported any anticipatory nausea [13]. The previously mentioned cross-sectional study performed in the Netherlands reported 9% of patients experienced anticipatory nausea. Interestingly, among patients who were considered to be MTX intolerant according to the

Table 1 Published prevalence rates of GI adverse effects associated with MTX in the treatment of JIA

Author	Year published	Study design	Number of subjects	Method of ascertainment	MTX-intolerance due to GI effects	Nausea with MTX	Vomiting with MTX	Anticipatory nausea
Bulatovic	2011	Cross-sectional	297 patients	MISS	51%	64%	27%	9%
van Dijkhuizen	2015	Cohort study of new MTX initiators	142 patients	MISS	42% (1 year incidence)	(n/a)	(n/a)	(n/a)
Ruperto	2004	Randomized clinical trial of MTX	80 patients	Direct questioning	(n/a)	21% (monthly)	11% (monthly)	(n/a)
Patil	2014	Survey	49 patients	Questionnaire	(n/a)	73%	43%	41%
Woo	2000	Randomized clinical trial of MTX	88 patients	Direct questioning	(n/a)	28% (monthly)	(n/a)	(n/a)
Mulligan	2013	Survey	171 parents	Questionnaire	(n/a)	~32% (weekly)	15% (weekly)	25% (weekly) >35% (any)
Amin	2015	Survey	84 physicians	Questionnaire	(n/a)	~25% in first year		(n/a)

MTX methotrexate, *GI* gastrointestinal, *MISS* methotrexate intolerance severity score

MISS, 18.7% reported anticipatory nausea, whereas no MTX tolerant patients reported anticipatory nausea. Anticipatory nausea can be difficult to treat and may result in non-adherence and treatment discontinuation. The best strategy appears to be to avoid the development of anticipatory nausea in the first place [18].

Assessing MTX-induced nausea

Bulatovic et al. developed the Methotrexate Intolerance Severity Score (MISS) instrument to measure MTX intolerance owing to GI-related symptoms [11]. The MISS includes items about stomachache, nausea, vomiting, and behavioral complaints and assesses both direct MTX effects as well as anticipatory or associative effects. With physician's opinion serving as the gold standard, the validation study determined that 90% of patients were correctly classified as being MTX intolerant using the MISS [11]. The MISS has subsequently been used to study adults with rheumatoid arthritis and psoriatic arthritis [19].

Another instrument to evaluate GI-related symptoms in JIA is the Gastrointestinal Symptom Scale for Kids (GISSK) [15]. This instrument was developed to assess for GI-related symptoms in general, not symptoms specifically related to treatment. It assesses dyspepsia, upper and lower abdominal pain, nausea, diarrhea, constipation, vomiting, and anorexia. The validation study identified the presence of GI symptoms in the majority (58%) of children with JIA, with 22% having nausea [15]. The GISSK does not specifically assess the temporal relationship between symptoms and medication administration, including anticipatory symptoms. Given its targeted development, the MISS is likely a superior method to assess MTX-associated nausea and intolerance in children with JIA, although the two instruments have not been compared directly in a study.

Folate supplementation for MTX-induced nausea

Folic acid (vitamin B9) and folinic acid (5-formyl tetrahydrofolate) are forms of folate that can be taken orally to attempt to reduce MTX toxicities. Both are able to function in biosynthetic pathways that are independent of the dihydrofolate reductase enzyme that MTX inhibits as part of its mechanism of action. It is thought that folic acid and folinic acid help to reduce the adverse effects of MTX by replenishing depleted intracellular folate levels that occur in hepatocytes and peripheral blood lymphocytes of patients treated with MTX. However, because the exact mechanisms of action of MTX in the treatment of arthritis are unknown, there is some concern that folate supplementation may reduce the efficacy of MTX, especially if the antirheumatic effects are mediated partially through folate antagonism [20].

Folate supplementation in JIA has been examined in a few published studies. In a randomized double blind placebo controlled crossover trial of 19 children with juvenile arthritis receiving MTX, each subject received either folic acid or placebo for 12 weeks to observe the impact of folic acid supplementation on the efficacy of MTX. It was determined that 1 mg/day of folic acid did not result in increased disease activity. The effects of folic acid on MTX-induced nausea were not assessed. A retrospective chart review of 43 children with juvenile arthritis who initiated folinic acid supplementation following the development of adverse effects of MTX demonstrated that folinic acid significantly reduced GI-associated symptoms from a mean of 1.09 episodes per patient-year to a mean 0.29 episodes per patient-year [21]. When starting MTX for the first time, 67% of respondents in the UK pediatric rheumatology provider survey reported always or often (>50% of the time) concurrently starting folic acid [14].

Folate supplementation in adult patients receiving methotrexate for rheumatoid arthritis was the subject of a recently published Cochrane Review [20]. A meta-analysis of 6 randomized controlled trials revealed a significant risk reduction for nausea, vomiting, or abdominal pain (RR 0.74 [95% CI 0.59 to 0.92]) with the use of folate supplementation compared to placebo. Folate supplementation did not appear to have any effect on the efficacy of MTX as measured by tender and swollen joint counts and physician global assessment scores. The results of the review did not show any definite clinical advantage of one form of folate supplementation over the other. However, because folic acid is considerably less expensive than folinic acid, folic acid is probably the more cost-effective therapy [20].

Subcutaneous MTX for nausea reduction

A common perception among rheumatologists is that the oral route of MTX administration is more likely to result in nausea and vomiting compared to the parenteral route, but the published evidence is challenging to interpret. In support of the common perception, a published retrospective review of 61 children with JIA treated with oral MTX identified 11 patients who were subsequently switched to SQ MTX because of nausea. Of these 11 patients, 9 (82%) experienced complete resolution of nausea and the other 2 experienced less severe nausea and were able to continue MTX therapy [22].

On the other hand, some studies have found the prevalence of MTX-induced nausea and vomiting to be greater in patients receiving parenteral MTX compared to those receiving oral MTX. The aforementioned survey of adolescents and adults with inflammatory arthritis reported that 77% of patients on parenteral MTX experienced nausea compared to 37% in the oral group ($p < 0.0001$) [10]. In a survey of 171 mothers of children with JIA, children receiving SQ MTX had higher adjusted odds of feeling sick before (OR 2.33 [95% CI 0.96-5.66]) but not necessarily after (OR 1.50 [95% CI 0.69 to 3.26]) MTX administration compared to those receiving oral MTX. Children receiving SQ MTX also had higher adjusted odds of vomiting after administration (OR 3.75 [95% CI 1.28-11.06]) compared to oral MTX [13]. Bulatović et al. found that the prevalence of nausea in patients receiving parenteral MTX was 61 versus 41% for oral MTX ($p = 0.002$), and patients receiving parenteral MTX had a higher adjusted odds of being MTX intolerant according to the MISS questionnaire compared to those receiving oral MTX (OR 1.9 [95% CI 1.01-3.58]) [11]. Importantly, these studies shared a major limitation: one of the primary reasons for children to switch from the oral to SQ route of administration is initial GI intolerance of the oral route, and this bias was not addressed.

A recently published cross-sectional study was conducted at several centers in Germany with the goal of assessing how the route of MTX administration affects MTX intolerance in patients with JIA [23]. The MISS questionnaire was used to compare MTX intolerance in 2 patient groups: 95 patients receiving oral MTX with no history of SQ MTX use and 46 patients receiving SQ MTX with no history of oral MTX use. The median methotrexate dose for the exclusively PO group and the exclusively SQ group was comparable at 11.8 mg/m2/week and 11.6 mg/m2/week, respectively. A greater proportion of patients receiving SQ MTX had MTX intolerance according to the MISS instrument compared to those receiving oral MTX (43 vs. 29%, OR: 3.4[95% CI 1.2-10.0]); however, there was no significant difference in the prevalence of nausea or vomiting between the 2 groups, and the significant differences between the groups lie in the behavioral components of intolerance.

Anti-emetics for MTX-induced nausea

Ondansetron is a 5-HT_3-receptor antagonist that is often used to treat nausea induced by chemotherapy in cancer patients. Ondansetron is an effective first-line antiemetic for children treated with chemotherapy and has been shown to be significantly more effective than metoclopramide and chlorpromazine in comparative studies [24]. More recently, ondansetron has been increasingly used to treat other causes of nausea. For example, a Cochrane Review analyzed the results of studies of ondansetron in the emergency department for vomiting related to acute gastroenteritis in children and found significant reductions in hospitalization rates and in the need for intravenous fluids [25]. In addition, ondansetron has been shown to be very well tolerated by children in the treatment of nausea for various indications. [18, 24–26].

Perhaps more relevant to the issue of MTX-induced nausea in children with JIA, ondansetron appears effective in pediatric patients with Crohn disease and MTX-induced nausea. In a retrospective study, researchers evaluated the occurrence of MTX-induced nausea among children with Crohn disease who received ondansetron pre-medication with the first dose of SQ MTX compared to those who did not initially receive ondansetron pre-medication [27]. Among the 50 children who initially received ondansetron pre-medication, only 1 (2%) experienced nausea in the 3 months after starting MTX, compared to 6 (60%) among the 10 children who did not initially receive ondansetron premedication ($p < 0.001$). Four of the 6 children who developed nausea without ondansetron premedication subsequently received ondansetron prior to weekly MTX doses and had no more complaints. The authors concluded that ondansetron was effective therapy for MTX-induced nausea associated with parenteral treatment in children with Crohn disease [27].

Ondansetron has also been shown to be effective in treating MTX-induced nausea in adults with rheumatoid arthritis. In an observational study, 9 adults with rheumatoid arthritis were given ondansetron because they had severe nausea that persisted despite receipt of the anti-emetic metoclopramide and switching MTX from oral to intramuscular administration [28]. Following initiation of ondansetron, the intensity and duration of nausea declined dramatically in all patients, and this improvement continued throughout the 24 weeks of follow-up.

Some pediatric rheumatologists are using ondansetron in clinical practice. Among the 84 respondents to the UK provider survey, 21% always or often (>50% of the time) start an anti-emetic concurrently when starting MTX for the first time. When prescribing an anti-emetic, ondansetron was the first choice for 88% of respondents [14].

Dosing recommendations for the use of ondansetron for the prevention of nausea and vomiting associated with emetogenic medications are provided by the manufacturer. For children ages 4 to 11 years, the recommended dose is 4 mg orally given 30 min prior to emetogenic medication. For children age 12 years or older, the recommended dose is 8 mg orally given 30 min prior to emetogenic medication [29]. Patients may take 1–2 additional doses of ondansetron every 8 h as needed for post-MTX nausea and vomiting.

Behavioral interventions for MTX-induced anticipatory nausea

Behavioral interventions may help increase tolerance to MTX and reduce the occurrence of associative and anticipatory nausea. In a retrospective chart review of children with JIA, investigators reported outcomes for 10 patients who were referred to a pediatric psychologist for behavioral therapy for anticipatory nausea (N = 6) and anxiety (N = 9) related to MTX [17]. Behavioral therapy was adapted to age. Children less than 10 years old received the "Magic Box" method based on systemic desensitization by distraction, and older children received cognitive behavioral therapy. The behavioral therapy intervention was found to be fully effective in 5 children (50%), moderately effective in 2 children (20%), and not effective in 3 children (30%) [17].

Alternative therapies to MTX

MTX-induced nausea can be intolerable and may lead to medication discontinuation. Fortunately for patients, there are alternative therapies available in cases of MTX intolerance.

Leflunomide is a non-biologic agent that is effective for the treatment of JIA. Leflunomide was directly compared to MTX in a randomized, blinded, placebo-controlled clinical trial of 94 children with polyarticular JIA who were naïve to both drugs [30]. At 16 weeks following randomization, a greater proportion of children in the MTX group achieved an ACR Pedi 30 response compared to the leflunomide group (89 versus 68%; p = 0.02). This observed result may have been partially attributable to differences in medication dosing, and other measures of effectiveness were similar between the two medications. In observational studies, children who initiated treatment with leflunomide owing to intolerance of MTX generally demonstrated good clinical responses and were not likely to discontinue leflunomide due to nausea [16, 30]. Taken together, these findings suggest that MTX may be more effective, but leflunomide is a possible alternative in the event that a patient cannot receive MTX for various reasons [30]. Because it is more expensive than MTX [31] and less well-studied, in clinical practice leflunomide is generally reserved for patients who have failed MTX owing to either intolerance or inefficacy [7].

Newer biologic agents, in particular the tumor necrosis factor inhibitors (TNFi), have been shown to be highly effective in the treatment of JIA [32]. MTX intolerance has been addressed in many patients by stopping MTX and initiating treatment with TNFi, although this practice has not been well-studied. A majority of the respondents (63%) in the UK survey reported more than 10% of their patients were switched from MTX to a biologic in response to MTX associated nausea and vomiting [14].

In contrast to current recommendations to use MTX prior to biologics [32], it appears that in clinical practice many patients receive TNFi without a trial of MTX use according to a recently published study of pharmacy records from the United States [8]. The reasons for this practice were unclear from this study, but the anticipated relatively high rate of MTX intolerance may play a role. Because TNFi and other newer therapeutic agents are considerably more expensive than MTX, increased tolerance of MTX among patients in whom it is effective could represent a significant cost-savings. In addition, because the combination of MTX and a biologic agent is generally more effective than a biologic agent alone [32], decreasing the impact of MTX-associated nausea would likely also benefit patients whose arthritis is refractory to MTX monotherapy.

Conclusions

MTX is an effective, relatively safe, and low-cost treatment for children with JIA, but its use is often limited by significant nausea. Various management approaches have been attempted and there is no clear single preferred method. Folate supplementation should likely be taken by all patients receiving MTX to help prevent nausea, as well as potentially counteract other adverse effects of MTX. Co-medication with anti-emetics, such as ondansetron, appears to be a highly effective approach, and behavioral therapies may be helpful with anticipatory nausea. There are alternative therapies to MTX in cases of intolerance, but initial prevention of intractable nausea is likely the best approach.

Abbreviations

DMARD: Disease modifying antirheumatic drug; GI: Gastrointestinal; GISSK: GI symptom scale for kids; JIA: Juvenile idiopathic arthritis; MISS: Methotrexate intolerance severity score; MTX: Methotrexate; PO: By mouth; SQ: Subcutaneous; TNFi: Tumor necrosis factor inhibitor; UK: United Kingdom

Acknowledgements

Not applicable.

Funding

Not applicable.

Author's contributions

SF, NI, and TB conceived and designed the study. SF, LS, and TB acquired and interpreted the data. SF, LS, and TB drafted the manuscript. All authors critically revised the manuscript and approved the final version.

Authors' information

Not applicable.

Competing interests

The authors declare that they have no competing interests.

Consent for publication

Not applicable.

Author details
[1]University of Mississippi School of Pharmacy, Oxford, USA. [2]Division of Pediatric Rheumatology, University of Alabama Birmingham, Birmingham, USA. [3]Children's Hospital at Montefiore, Albert Einstein College of Medicine, Bronx, USA.

References

1. Petty RE, Southwood TR, Manners P, Baum J, Glass DN, Goldenberg J, et al. International league of associations for rheumatology classification of juvenile idiopathic arthritis: second revision, Edmonton, 2001. J Rheumatol. 2004;31(2):390–2.
2. Gowdie PJ, Tse SM. Juvenile idiopathic arthritis. Pediatr Clin N Am. 2012;59(2):301–27.
3. Giannini EH, Brewer EJ, Kuzmina N, Shaikov A, Maximov A, Vorontsov I, et al. Methotrexate in resistant juvenile rheumatoid arthritis. Results of the U.S.A.-U.S.S.R. double-blind, placebo-controlled trial. The Pediatric rheumatology collaborative study group and the cooperative Children's study group. N Engl J Med. 1992;326(16):1043–9.
4. Woo P, Southwood TR, Prieur AM, Dore CJ, Grainger J, David J, et al. Randomized, placebo-controlled, crossover trial of low-dose oral methotrexate in children with extended oligoarticular or systemic arthritis. Arthritis Rheum. 2000;43(8):1849–57.
5. Klein A, Kaul I, Foeldvari I, Ganser G, Urban A, Horneff G. Efficacy and safety of oral and parenteral methotrexate therapy in children with juvenile idiopathic arthritis: an observational study with patients from the German Methotrexate registry. Arthritis Care Res (Hoboken). 2012;64(9):1349–56.
6. Ruperto N, Murray KJ, Gerloni V, Wulffraat N, de Oliveira SK, Falcini F, et al. A randomized trial of parenteral methotrexate comparing an intermediate dose with a higher dose in children with juvenile idiopathic arthritis who failed to respond to standard doses of methotrexate. Arthritis Rheum. 2004;50(7):2191–201.
7. Beukelman T, Ringold S, Davis TE, DeWitt EM, Pelajo CF, Weiss PF, et al. Disease-modifying antirheumatic drug use in the treatment of juvenile idiopathic arthritis: a cross-sectional analysis of the CARRA registry. J Rheumatol. 2012;39(9):1867–74.
8. Mannion ML, Xie F, Curtis JR, Beukelman T. Recent trends in medication usage for the treatment of juvenile idiopathic arthritis and the influence of tumor necrosis factor inhibitors. J Rheumatol. 2014;41(10):2078–84.
9. Hashkes PJ, Becker ML, Cabral DA, Laxer RM, Paller AS, Rabinovich CE, et al. Methotrexate: new uses for an old drug. J Pediatr. 2014;164(2):231–6.
10. Patil P, Parker RA, Rawcliffe C, Olaleye A, Moore S, Daly N, et al. Methotrexate-induced nausea and vomiting in adolescent and young adult patients. Clin Rheumatol. 2014;33(3):403–7.
11. Bulatovic M, Heijstek MW, Verkaaik M, van Dijkhuizen EH, Armbrust W, Hoppenreijs EP, et al. High prevalence of methotrexate intolerance in juvenile idiopathic arthritis: development and validation of a methotrexate intolerance severity score. Arthritis Rheum. 2011;63(7):2007–13.
12. van Dijkhuizen EH, Bulatovic Calasan M, Pluijm SM, de Rotte MC, Vastert SJ, Kamphuis S, et al. Prediction of methotrexate intolerance in juvenile idiopathic arthritis: a prospective, observational cohort study. Pediatr Rheumatol Online J. 2015;13:5.
13. Mulligan K, Kassoumeri L, Etheridge A, Moncrieffe H, Wedderburn LR, Newman S. Mothers' reports of the difficulties that their children experience in taking methotrexate for juvenile idiopathic arthritis and how these impact on quality of life. Pediatr Rheumatol Online J. 2013;11(1):23.
14. Amin TS, Shenton S, Mulligan K, Wedderburn LR, Wood M, VanRooyen V, et al. Strategies for the prevention and management of methotrexate-related nausea and vomiting in juvenile idiopathic arthritis: results of a UK paediatric rheumatology prescriber survey. Rheumatology (Oxford). 2015;54(11):2108–9.
15. Brunner HI, Johnson AL, Barron AC, Passo MH, Griffin TA, Graham TB, et al. Gastrointestinal symptoms and their association with health-related quality of life of children with juvenile rheumatoid arthritis: validation of a gastrointestinal symptom questionnaire. J Clin Rheumatol. 2005;11(4):194–204.
16. Foeldvari I, Wierk A. Effectiveness of leflunomide in patients with juvenile idiopathic arthritis in clinical practice. J Rheumatol. 2010;37(8):1763–7.
17. van der Meer A, Wulffraat NM, Prakken BJ, Gijsbers B, Rademaker CM, Sinnema G. Psychological side effects of MTX treatment in juvenile idiopathic arthritis: a pilot study. Clin Exp Rheumatol. 2007;25(3):480–5.
18. Zoubek A, Kronberger M, Puschmann A, Gadner H. Ondansetron in the control of chemotherapy-induced and radiotherapy-induced emesis in children with malignancies. Anti-Cancer Drugs. 1993;4(Suppl 2):17–21.
19. Calasan MB, van den Bosch OF, Creemers MC, Custers M, Heurkens AH, van Woerkom JM, et al. Prevalence of methotrexate intolerance in rheumatoid arthritis and psoriatic arthritis. Arthritis Res Ther. 2013;15(6):R217.
20. Shea B, Swinden MV, Tanjong Ghogomu E, Ortiz Z, Katchamart W, Rader T, et al. Folic acid and folinic acid for reducing side effects in patients receiving methotrexate for rheumatoid arthritis. Cochrane Database Syst Rev. 2013;5:CD000951.
21. Ravelli A, Migliavacca D, Viola S, Ruperto N, Pistorio A, Martini A. Efficacy of folinic acid in reducing methotrexate toxicity in juvenile idiopathic arthritis. Clin Exp Rheumatol. 1999;17(5):625–7.
22. Alsufyani K, Ortiz-Alvarez O, Cabral DA, Tucker LB, Petty RE, Malleson PN. The role of subcutaneous administration of methotrexate in children with juvenile idiopathic arthritis who have failed oral methotrexate. J Rheumatol. 2004;31(1):179–82.
23. van Dijkhuizen EH, Pouw JN, Scheuern A, Hugle B, Hardt S, Ganser G, et al. Methotrexate intolerance in oral and subcutaneous administration in patients with juvenile idiopathic arthritis: a cross-sectional, observational study. Clin Exp Rheumatol. 2016;34(1):148–54.
24. Culy CR, Bhana N, Plosker GL. Ondansetron: a review of its use as an antiemetic in children. Paediatr Drugs. 2001;3(6):441–79.
25. Fedorowicz Z, Jagannath VA, Carter B. Antiemetics for reducing vomiting related to acute gastroenteritis in children and adolescents. Cochrane Database Syst Rev. 2011;9:CD005506.
26. Cheng A. Emergency department use of oral ondansetron for acute gastroenteritis-related vomiting in infants and children. Paediatr Child Health. 2011;16(3):177–82.
27. Kempinska A, Benchimol EI, Mack A, Barkey J, Boland M, Mack DR. Short-course ondansetron for the prevention of methotrexate-induced nausea in children with Crohn disease. J Pediatr Gastroenterol Nutr. 2011;53(4):389–93.
28. Blanco R, Gonzalez-Gay MA, Garcia-Porrua C, Ibanez D, Garcia-Pais MJ, Sanchez-Andrade A, et al. Ondansetron prevents refractory and severe methotrexate-induced nausea in rheumatoid arthritis. Br J Rheumatol. 1998;37(5):590–2.
29. Lexicomp Online®, Pediatric & Neonatal Lexi-Drugs®, Hudson, Ohio: Lexi-Comp, Inc.; 2015.
30. Silverman E, Mouy R, Spiegel L, Jung LK, Saurenmann RK, Lahdenne P, et al. Leflunomide or methotrexate for juvenile rheumatoid arthritis. N Engl J Med. 2005;352(16):1655–66.
31. Benucci M, Saviola G, Manfredi M, Sarzi-Puttini P, Atzeni F. Cost effectiveness analysis of disease-modifying antirheumatic drugs in rheumatoid arthritis. A systematic review literature. Int J Rheumatol. 2011;2011:845496.
32. Beukelman T, Patkar NM, Saag KG, Tolleson-Rinehart S, Cron RQ, DeWitt EM, et al. 2011 American College of Rheumatology recommendations for the treatment of juvenile idiopathic arthritis: initiation and safety monitoring of therapeutic agents for the treatment of arthritis and systemic features. Arthritis Care Res (Hoboken). 2011;63(4):465–82.

4

Cross sectional, qualitative thematic analysis of patient perspectives of disease impact in juvenile idiopathic arthritis-associated uveitis

Ethan S. Sen[1,2], Michelle J. Morgan[3], Rachael MacLeod[4], Helen Strike[1], Ann Hinchcliffe[5], Andrew D. Dick[2,5,6], Brinda Muthusamy[7] and Athimalaipet V. Ramanan[1,2*]

Abstract

Background: Chronic health conditions in children can have a significant impact on their quality of life. The aim of this study was to explore the subjective experience of children and young people being treated for chronic, non-infectious uveitis associated with a systemic disease such as juvenile idiopathic arthritis.

Methods: A semi-structured interview was conducted with 10 children and young people aged between 6 and 18 years of age and their parents.

Results: Preliminary thematic analysis indicated that both the treatment and complications of the disorder have a significant impact on the quality of life and emotional well-being of patients, not only in terms of the discomfort experienced but also in perceptions of social isolation, anxiety and sense of injustice.

Conclusion: This study shows that themes including "impact on school", "social factors" and "emotional reactions" are important domains influencing health-related quality of life (HRQoL) in children with chronic uveitis. Inclusion of questions relating to these domains should be considered in future uveitis-specific tools examining HRQoL in these patients.

Keywords: Juvenile idiopathic arthritis, Uveitis, Quality of life, Patient-reported outcome measures

Background

The importance of measuring health-related quality of life (HRQoL) in children with chronic health conditions is widely acknowledged [1, 2]. Multiple generic, organ- and disease-specific patient-reported outcome measures (PROMs) of HRQoL in children exist, including tools that combine generic and specific measures [3–8]. HRQoL is known to result from a complex interaction of physical, social and cultural factors, with severity of illness or disability not necessarily being associated with worse HRQoL, as exemplified by the disability paradox [3, 9, 10].

Understandably, the HRQoL of children with visual impairment can be significantly reduced [3, 4, 6]. In recent years, a number of vision- and disease-specific HRQoL PROMs for children have been developed, beginning to populate a landscape that previously was largely void of such tools, although it is still felt that there is a lack of instruments to measure vision-related function and QoL in children overall [3, 4, 6–8, 11, 12]. Amongst these tools is the Effects of Youngsters' Eyesight on Quality of Life Questionnaire (EYE-Q), which has been validated as a uveitis-specific measure, both for uveitis alone, and uveitis associated with chronic illness, such as juvenile idiopathic arthritis (JIA) [4]. The EYE-Q comprises 19 items, including 4 regarding QoL.

Chronic anterior uveitis (CAU), the persistent inflammation of the anterior segment of the eye, is the most frequent extra-articular manifestation of JIA. Often

* Correspondence: avramanan@hotmail.com
[1]Department of Paediatric Rheumatology, Bristol Royal Hospital for Children, Upper Maudlin Street, Bristol BS2 8BJ, UK
[2]School of Clinical Sciences, University of Bristol, Bristol, UK

clinically silent, CAU can lead to visually-disabling complications including cataracts, glaucoma, band keratopathy and macular oedema, both as a result of chronic disease activity and treatment, which can be burdensome [13, 14]. Treatment includes topical and systemic glucocorticoids as well as systemic immunosuppressive therapies, including methotrexate, and newer biological therapies, with a move to introducing these sooner to minimise glucocorticoid use [14, 15].

This study aims to develop an understanding of the subjective experience of the impact of both uveitis treatment and its complications on the HRQoL of children, incorporating parent perceptions, with a view to ascertaining if any important additional topics are worth considering for inclusion in future PROMs of QoL in children with uveitis.

Methods

This cross-sectional interview study was sponsored by the University Hospitals Bristol NHS Foundation Trust and approved by the South West Research Ethics Committee (Reference [11]/SW/0109, Protocol number CH/2010/3587, IRAS project ID 61606). This study included both child and parent perspectives, as there is often discordance between the two, with the parent proxy of cognitive and emotional reactions to various disorders differing from child reports [1, 16]. Both the children and their parents provided written informed consent/assent to participate in the study.

Ten subjects aged 6 to 18 years old and their parents were selected by purposive sampling from the records of the multi-disciplinary paediatric rheumatology and uveitis clinic. The sample was stratified by age, gender and uveitis severity in order to achieve a representative group for analysis. Two age bands were used for sampling: 6 to 12 years and 13 to 18 years with five participants in each age band. Five participants were male and five were female. The two categories of disease severity (moderate and severe uveitis) were equally represented in the sample. The severity of the uveitis was determined by the treating ophthalmologist using the Standardisation of Uveitis Nomenclature (SUN) anterior chamber (AC) cell grade, AC flare and vitreous haze together with ocular co-morbidities and the number of systemic therapies in preceding years [17, 18]. Nine children had JIA-associated uveitis and one child was diagnosed with Blau syndrome and uveitis. Children under 6 years old and those with significant learning difficulties were excluded due to restriction in cognitive and verbal skills [16].

A Consultant Clinical Psychologist conducted a 30 min, audio-taped, semi-structured interview covering six principal domains and a general section with each participant. The six domains included: treatment received, ocular complications, impact on school activities, impact on out-of-school activities, social impact and emotional reactions. The general section comprised further open-ended questions to elicit items that either the children or their parents felt were indicative of the impact of the disease on the child's life but had not been previously covered. Whenever possible, children and parents were interviewed separately with the interview schedules covering the same domains but with the wording of questions adapted to the appropriate developmental level.

The audiotapes of the discussions were transcribed verbatim. Responses were analysed using inductive thematic analysis [19–21]. First the data were read carefully to identify meaningful units of text relevant to the research topic. Second, units of text dealing with the same issue were grouped together in analytic categories and given provisional labels. Finally, the data were reviewed to ensure that sets of data to support each label were identified.

Results

A total of 10 children / young people were included in this study. Three patients, at their request, were interviewed together with their parents. In the remaining seven cases, the patients and parents were interviewed separately. The results, therefore, represent the outcomes from 17 different interviews.

Patient demographics and disease characteristics are shown in Table 1. As expected from the purposive sampling strategy, males and females, and ages above and below 12 years, were equally represented. The duration of uveitis ranged from 1.5 to over 8 years. There was a variety of disease severity: one patient had uncomplicated disease controlled with topical corticosteroid drops and subcutaneous methotrexate; other patients had ongoing active disease, previous treatments with four or five systemic therapies and surgery for cataracts or glaucoma.

The study has identified multiple important themes across the six principal domains of "impact of treatment", "complications", "impact on school", "impact outside of school", "social factors" and "emotional reactions" (Table 2).

In the "impact of treatment" domain, the direct effects of therapeutic interventions such as painful injections, nausea and difficulties swallowing tablets were highlighted. These, in turn, led to both anticipatory nausea in some patients and avoidance behaviour in others, with negative emotional reactions to treatment being a frequently occurring theme:

> "On some occasions it would take up to two hours to administer the injection because he would cry and scream and throw a general wobbly...he ended up

Table 1 Patient demographics, immunosuppressive treatments and disease characteristics at the time of interview

Gender	Age (years)	Diagnosis	Duration of arthritis / uveitis (years)	Previous treatment	Treatment at time of interview	Active joints	Uveitis complications	Ophthalmic surgery	Eye	Visual acuity (LogMAR)	Anterior chamber cells (SUN grade)
M	6	Extended oligo JIA Left anterior uveitis	6 / 3.5	TS, MTX sc, ETA (stopped after onset of uveitis), ADA	MTX sc, ADA	nil	Posterior synechiae, cataract, band keratopathy	Orbital floor steroid injection	RE	0.000	0
									LE	0.150	0.5
F	7	RF-ve poly JIA Bilateral anterior uveitis	5 / 1.5	TS, MTX sc	MTX sc, ADA	nil	Glaucoma	Nil	RE	0.000	0
									LE	0.050	0
F	7	Persistent oligo JIA Bilateral anterior uveitis	2 / 2	TS, MTX sc	TS, MTX sc	nil	nil	nil	RE	−0.100	0
									LE	−0.100	0
F	10	Extended oligo JIA Bilateral anterior uveitis	5 / 5	TS, IVMP, MTX, MMF, INF, ADA	TS, MMF, ADA	nil	Posterior synechiae cataract, glaucoma	Cataract surgery BE, glaucoma surgery BE	RE	0.075	0
									LE	0.025	0.5
F	10	RF-ve poly JIA Bilateral anterior uveitis	9 / 5	TS, MTX sc, IVMP, INF, MMF, ADA	TS, MTX sc, ADA	Left ankle	Posterior synechiae, cataract, glaucoma, CMO, band keratopathy	Cataract surgery BE, Trabeculectomy BE	RE	0.125	0.5
									LE	0.175	0.5
M	13	RF-ve poly JIA Bilateral anterior uveitis	>8 / 6	IVMP, INF, MTX sc, ADA, MMF, ABA	MTX, MMF, ABA	nil	Posterior synechiae, cataract	Cataract surgery RE	RE	0.050	2
									LE	−0.100	3
F	14	Extended oligo JIA Bilateral anterior uveitis	>8 / >8	TS, MTX sc, INF	TS, MTX sc, ADA	Left hip, right knee	Cataract, glaucoma	Cataract surgery BE, glaucoma surgery BE	RE	−0.100	0.5
									LE	HM	0.5
M	16	Blau syndrome Bilateral panuveitis	15 / 8	TS, MTX sc, ADA	TS, MTX sc, MMF, IVMP, INF	nil	Posterior synechiae, cataract, chorioretinal scars, vitritis	nil	RE	0.850	1
									LE	0.100	1
M	16	Psoriatic JIA Bilateral anterior uveitis	>8 / >8	MTX sc, INF	MTX sc, ADA	nil	nil	nil	RE	0.000	0
									LE	−0.075	0
M	17	Extended oligo JIA Bilateral panuveitis	9 / 8	TS, MTX sc	TS, MTX sc	nil	Cataract, glaucoma	ST steroid injection RE	RE	0.125	0.5
									LE	−0.200	2

Legend: *ABA* Abatacept, *ADA* Adalimumab, *BE* Both eyes, *CMO*, Cystoid macular oedema, *ETA* Etanercept, *HM* Hand motion, *INF* Infliximab, *IVMP* Intravenous methylprednisolone, *JIA* Juvenile idiopathic arthritis, *LE* Left eye, *MMF* Mycophenolate mofetil, *MTX* Methotrexate, *oligo* Oligoarticular, *poly* Polyarticular, *RE* Right eye, *RF* Rheumatoid factor, *sc* Subcutaneously, *ST* Sub-Tenon's capsule, *SUN* Standardisation of Uveitis Nomenclature, *TS* Topical steroids

Table 2 Themes identified across the six domains in the semi-structured interview

THEME	Frequency (n = 17 interviews)
DOMAIN 1: Impact of treatment	
Negative emotional reactions to treatment	10
Missing school for treatment	7
Anxiety about improvement	5
Avoidance	5
Side Effects	5
Anticipatory nausea	4
Painful Injections	4
Difficulty swallowing tablets	3
DOMAIN 2: Complications	
Cataract removal	6
Poor vision/blurring	6
Glaucoma surgery	3
DOMAIN 3: Impact on School	
Difficulties reading information	9
Upset at missing lessons	8
Teachers forgetting	7
Anxiety about catching up with missed work	5
Difficulties seeing the ball in PE	4
Upset at missing friends/activities at school	4
DOMAIN 4: Impact outside school	
Needing adaptations in order to participate	5
Not able to see bus numbers readily	4
DOMAIN 5: Social Factors	
Being excluded	8
Not chosen as team member	6
Bullying	4
Self-exclusion	2
DOMAIN 6: Emotional Reactions	
Distress/sadness about illness	11
Fear	9
Anger	8
Worry about deterioration	7
Worry about going blind	7
Worry about the future/careers	6
Why me?	2

developing a phobia of all things yellow because the sharps bins were yellow and methotrexate is yellow".

The indirect effects of receiving treatment, such as missing school for appointments and treatment were important to both children and young people. Additionally, anxiety about perceived lack of symptom improvement despite treatment was identified as a significant concern by one patient:

"I can get agitated as I don't really see it getting any better".

This lack of perceived improvement also exacerbated avoidance of treatments and caused difficulties between parents and children regarding adherence to treatment regimes. Patterns of non-adherence followed by "nagging" on the part of the parent were described. Unfortunately, adjustment to medication does not necessarily follow and some families indicated that the negative emotional reaction actually increased over time:

"She has got more upset about having her injection than she used to be".

There were a number of themes identified in the "impact on school" domain. Upset at missing lessons and subsequent anxiety was a strong theme:

"I usually miss out on the understanding of some of the lessons because I wasn't there for it – it makes you feel worried because I don't know what I am doing".

The pressure to catch up with missed schoolwork is an additional stress for these children, and parents are aware that progress can be patchy, often in relation to the child's interests and motivation. There were also practical issues for those experiencing visual problems such as not being able to read the board in class, especially if placed at the rear of the classroom, or not being able to participate fully in Physical Education (PE):

"I'm always the last one to get ready for PE and everyone else is waiting on the carpet for me. I feel embarrassed and lonely".

Even when adaptations are made by the school, they are not always successful, with young people commenting on laptop computers not being available at the beginning of each school year or examinations being printed on large sheets of paper that would not fit onto the desk. Furthermore, young people felt that teachers did not always remember the visual difficulties they had and they were reluctant to inform or remind teaching staff as they did not wish to appear different from their peers:

"I don't really tell the teachers about my medical stuff ....I don't want to sit in another place to other people because that can be embarrassing".

There were fewer themes identified in the "impact outside of school" domain. The most commonly reported adaptations were sitting close to the television and holding hand held consoles or books close to the face. The zoom function on many IT tablets was reported as being very useful. Children and young people reported not being able to see the numbers on buses until they were quite close. Occasionally activities were dropped due to problems with eyesight which saddened young people.

In the "social factors" domain, the impact of both the treatment and complications of uveitis ranged from not feeling included or being the last person selected for a team or activity, to being actively bullied:

> "I was bullied every day in Year 9 [age 13-14 years]...They found out I had had eye surgery and they called me 'eye surgery gone wrong'. They said I was diseased or contagious and wouldn't go near me".

In addition to peer rejection, self-exclusion from activities was also reported. In older teenagers, restrictions imposed by treatment also led to feelings of being left out, especially when medication contraindicated alcohol consumption.

A range of almost universally negative emotional reactions both to the treatment and complications of uveitis were described. Reactions included anger, fear, embarrassment, isolation and low mood.

> "...when I used to go to [hospital] for my cataracts and see the people in there and I was the youngest by at least half a century ...it gets a bit depressing".

Much of the anxiety and worry surrounded possible visual deterioration and the unpredictability of the disease. Fears about the future were apparent, especially in relation to possible careers. Those who had identified potential careers for themselves were particularly concerned about the impact that eyesight problems would have. Some children and young people were explicit about their fear of going blind:

> "I am scared I am going to go blind".

Many of the children and young people involved in the study expressed distress, anger and resentment of the condition. There were reports of being frustrated and angry about the restrictions and limitations imposed by the condition, feelings often associated with questions about why this had happened to them. In more extreme cases, children and young people reported feeling that life was not worth living.

> "I used to feel, well I still feel like 'why me?' and all that kind of stuff, because it can feel unfair"

Discussion

Our study has identified multiple important themes across all 6 domains. As expected, within Domain 1, "impact of treatment", the greatest number of themes for any single domain were identified. The themes most strongly represented were negative emotional reactions to treatment, missing school for treatment, side effects and treatment avoidance. Within Domain 2, "complications of uveitis and treatment", the themes most frequently occurring were concerns regarding cataract removal and poor vision or visual blurring.

Domain 3, "impact on school", also highlighted several important themes, primarily difficulties reading information, upset at missing lessons, teachers forgetting about their condition, anxiety about catching up with missed work and upset at missing friends. It was also apparent that it is more difficult for children to spend free time catching up with subjects that they dislike, leading to additional resentment about missed school. Furthermore, for many children and young people, school is the main opportunity to socialise with their peers, and interruption of peer interaction was raised as an important concern, as was re-integrating into the peer group following periods of absence. The social importance of school was demonstrated in several strong themes coming from Domain 5, "social factors", including bullying, being excluded and not being chosen as a team member. Such bullying can lead to school avoidance, potentially further impairing the academic achievements of a young person already regularly absent from school due to hospital appointments and illness.

The "impact outside of school", Domain 4, developed fewer themes, with the requirement of adaptations in order to participate in activities and the inability to see bus numbers with ease being identified.

In view of the distress and difficulty apparent from the themes discussed above, it is unsurprising perhaps that Domain 6 "emotional reactions" produced some very strong themes, primarily distress and sadness about the illness, fear, anger and worry about deterioration, going blind and the future. This implies that although specific practical and social difficulties are problematic, the combination of these issues, compounded by the frightening nature of a vision-threatening condition, can result in a heavy emotional burden.

The only current validated uveitis-specific QoL measure in children, the EYE-Q, comprises 19 items measuring near, far, colour and night vision, photosensitivity, and functionality. There are four QoL items enquiring about feelings regarding the use of medications, missing school for appointments, and "laboratory draws". One question enquires about the presence of common uveitis symptoms, and there is an item that enquires about visual aids [4]. An early version was felt to be more a measure of visual function than QoL, demonstrated by EYE-Q scores being weakly associated with HRQoL measured using the generic PedsQL tool, however the most recent version, which included the 4 QoL questions, shows moderate correlation with PedsQL [4, 11, 22]. The topics include two important issues identified in Domain 1, "impact of treatment", one from Domain 2, "complications" and one from Domain 4 "impact outside school". However, no themes from Domains 3, 5 or 6, "impact on school", "social factors" and "emotional reactions" are covered, topics we found to be of significant concern to children in our study.

Other tools, generic, vision and disease-specific, measuring QoL in children have good coverage of these important themes (Table 3).

The PedsQL, a validated measure of general HRQoL in children aged 2–18 years, covers 4 core scales: physical functioning, emotional functioning, social functioning and school functioning, with 5 questions in each [5]. It thoroughly covers three domains we also found to be important: "impact on school", "social factors" and "emotional reactions". It is the standard against which other QoL tools are correlated [3, 4, 11].

The Impact of Vision Impairment on Children (IVI_C) is a 24 question, psychometrically valid vision-specific QoL measure, for use in vision-impaired children aged 8 to 18 years who have no additional disabilities. It includes themes identified in Domains 3, 4, 5 and 6, with a heavy emphasis on the impact on school and social functioning. It has been shown to have construct, face and content validity, as well as internal consistency and good test re-test reliability [8, 11]. A second vision-specific instrument, the VQoL_CYP, is an age-appropriate, vision related quality of life instrument for self-reporting by children with visual impairment, consisting of a 35 item scale [3]. It covers Domain 3 and has extensive coverage of Domains 4 and 5, with a focus on "social factors" and "emotional reactions" in particular. A strong correlation between VQoL_CYP and PedsQL Total Summary Score, particularly its psychosocial health scale has been shown. The correlation of VQoL_CYP with the PedsQL psychosocial summary score was found to be greater than the moderate correlation with PedsQL physical health summary score, providing evidence for strong psychosocial component of the VQoL_CYP [3].

A disease-specific tool, the Intermittent Exotropia Questionnaire (ITXQ), is a 3-part, patient-derived HRQoL questionnaire for children with intermittent exotropia (IXT) and their parents, comprising child, proxy and parent questionnaires with 12 questions in each part [23]. It especially examines "emotional concerns", Domain 6, and some "social factors", Domain 5. Although the ITXQ was not directly compared with another measure of HRQoL, during validity studies, children with ITX were shown to have worse HRQoL than controls. This finding is reinforced by previous studies showing children with ITX had worse HRQoL compared to controls, when measured by PedsQL [23]. A second disease-specific tool, the Quality of Life in Children with Vernal Keratoconjunctivitis (QUICK) questionnaire is for children aged 5 to 12 years with chronic keratoconjunctivitis [7]. It consists of 16 items and primarily enquires about symptoms and the social impact of disease, Domain 5. It showed internal validity and consistency, with significant correlations to the KINDL, a generic instrument for assessing HRQoL in children and adolescents aged 3 years and older and an alternative to PedsQL [24].

This study has included patients of a variety of ages and with a range of uveitis disease severity. Patients were recruited through a joint Paediatric Rheumatology / Ophthalmology clinic at a tertiary referral hospital and those included had moderate or severe disease. The results may not, therefore, be representative of patients with mild, uncomplicated disease controlled with a single agent. One included patient had Blau syndrome with panuveitis, predominantly anterior uveitis. One of the patients with JIA-associated uveitis had panuveitis and another also had macular involvement (Table 1). It is unlikely that the impact of uveitis and its treatment in

Table 3 Coverage of QoL domains by tool

	Quality of Life tool					
Domain	EYE-Q [4]	Peds-QL [5]	IVI-C [8]	VQoL-CYP [3]	ITXQ [23]	QUICK [7]
1: Impact of treatment	X					
2: Complications	X					
3: Impact on school		X	X	X		
4: Impact outside school	X		X	X		
5: Social factors		X	X	X	X	X
6: Emotional reactions		X	X		X	

Legend: *EYE-Q* Effects of Youngsters' Eyesight on Quality of Life Questionnaire, *ITXQ* Intermittent exotropia questionnaire, *IVI-C* Impact of Vision Impairment for Children, *PedsQL* Pediatric Quality of Life Inventory, *QUICK* Quality of Life in Children with Vernal Keratoconjunctivitis, *VQoL_CYP* Vision-related Quality of Life Instrument for Children and Young People

the patient with Blau syndrome is very dissimilar to those with JIA.

The study has identified themes within three domains ("impact on school", "social factors" and "emotional reactions") which are affected specifically by uveitis disease and treatment but are not covered by the EYE-Q. Questions which address these domains are included in other generic and ophthalmology disease-specific HRQoL tools for children (Table 3). In the future, it will be important to develop uveitis-specific HRQoL tools covering all these domains, and to include patients with other similar diseases and healthy controls as part of the validation process.

Clinical trials of treatments for JIA-associated uveitis are ongoing, including APTITUDE, a phase II trial of tocilizumab in anti-tumour necrosis factor (TNF) refractory patients [25] and studies of other biologic drugs are likely in the coming years. HRQoL measures are increasingly important as part of health economic evaluation of novel treatments [26]. These form a critical part of the recommendations of organisations advising health services about clinical and cost effectiveness such as the National Institute for Health and Care Excellence (NICE) in the UK. Similarly, being able to demonstrate effectiveness of treatment of JIA-associated uveitis using not only SUN criteria but also PROMs and HRQoL will provide additional patient-centred outcomes [27].

Conclusion

Multiple vision and disease-specific measures of HRQoL include questions on domains that this study has shown to be important factors influencing HRQoL in children with chronic anterior uveitis, such as "impact on school", "social factors" and "emotional reactions". This study suggests that the inclusion of these domains should be considered in future uveitis-specific tools examining HRQoL in children.

Abbreviations

CAU: Chronic anterior uveitis; CVFQ: Children's Visual Function Questionnaire; EYE-Q: Effects of Youngsters' Eyesight on Quality of Life Questionnaire; HRQoL: Health related quality of life; ITX: Intermittent exotropia; ITXQ: Intermittent exotropia questionnaire; IVI-C: Impact of Vision Impairment for Children; JIA: Juvenile idiopathic arthritis; PedsQL: Pediatric Quality of Life Inventory; PROM: Patient-reported outcome measure; QoL: Quality of life; QUICK: Quality of Life in Children with Vernal Keratoconjunctivitis; SUN: Standardisation of uveitis nomenclature; VQoL_CYP: Vision-related Quality of Life Instrument for Children and Young People

Acknowledgements

The authors would like to thank all patients and families for participation in this study.

Funding

There was no funding specifically for this study. ESS is funded by a National Institute for Health Research (NIHR) Rare Disease Translational Research Collaboration (RD-TRC) Clinical Research Fellowship. The views expressed are those of the authors and not necessarily those of the NHS, the NIHR or the Department of Health.

Authors' contributions

ESS collected and analysed clinical data, conducted a literature review, drafted and revised the manuscript. MJM interviewed participants, analysed recordings and revised the manuscript. RM conducted a literature review, drafted and revised the manuscript. HS and AH identified and recruited participants. BM designed and developed the study and revised the manuscript. ADD and AVR developed the study, identified participants and revised the manuscript. All authors read and approved the final manuscript.

Consent for publication

Not applicable.

Competing interests

All authors declare no competing interests.

Author details

[1]Department of Paediatric Rheumatology, Bristol Royal Hospital for Children, Upper Maudlin Street, Bristol BS2 8BJ, UK. [2]School of Clinical Sciences, University of Bristol, Bristol, UK. [3]Sirona Care & Health, Community Children's Health Partnership, Bristol, UK. [4]Department of Paediatrics, Bristol Royal Hospital for Children, Bristol, UK. [5]Retinal Treatment and Research Unit, Bristol Eye Hospital, Bristol, UK. [6]National Institute for Health Research Biomedical Research Centre at Moorfields Eye Hospital NHS Foundation Trust and UCL Institute of Ophthalmology, London, UK. [7]Department of Ophthalmology, Cambridge University Hospitals NHS Foundation Trust, Cambridge, UK.

References

1. Eiser C, Jenney M. Measuring quality of life. Arch Dis Child. 2007;92:348–50.
2. Bullinger M, Ravens-Sieberer U. Health related quality of life assessment in children: a review of the literature. Eur Rev Appl Psychol. 1995;45:245–56.
3. Tadić V, Cooper A, Cumberland P, Lewando-Hundt G, Rahi JS, Vision-related Quality of Life (VQoL) group. Measuring the quality of life of visually impaired children: first stage psychometric evaluation of the novel VQoL_CYP instrument. PLoS One. 2016;11:e0146225.
4. Angeles-Han ST, Yeh S, McCracken C, Jenkins K, Stryker D, Myoung E, et al. Using the effects of Youngsters' eyesight on quality of life questionnaire to measure visual outcomes in children with Uveitis. Arthritis Care Res. 2015;67: 1513–20.
5. Varni JW, Seid M, Kurtin PS. PedsQL 4.0: reliability and validity of the pediatric quality of life inventory version 4.0 generic core scales in healthy and patient populations. Med Care. 2001;39:800–12.
6. Birch EE, Cheng CS, Felius J. Validity and reliability of the Children's visual function questionnaire (CVFQ). J AAPOS. 2007;11:473–9.
7. Sacchetti M, Baiardini I, Lambiase A, Aronni S, Fassio O, Gramiccioni C, et al. Development and testing of the quality of life in children with vernal keratoconjunctivitis questionnaire. Am J Ophthalmol. 2007;144:557–63.
8. Cochrane GM, Marella M, Keeffe JE, Lamoureux EL. The impact of vision impairment for children (IVI_C): validation of a vision-specific pediatric quality-of-life questionnaire using Rasch analysis. Invest Ophthalmol Vis Sci. 2011;52:1632–40.
9. The World Health Organization Quality of Life assessment (WHOQOL): Position paper from the World Health Organization. Soc Sci Med. 1995; 41:1403-1409.
10. Albrecht GL, Devlieger PJ. The disability paradox: high quality of life against all odds. Soc Sci Med. 1999;48:977–88.
11. Tadic V, Hogan A, Sobti N, Knowles RL, Rahi JS. Patient-reported outcome measures (PROMs) in paediatric ophthalmology: a systematic review. Br J Ophthalmol. 2013;97:1369–81.
12. Angeles-Han ST. Quality-of-life metrics in pediatric uveitis. Int Ophthalmol Clin. 2015;55:93–101.
13. Clarke SL, Sen ES, Ramanan AV. Juvenile idiopathic arthritis-associated uveitis. Pediatr Rheumatol Online J. 2016;14:27.
14. Carvounis PE, Herman DC, Cha S, Burke JP. Incidence and outcomes of uveitis in juvenile rheumatoid arthritis, a synthesis of the literature. Graefes Arch Clin Exp Ophthalmol. 2006;244:281–90.

15. Sen ES, Dick AD, Ramanan AV. Uveitis associated with juvenile idiopathic arthritis. Nat Rev Rheumatol. 2015;11:338–48.
16. Ravens-Sieberer U, Erhart M, Wille N, Wetzel R, Nickel J, Bullinger M. Generic health-related quality-of-life assessment in children and adolescents: methodological considerations. PharmacoEconomics. 2006;24:1199–220.
17. Trusko B, Thorne J, Jabs D, Belfort R, Dick A, Gangaputra S, et al. The standardization of Uveitis nomenclature (SUN) project. Development of a clinical evidence base utilizing informatics tools and techniques. Methods Inf Med. 2013;52:259–65. S1-6
18. Jabs DA, Nussenblatt RB, Rosenbaum JT, Standardization of Uveitis Nomenclature (SUN) Working Group. Standardization of uveitis nomenclature for reporting clinical data. Results of the first international workshop. Am J Ophthalmol. 2005; 140:509–16.
19. Hayes N. Doing psychological research. Buckingham: Open University Press; 2000.
20. Joffe H. Thematic analysis. In: Harper D, Thompson AR, editors. Qualitative research methods in mental health and psychotherapy. Chichester: John Wiley & Sons, Ltd; 2011. p. 209–23.
21. Braun V, Clarke V. Using thematic analysis in psychology. Qual Res Psychol. 2008;3:77–101.
22. Angeles-Han ST, Griffin KW, Harrison MJ, Lehman TJ, Leong T, Robb RR, et al. Development of a vision-related quality of life instrument for children ages 8-18 years for use in juvenile idiopathic arthritis-associated uveitis. Arthritis Care Res. 2011;63:1254–61.
23. Hatt SR, Leske DA, Yamada T, Bradley EA, Cole SR, Holmes JM. Development and initial validation of quality-of-life questionnaires for intermittent exotropia. Ophthalmology. 2010;117:163–8.e1.
24. Ravens-Sieberer U, Bullinger M. Assessing health-related quality of life in chronically ill children with the German KINDL: first psychometric and content analytical results. Qual Life Res. 1998;7:399–407.
25. A phase II trial of tocilizumab in anti TNF refractory patients with JIA associated uveitis (APTITUDE study). BioMed central. 2015 [cited 22 DEC 2015]. Available from: http://www.isrctn.com/ISRCTN95363507.
26. Whitehead SJ, Ali S. Health outcomes in economic evaluation: the QALY and utilities. Br Med Bull. 2010;96:5–21.
27. Heiligenhaus A, Foeldvari I, Edelsten C, Smith JR, Saurenmann RK, Bodaghi B, et al. Proposed outcome measures for prospective clinical trials in juvenile idiopathic arthritis-associated uveitis: a consensus effort from the multinational interdisciplinary working group for uveitis in childhood. Arthritis Care Res. 2012;64:1365–72.

5

Immunogenicity and safety of influenza vaccination in patients with juvenile idiopathic arthritis on biological therapy using the microneutralization assay

M. S. Camacho-Lovillo[1], A. Bulnes-Ramos[2], W. Goycochea-Valdivia[1], L. Fernández-Silveira[1], E. Núñez-Cuadros[3], O. Neth[1*] and P. Pérez-Romero[2]

Abstract

Background: Seasonal influenza virus vaccination should be considered in all pediatric patients with rheumatic diseases. Few studies have addressed influenza vaccination safety and efficacy in this group. We aim to prospectively evaluate immunogenicity and safety of the trivalent inactivated influenza vaccine including A/H1N1, A/H3N2 and B strains in children with juvenile idiopathic arthritis (JIA) receiving biological therapy.

Methods: Thirty-five children diagnosed with JIA and 6 healthy siblings were included. Serum samples were collected prior to, 4-8 weeks and one year after vaccination. Microneutralization assays were used to determine neutralizing antibody titers. The type and duration of therapy were analyzed to determine its effect on vaccine response. Clinical data of the participants were collected throughout the study including severe adverse events (SAE) and adverse events following immunization (AEFI).

Results: Twenty-five patients (74.3%) received biological treatment for JIA; anti TNF-α was prescribed in 15, anti IL-1 receptor in 4 and anti IL-6 receptor therapy in 6 children. The seroprotection rate 4-8 weeks after vaccination in the JIA group was 96% for influenza A/(H1N1)pdm and influenza A/H3N2, and 88% for influenza B. No differences were found in GMT, seroprotection and seroconversion rates for the three influenza strains between the control group and patients receiving biological therapy. Furthermore, long-term seroprotection at 12 months after vaccination was similar in patients receiving either biological or non-biological treatments. No SAEs were observed.

Conclusions: In this study, influenza vaccination was safe and immunogenic in children with JIA receiving biological therapy.

Background

Children and adolescents with rheumatic diseases (RD) are at increased risk of infection compared to age- and gender-matched subjects without RD due to their aberrant immunity and frequent use of immunosuppressive drugs [1]. Annual vaccination against influenza is recommended for immunocompromised patients [2]. Efficacy and safety of vaccination remain to be defined in rheumatologic patients with immunomodulatory therapy, including high doses of steroids. Recommendations for vaccination in pediatric patients with RD were published in 2011 by the European League Against Rheumatism (EULAR). Seasonal influenza virus vaccination should be considered in all pediatric patients with RD [3, 4]. Few studies have addressed influenza vaccination safety and efficacy in this group, most of which have small sample sizes, include a wide variety of rheumatic diseases and have scarce data on new biological therapies [3–6].

Juvenile idiopathic arthritis (JIA) is the most common inflammatory rheumatic chronic disease of childhood,

* Correspondence: oneth-ibis@us.es
M. S. Camacho-Lovillo and A. Bulnes-Ramos shared 1st authors.
O. Neth and P. Pérez-Romero shared last authors.
[1]Unidad de Enfermedades Infecciosas e Inmunopatologías Pediátrica, Hospital Universitario Virgen del Rocío/Instituto de Biomedicina de Sevilla (IBIS), Sevilla, Spain

with a prevalence of approximately 1 per 1000. JIA is defined as arthritis of unknown etiology beginning prior the age of 16 years persisting for at least 6 weeks with other known conditions excluded [7]. The incidence of influenza infection in this patient group is unknown and evidence is lacking whether children with JIA have an increased risk of severe influenza infection or its associated complications. However, influenza virus can trigger disease flare, treatment interruption and the use of antibiotic therapy for suspected bacterial co-infection, all of which are associated with unnecessary medical revisions, thus reducing the quality of life of these children and their families [8]. The development of therapeutic biological agents including anti IL-6 and anti IL-1 receptor (R) therapy, has markedly altered treatment strategies for RD and greatly improved the prognosis of affected individuals [9]. Whilst influenza vaccination in children with RD receiving non biological immunosuppressive agents results in similar serum antibody titers compared to those of healthy children, few data exist on the impact of biological therapy [10]. Here, we describe the immunogenicity and safety of influenza vaccination and long term seroprotection on a pediatric cohort diagnosed with JIA receiving immunomodulatory therapy including anti IL-6 and anti IL-1R therapy and review the published literature.

Methods

Patient inclusion

We performed a prospective, longitudinal study of children with JIA receiving the influenza vaccine in two consecutive influenza seasons 2013/2014 and 2014/2015 at the University Hospital Virgen del Rocío, Seville. Diagnosis of JIA was made according to the recommendations of the International League of Associations for Rheumatology [7]. Patients (aged 1-18 years) and healthy siblings, as controls, were included once and consecutively after the legal guardians signed informed consent. Exclusion criteria for this study included acute infection at the time of vaccination, history of previous adverse reaction or anaphylaxis to chicken egg protein or any other vaccine, demyelinating disease or parents refusing to sign the informed consent. The Ethics Committee for Clinical Research of the local Hospital approved the study.

Samples

Serum samples were collected from each patient at the time of vaccination (baseline), at 4-8 weeks post vaccination (Tpv) and one year after vaccination (before the new seasonal vaccine immunization). Samples were stored at −80 °C for further analysis.

Clinical and laboratory data

Demographic data, including sex, age, time of diagnosis, JIA subtype, type of treatment, previous influenza vaccination, date of vaccination, activity of disease using the Juvenile Arthritis Disease Activity Score (JADAS) including 4 criteria (physician global assessment of disease activity, parent/patient global assessment of well-being, active joint count, and erythrocyte sedimentation rate), full blood count, immunoglobulin levels, Rheumatoid factor (RF), antinuclear antibodies (ANA), immunological and clinical response were collected [11]. Patients diagnosed with JIA were stratified according to the treatment received at time of vaccination (biological treatment and non-biological treatment including methotrexate (MTX) only or no treatment).

Safety assessment

Patients were followed-up during a six-month period to collect and record adverse events following immunization (AEFI). International guidelines for AEFI reporting and causality assessment were used according to the WHO, Global Vaccine Safety Initiative (GVSI) [12]. AEFI were monitored using a questionnaire given to patients on the vaccination day, and every 3 months in the follow-up visits, whilst serious adverse events (SAEs) and adverse events of special interest (AESI) were actively monitored during trial duration. AESI included were flare and worsening of the JADAS [11]. A flare was defined as a worsening of 40% in at least 2 of the 6 disease activity parameters of the American College of Rheumatology (ACR) pediatric core set, without a simultaneous improvement of 30% or more in at least 2 of the remaining parameters [13].

Vaccines

Patients received one dose of the trivalent non-adjuvanted inactivated vaccine in 2013/2014 (Sanofi, Sanofi- Pasteur MSD) containing the following strains: influenza A/California/7/2009-H1N1 (A/(H1N1)pdm), influenza A/Victoria/361/2011-H3N2 (A/H3N2) and B/Massachusetts/2/2012 and in 2014/2015 containing the following strains: A/California/7/2009 (H1N1)pdm; A/Texas/50/2012 (H3N2); B/Massachusetts/2/2012. Children under the age of nine, who were vaccinated for the first time against influenza, received a second dose of vaccine after one month.

Microneutralization assay

As described previously [14], two-fold serial dilutions of the inactivated human sera (from 1:5 to 1:2560) were incubated for 2 h at 37 °C with a multiplicity of infection (MOI) of 0.25 for A/(H1N1)pdm, 1.4 MOI for A/H3N2, and 0.05 MOI for B. Four wells with infected cells were used as positive controls and wells with only cells were used as negative controls. One hundred microliters containing 1.5×10^5 Madin–Darby canine kidney (MDCK) cells/ml were added to each well of a 96-well dish and incubated for 24 h at 37 °C. Primary antibodies for influenza A nucleoprotein (Anti-Influenza A nucleoprotein Bioporto Bionova, Gentofte, Denmark) diluted 1:1500 or influenza B nucleoprotein (Anti-Influenza B nucleoprotein Bioporto from Bionova, Gentofte, Denmark) diluted 1/1000 were used, followed by a HRP-conjugated anti-mouse IgG antibody diluted 1:1000 (Sigma-Aldrich). One-hundred microliters of peroxidase substrate (3, 3′, 5, 5′-Tetramethyl-benzidine substrate, supersensitive, for ELISA; Sigma-Aldrich) were added to each well and absorbance was measured at 450 nm. The average absorbance ($A450$) from the quadruplicate wells of virus-infected (VC) and uninfected (CC) control wells was determined, and the neutralizing endpoint was determined by using a 50% specific signal calculation. The endpoint titer was expressed as the reciprocal of the highest dilution of serum with $A450$ value less than X, where X = [(average $A450$ of VC wells) - (average $A450$ of CC wells)]/2 [14]. Sera were considered positive if titers were ≥40 obtained in at least two independent assays. Vaccination immunogenicity parameters were based on the following international EMEA/CPMP 1997 criteria described for the hemagglutination inhibition assay, which have shown correlation with antibody titres measured by microneutralization assay [15, 16]. Seroprotection was considered as a post-vaccination serum antibody titer >1:40. Seroconversion was considered when a 4-fold antibody titer increase from baseline was achieved. Geometric mean titers (GMT) defined as mean antibody titer in the group of vaccinated individuals; seroprotection rate defined as the proportion of vaccinated individuals with antibody titers ≥1:40; seroconversion rate as the percentage of subjects showing seroconversion; and geometric mean ratio (GMR) defined as seroconversion factor post to prevaccination.

Statistical analysis

A descriptive statistical analysis was performed. Continuous variables were expressed as median and interquartile range or mean ± standard deviation if adjusted to normal distribution, and evaluated by Shapiro-Wilk or Kolmogorov-Smirnov tests when appropriate. The main primary outcome for the analysis was seroprotection. Secondary outcomes were seroconversion, GMT after vaccination, and safety. For bivariate analysis, the chi-square test, Fisher's exact test or the McNemar test were used for categorical variables. For quantitative variables, the Mann-Whitney test or Student's t test were used. If the variance was not homogeneous the Welch test was applied, in case of homogeneity of variances, ANOVA was applied.

For immunogenicity analysis, GMT at each time point was used. Relative risk and 95% confidence interval (CI) were calculated by taking the exponent of natural logarithm of the mean and 95% CI. Results were analyzed by PASW Statistic 18.0.1 software. Statistical significance was established as a p value of <0.05. All reported p values were based on two-tailed tests. Bivariate analysis was an exploratory outcome and adjustment for multiplicity was done for this analysis using the Bonferroni method (adjusted p value <0.002).

Results

Patient cohort

Baseline clinical parameters and demographic characteristics of the patients are shown in Table 1. A total of 41 subjects were included in the study. Three patients received two vaccine doses. 35 (83.3%) patients were diagnosed with JIA (experimental group), median age of 10.6 years (IQR 8.8-12.7), 12 (35.3%) were male and 25 (74.3%) were receiving biological treatment for JIA; 15 patients anti-TNFα (11 etanercept and 4 adalimumab), 4 anti-IL-1R (anakinra) and 6 anti-IL-6R (tocilizumab). Six (14.2%) children were healthy individuals (control group), with a median age of 11.6 years (IQR 9.8-14.6) and two (33.3%) male.

Immunological response to influenza vaccination

Overall, control and experimental, groups together achieved an adequate seroprotection rate at Tpv: 97.8% for influenza A/(H1N1)pdm, 95.6% for influenza A/H3N2 and 91.1% for influenza B. Median Tpv was 5.4 weeks IQR (4.6-6.1). Immunological response to vaccination was analyzed in the experimental group and compared with the control group. No differences were found in GMT, seroprotection and seroconversion rates at Tpv for the three influenza strains (A/(H1N1)pdm, A/H3N2 and B) (Table 2). Children diagnosed with JIA were stratified according to receiving biological treatment and again no differences were observed in the antibody response to vaccination based on treatment (Table 2). There were no differences for A/(H1N1)pdm and A/H3N2 postvaccination seroprotection rates between children receiving biological treatment and those receiving no biological therapy (96% vs. 100%; p = 0.521); neither for influenza B strain (88% vs. 90%; p = 0.867). Similarly, receiving biological treatment was not associated with differences in the post-vaccination GMT or in seroconversion for the three vaccine strains. Two of the patients receiving biological treatment had concomitant systemic steroids, however no differences were found in pre- or post-vaccination seroprotection or antibody titers compared with patients on biological treatment with no steroids.

Within the experimental group, patients were stratified according to the type of biological treatment and no differences were found in the antibody response against the three influenza strains (Additional file 1: Table S1).

Three children received two vaccine doses and showed, post-vaccination seroprotection after the second dose,

Table 1 Baseline clinical and laboratory parameters

Variables	Control group (n = 6)	JIA group (n = 35)	Biological therapy (n = 25)	Non biological therapy (n = 10)
Female n (%)	4 (66.6)	23 (65.7)	17 (68)	6 (60)
Age in y (IQR)	11.6 (9.8-14.6)	10.6 (8.8-12.7)	11.4 (8.9-13.0)	11.4 (4.7-12.3)
Previous seasonal vaccination n (%)	2 (33)	22 (62.8)	18 (72)	4 (40)
Duration of JIA in y (IQR)		4.9 (2.7-8.3)	5.99 (3.0-8.6)	3.94 (2.5-4.7)
JIA category n (%)				
Persistent oligoarthritis		13 (37.1)	7 (28)	6 (60)
Extended oligoarthritis		6 (17.1)	5 (20)	1 (10)
Polyarthritis RF negative		6 (17.1)	4 (16)	2 (20)
Polyarthritis RF positive		0 (0)	0 (0)	0 (0)
Systemic onset arthritis		7 (20)	7 (28)	0 (0)
Enthesitis related arthritis		3 (8.5)	2 (8)	1 (10)
Psoriatic arthritis		0	0	0
Undifferentiated arthritis		0	0	0
Treatment n (%) [(a)]				
Without therapy		3 (8.5)	–	3 (30)
Systemic corticosteroids (concomitant MTX + tocilizumab)		2 (5.7)	2 (8)	
Methotrexate monotherapy		7 (20)	–	7 (70)
Biological monotherapy		16 (45.7)	16 (64)	–
Biological therapy + methotrexate		9 (25.7)	9 (36)	–
Duration of biological therapy in years (IQR)	NA	NA	3.1 (1.8-4.8)	NA
JADAS 71 (IQR)		1 (0-5)	3 (0-7)	2 (0.25-6.75)
IgG mg/dl (IQR)		1036 (888-1243)	1021 (880-1249)	1143 (965-1205)
Leukocytes $\times 10^9$/L (IQR)	6.5 (3.7-8.2)	6.0 (5.2-7.4)	5.8 (5.0-6.9)	7.5 (5.9-9.1)
Lymphocytes $\times 10^9$/L	2.3 (1.3-2.5)	2.2 (1.6-2.8)	2.2 (1.6-2.8)	2.283 (1.9-3.1)
Neutrophils $\times 10^9$/L	3.4 (2.0-4.7)	3.1 (2.7-3.9)	3.1 (2.5-3.6)	3.9 (3.0-4.7)
Hemoglobin g/L (IQR)	13.3 (12.8-13.6)	13.3 (12.7-13.6)	13.3 (12.8-14.2)	13.1 (12.2-13.3)
Platelets $\times 10^9$/L (IQR)	305 (289-376)	263 (234-320)	255 (227-318)	275 (251-356)
ESR mm/h (IQR)	5 (4.0-9.5)	8 (4.0-10.5)	6 (4.0-9.0)	8.5 (6.5-10.8)

Values are expressed as median unless stated otherwise; *IQR* interquartile range, *JIA* juvenile idiopatic arthritis; *y* years; *MTX* methotrexate, *IgG* immunoglobulin G, *ESR* erythrocyte sedimentation rate, *NA* not applicable

[(a)]Methotrexate was given at a dose of 10-15 mg/m^2/week (35% received lower doses due to clinical remission). Systemic corticosteroids included oral 0.1 mg/kg/day in a patient and 10 mg/kg/dose iv in the remaining patients. Biological therapy included: tocilizumab 8 mg/kg/dose monthly or fortnightly (polyarticular or systemic JIA respectively), anakinra 2-4 mg/kg/day, etanercept 0.8 mg/kg/week and adalimumab 24 mg/kg/m^2 (52% of patients received lower doses due to clinical remission). Biological therapy was administered simultaneously with the influenza vaccination

however antibody titers did not differ from those receiving one dose only (data not shown).

Long-term seroprotection rates after vaccination

In the JIA group 12 individuals had serum samples available one year after vaccination, six (50%) of them received biological treatment, and long-term seroprotection after vaccination was analyzed. Overall no differences in humoral responses were observed for the three strains analyzed. All 12 patients (100%) were seroprotected at Tpv vs. 91.7% one year after vaccination against A(H1N1)pdm (p = 0.327); 81.8% vs. 91.7% were protected against A/H3N2 (p = 0.070), and 91.7% vs. 91.7% (p = 0.500) against influenza B at Tpv vs. one year after vaccination.

Similarly, the type of treatment (biological or non-biological) did not influence long-term antibody response. In patients with biological treatment (n = 6), seroprotection at one-year post vaccination was 100% (100% at Tpv) for influenza A/H1N1 (p = 0.999), 66.7% (83.3% at Tpv) for H3N2 (p = 0.999) and 100% (100% at Tpv) for influenza B (p = 0.999).

Bivariate analysis

The analysis of confounding factors associated with antibody response to vaccination in patients with JIA

Table 2 Influenza A/(H1N1)pdm, A/H3N2 and B virus antibody response in JIA patients receiving or not biological therapy

	Control group (n = 6)	JIA group (n = 35)	p-value	Biological therapy (n = 25)	No biological therapy (n = 10)	p-value
A/H1N1						
GMT						
Pre-vaccine (range)	31.7 (10 -160)	47.8 (5-1280)	*0.388*	45.9 (5 -320)	52.7 (5 -1280)	*0.504*
Post-vaccine (range)	320 (160-1280)	273.1 (20-2560)	*0.684*	242.5 (20-2560)	367.5 (40-2560)	*0.535*
GMR mean (range)	6.10 (2.7-22.3)	5.1 (2.7-85.2)	*0.646*	4.89 (2.71-85.2)	5.99 (2.71-30.2)	*0.510*
Seroprotection						
Pre-vaccine- n (%)	3 (50)	24 (68.6)	*0.375*	18 (72.0)	6 (60)	*0.490*
Post-vaccine- n (%)	6 (100)	34 (97.1)	*0.675*	24 (96)	10 (100)	*0.521*
Seroconversion- n(%)	5 (83.3)	23 (65.7)	*0.391*	15 (60)	8 (80)	*0.260*
A/H3N2						
GMT						
Pre-vaccine (range)	22.44 (5-80)	38.44 (5-2560)	*0.562*	34.82 (5-80)	49.2 (5-2560)	*0.334*
Post-vaccine (range)	320 (80-2560)	233.0 (20-2560)	*0.684*	199.7 (20-2560)	342.9 (80-2560)	*0.565*
GMR mean (range)	8.0 (3.1-35.0)	4.9 (2.7-22.3)	*0.079*	4.70 (2.7-13.7)	5.66 (2.7-22.4)	*0.383*
Seroprotection						
Pre-vaccine- n (%)	3 (50)	22 (62.9)	*0.551*	17 (68.0)	5 (50.0)	*0.319*
Post-vaccine- n(%)	6 (100)	34 (97.1)	*0.675*	24 (96)	10 (100)	*0.521*
Seroconversion- n(%)	5 (83.3)	22 (62.9)	*0.328*	15 (60)	7 (70)	*0.580*
Flu B						
GMT						
Pre-vaccine (range)	63.4 (40-80)	40.8 (5-640)	*0.114*	26.1 (5-640)	37.3 (5-320)	*0.912*
Post-vaccine (range)	640 (40-2560)	118.9 (20-1280)	*0.396*	91.9 (20-1280)	226.2 (20-1280)	*0.871*
GMR mean (range)	4.7 (2.7-8.3)	3.8 (2.7-9.8)	*0.235*	3.6 (2.7-9.9)	4.7 (3.06-6.70)	*0.038*
Seroprotection						
Pre-vaccine n (%)	6 (100)	24 (68.6)	*0.108*	17 (68.0)	7 (70)	*0.908*
Post-vaccine n (%)	6 (100)	31 (88.6)	*0.383*	22 (88.0)	9 (90.0)	*0.867*
Seroconversion n (%)	4 (66.7)	17 (48.6)	*0.413*	9 (36)	8 (80)	*0.019*

Parameters were compared by multiple comparison chi-square test or linear regression. *GMR* geometric mean ratio, *GMT* geometric mean titer

(Additional file 2: Table S2), revealed seroprotected patients to Tpv A/H1N1 to have lower platelet levels and ESR at baseline compared with non-seroprotected individuals (286 vs. 594 × 10 [9]/L, p = 0.001 and 7.2 vs 18 mm/h, p = 0.009). When adjusted for multiplicity (p < 0.002), only platelet level was significantly lower in seroprotected patients to Tpv for A/H1N1.

Safety of influenza vaccination

There was no follow-up loss of any of the subjects in the study. Overall no SAEs were observed. Seven out of 41 (17%) children showed adverse drug local reactions (six with local skin inflammation and one hematoma), whilst two out of 41 (4.9%; one each in the control and biological therapy group) had systemic adverse drug reactions (general malaise and fever >24 h). During the 6-month follow-up, 16 febrile episodes, not related to vaccination, were reported in 11 patients (four in the non-biological and seven in the biological therapy group), 10 of which were treated with oral antibiotic therapy. JADAS score increased in 6 patients at Tpv compared with baseline, in three of them from a low or no activity to moderate [17]. However, none of them had a flare based on the mentioned criteria [13].

Discussion

In this cohort of children with JIA receiving immunomodulatory therapy, influenza vaccination was safe and immunogenic; and the neutralizing antibody response was independent of the type of treatment. To date few influenza vaccine studies have included children with JIA, and biological therapy was specifically studied in only five of them (Table 3). In all but one (Toplak et al. [18]) the hemagglutination inhibition test (HAI) was used to determine antibody response to vaccination, which is known for its overall poor sensitivity, thereby

Table 3 Summary of published reports describing pediatric patients with JIA receiving influenza vaccine

Article	Vaccination season Vaccine type	Methodology antibody response	Number of JIA patients	Number of controls	Number of JIA patients on biological therapy	Adverse events (AE)	Efficacy (seroprotection) according to group and vaccine type	Time post-vaccination
Toplak et al. [18]. 2012 Slovenia	2008/2009 A/(H1N1) pdm, H3N2,B	Virus neutralization test	31	14	anti-TNFα 4	Short-term AE: JIA 35% Control 36% Pain at injection site: JIA 32% Control 21% Malaise and headache: JIA 3% Control 14% No severe AE	JIA 100%H1N1 100% H3N2 84%B anti-TNFα 75%H1N1 75%H3N2 10% B Control 100% H1N1 100%H3N2 78%B	1 month
Malleson et al. [6]. 1993 Canada	1991/1992-2008/2009 A/(H1N1)pdm, H3N2,B	HAI	26	13	0	Soreness and redness at injection site: JIA 69% and 15% Control 69% and 8% Fever and feeling unwell: JIA 19% and 46% Control 8% and 26% No severe AE	JIA 100% H1N1 97% H3N2 97% B Control 90% H1N1 90% H3N2 90% B	4 - 6 week
Dell' Era et al. [25]. 2012 Italy	2010/2011-2008/2009 A/(H1N1)pdm, H3N2,B	HAI	60	30	Etanercept 30	Local AE: JIA with DMARD 43.3% JIA with Etanercept 36.7% Control 40% Systemic AE: JIA with DMARD 30% JIA with Etanercept 26.7% Control 26.7% Severe AE: JIA with DMARD 3.3% JIA with Etanercept 3.3%	JIA with DMARD 100% H1N1 100% H3N2 83.3% B JIA with Etanercept 100% H1N1 100% H3N2 30% B Control 100% H1N1 100% H3N2 93,3% B	1 month
Aikawa et al. [26]. 2013 Brazil	2009 A/(H1N1)pdm	HAI	95	91	anti-TNFα 16	Local pain: JIA 21.1% Control 23.1% No severe AE	JIA 88.4% H1N1 anti-TNFα 100% H1N1 Control 95.6% H1N1	3 weeks
Shinoki et al. [9]. 2012 Japan	2007/2008 A/(H1N1) pdm, H3N2,B	HAI	27	17	Tocilizumab 27	Local AE: JIA14.8% Control 0%	JIA 88.9% H1N1 85.2% H3N2 40.7% B	4 -7 weeks

Table 3 Summary of published reports describing pediatric patients with JIA receiving influenza vaccine *(Continued)*

						No severe AE	Control 76.5% H1N1 100% H3N2 35.3% B	
Miraglia et al. [5]. 2011 Brazil	2009 A/(H1N1)pdm	HAI	83	-	Not specified	1.3% redness, 20% malaise JIA No severe AE	JIA 85.5% H1N1	3 weeks
Carvalho et al. [8]. 2013 Brazil	2008 A/(H1N1)pdm, H3N2,B	HAI	44	10	anti-TNFα 5	Local pain JIA 13.6% Control 10% Other local change JIA4.5% Control 10%	JIA 100% H1N1 93% H3N2 95% B Anti TNFα 60% H1N1 100% H3N2 80% B Control 100% H1N1 80% H3N2 100 B	30-40 days

HAI hemagglutination inhibition, *DMARDS* disease-modifying anti-rheumatic drugs. Severe AE: defined as patients requiring hospitalization or iv treatment

potentially underestimating the seroprevalence in a given population [19]. The microneutralization assay, which was used in the present study, has been shown to enhance sensitivity and specificity [14]. No correlate of protection has been defined for microneutralization, but good correlation with HAI defined protection thresholds has been reported [16]. Furthermore, it has been proposed that HAI antibody seroprotection cut-offs in children aged 6-72 months may be 1:110 to achieve 50% protection [20], thus it is possible that children with RD may need antibody titers equal to or higher than those described. There is a need to review the current practice of evaluating vaccine responses and should include more advanced techniques to evaluate immunogenicity such as microneutralization assay, which identifies functional antibodies, rather than quantitative tests only [21].

Blockade of the IL-6R has been shown to decrease lymphocyte activation and to restore B and T cell homoeostasis in patients with SLE [22]. Anti-IL-6R treatment may diminish influenza vaccine antibody responses since IL-6 induces B cell differentiation into antibody-forming cells and T cells into effectors cells [22]. However, Shinoki et al. studied JIA patients treated with tocilizumab (anti IL-6R) and demonstrated that influenza vaccination was immunogenic and safe, as was the case in our study (Table 3) [9]. Whilst in healthy subjects therapy with anti-IL-1 did not affect the antibody responses after vaccination with influenza vaccine [23], the impact of its use in children with JIA is unknown. To the best of our knowledge, this is the first study evaluating influenza vaccine in children receiving IL-1R antagonist (anakinra) for JIA and was found to be safe and immunogenic. However, further studies are needed to confirm its safety in pediatric patients, as only four patients were included here.

Anti-TNF-α therapy in rheumatoid arthritis inhibits germinal center reactions, thereby leading to decrease peripheral blood memory B cell levels, potentially contributing to a poor response to vaccination [24]. Four pediatric studies (Table 3) have evaluated influenza vaccine in JIA patients receiving anti-TNF-α therapy. Antibody titers against A(H1N1), A(H3N2), and B vaccine viruses were found to be reduced in patient receiving anti-TNF-α although only four children were enrolled [18]. In another study, 30 JIA patients treated with anti-TNF-α showed significantly lower GMTs against the A/H1N1 strain compared to those treated with disease-modifying antirheumatic drugs (DMARD) and healthy controls. Furthermore, sero-conversion and -protection rates were significantly lower in patients receiving anti-TNF-α [25], as was also reported by Carvalho et al. in 5 patients and only for the A/H1N1 strain [8]. In the Aikawa et al. study, no differences were observed in immunogenicity parameters between patients with or without anti-TNF-α blockers however, the seroconversion rate for the A/H1N1 strain was significantly lower in JIA patients compared to controls (83.2% vs. 95.6%, p = 0.008) [26]. In our study, no differences between the control group and patients with or without biological therapy were observed, thus biological therapy plus MTX did not alter the vaccine response. Although lack of differences between groups could be due to the small sample size, these findings are in contrast with previous results, where the use of anti-TNF-α blockers was associated with a reduced vaccine response [25, 26]. One year after vaccination seroprotection rates were similar with a slight and expectable reduction for all strains but A/H3N2, which was higher. This could be due to natural exposition to the virus, or test precision variability. Although it was evaluated in only few patients, biological treatment seems not to influence in long-term seroprotection rates after vaccination.

Like in other studies in children with RD, no SAEs were reported and vaccination using an inactivated influenza vaccine was shown to be safe with mild systemic and local reactions as most reported AEFI [26, 27]. Our patients remained clinically stable (JADAS-71:1 (0-5)) during the study period with only two patients receiving systemic corticoids at the time of vaccination. Lack of active inflammation at the time of vaccination could have influenced the safety and immunogenicity outcomes in our cohort. This is supported by the study of Toplak et al., where only 42% of the children had inactive disease at the time of vaccination and all children suffering from a flare post vaccination, had at least one criterion for active disease prior to vaccination [18]. This is important as high dose steroid therapy is known to be associated with a reduced immnunogenicity of the influenza vaccine resulting in lower antibody titers [28, 29]. We observed seroprotected patients to have lower inflammatory markers such as platelet count and ESR compared to non-seroprotected children. A low inflammatory state may result in an enhanced cellular immune response (Th1 vs Th2) thereby supporting B and T cell differentiation with subsequent improved vaccine response [30, 31]. In contrast to the studies of Dell' Era and Toplak et al. where only 8.3% and 13% of the patients were previously vaccinated, 62.8% of children with JIA (and 72% of those receiving biological treatment) received the influenza vaccine the season prior to this study, and that has likely contributed to the overall high vaccine response shown here. This is also supported by previous results suggesting that baseline seroprotection promotes significantly higher GMT after vaccination [32]. Whilst over 60% (H1N1 68.6%, H3N2 62.9% and Flu B 68.6%) of our JIA children were seroprotected prior vaccination, only 20% of the patients described by Toplak and Aikawa et al. showed pre-vaccine seroprotection, further supporting the benefit of seasonal influenza vaccination. However, differences between participant's age and previous exposure to the virus could alter pre-vaccination seroprotection rates. A limitation of this study is the overall low number of patients and healthy controls included, which may have limited the power to detect differences, especially when performing subgroup analysis. Although clinical, laboratory baseline parameters and GMT baseline titers were similar in the groups; there was heterogeneity in the treatment used and likely in the previous influenza exposure (artificial or natural) of the included patients. Further studies evaluating vaccine efficacy and effectiveness are necessary.

Conclusions

In this prospective study of children with JIA, the use of the trivalent inactivated influenza vaccine including A/H1N1, A/H3N2 and B strains was shown to be safe and immunogenic. The type of immunomodulatory therapy did not alter vaccine response. This patient group would likely benefit from seasonal influenza vaccination thereby supporting the annual immunization program.

Abbreviations

AEFI: adverse events following immunization; AESI: Adverse events of special interest; EULAR: European League Against Rheumatism; GMR: Geometric mean ratio; GMT: Geometric mean titers; GVSI: Global Vaccine Safety Initiative; JADAS: Juvenile Arthritis Disease Activity Score; JIA: juvenile idiopathic arthritis; SAE: severe adverse events; Tpv: time post vaccination

Acknowledgements

We thank all patients, siblings and their parents for participating in this study.

Funding

This work was supported by the

- Instituto de Salud Carlos III-Fondo de Investigación Sanitaria [PI1101537], Consejería de Economía e Innovación [CTS-2012-1909] and Ministerio de Sanidad y Consumo, Instituto de Salud Carlos III-FEDER, Spanish Network for the Research in Infectious Diseases [REIPI RD06/0008/0000].
- CLMS was supported by Sociedad Española de Reumatología Pediátrica (SERPE)
- PRP is supported by the Ministerio de Economía y Competitividad of Spain (CP11/00314) co-financed by the Programa Nicolás Monardes (RC-0005-2015) Servicio Andaluz de Salud, Junta de Andalucía.
- CLMS and NCE are members of PRINTO, SHARE y SERPE

Authors' contributions

CLMS, BRA, NO, PRP participated in the design of the study. CLMS, BRA, GVW performed the statistical analysis. CLMS, FSL, NCE recruited patients and included clinical data. BRA, PRP performed microneutralization assay. All authors participated in the coordination of the study and helped to draft the manuscript lead by CLMS, BRA, NO, PRP. All authors read and approved the final manuscript.

Consent for publication

Not applicable.

Competing interests

The authors declare that they have no competing interests.

Author details

[1]Unidad de Enfermedades Infecciosas e Inmunopatologías Pediátrica, Hospital Universitario Virgen del Rocío/Instituto de Biomedicina de Sevilla (IBIS), Sevilla, Spain. [2]Instituto de Biomedicina de Sevilla (IBIS), University Hospital Virgen del Rocío/CSIC/University of Sevilla, Unidad Clínica de Enfermedades Infecciosas, Microbiología y Medicina Preventiva, Sevilla, Spain. [3]Unidad de Reumatología Pediátrica, Hospital Materno Infantil, Hospital Regional Universitario de Málaga, Málaga, Spain.

References

1. Dell' Era L, Esposito S, Corona F, Principi N. Vaccination of children and adolescents with rheumatic diseases. Rheumatology (Oxford) [Internet]. 2011; 50(8):1358–1365. Available from: http://www.ncbi.nlm.nih.gov/pubmed/21482543.
2. Rubin LG, Levin MJ, Ljungman P, Davies EG, Avery R, Tomblyn M, et al. 2013 IDSA Clinical Practice Guideline for Vaccination of the Immunocompromised Host. Clin Infect Dis. 2014;58:e44–100.
3. Heijstek MW, Ott de Bruin LM, Borrow R, van der Klis F, Koné-Paut I, Fasth A, et al. Vaccination in paediatric patients with auto-immune rheumatic diseases: A systemic literature review for the European League against Rheumatism evidence-based recommendations. Autoimmun Rev. 2011;11(2):112–22.
4. Heijstek MW, Ott de Bruin LM, Bijl M, Borrow R, F K-PI v d K. EULAR recommendations for vaccination in paediatric patients with rheumatic diseases. Ann Rheum Dis. 2011;70(10):1704–12.
5. Miraglia JL, Abdala E, Hoff PM, Luiz AM, Oliveira DS, Saad CGS, et al. Immunogenicity and reactogenicity of 2009 influenza a (H1N1) inactivated monovalent non-adjuvanted vaccine in elderly and immunocompromised patients. PLoS One. 2011;6(11):e27214.
6. Malleson PN, Tekano JL, Scheifele DWWJ. Influenza immunization in children with chronic arthritis: a prospective study. J Rheumatol. 1993;Oct;20(10):1769–7.
7. Petty RE, Southwood TR, Manners P, Baum J, Glass DN, Goldenberg JHX, Maldonado-Cocco J, Orozco-Alcala J, Prieur AM, Suarez-Almazor MEWP, Rheumatology. IL of A for. International League of Associations for Rheumatology classification of juvenile idiopathic arthritis: second revision, Edmonton, 2001. J Rheumatol. 2004;31(2):390–2.
8. Carvalho LM, De Paula FE, Silvestre RVD, Roberti LR, Arruda E, Mello WA, et al. Prospective surveillance study of acute respiratory infections, influenza-like illness and seasonal influenza vaccine in a cohort of juvenile idiopathic arthritis patients. Pediatr Rheumatol. 2013;11:10.
9. Shinoki T, Hara R, Kaneko U, Miyamae T, Imagawa T, Mori M, et al. Safety and response to influenza vaccine in patients with systemic-onset juvenile idiopathic arthritis receiving tocilizumab. Mod Rheumatol. 2012;22(6):871–6.
10. Ogimi C, Tanaka R, Saitoh A, Oh-Ishi T. Immunogenicity of Influenza Vaccine in Children With Pediatric Rheumatic Diseases Receiving Immunosuppressive Agents. Pediatr Infect Dis J. 2011;30(3):208–11.
11. Consolaro A, Ruperto N, Bazso A, Pistorio A, Magni-Manzoni S, Filocamo G, et al. Development and Validation of a Composite Disease Activity Score for Juvenile Idiopathic Arthritis. Arthritis Care Res. 2009;61(5):658–66.
12. The Global Vaccine Safety Initiative (GVSI [Internet]. Available from: http://www.who.int/vaccine_safety/initiative/en. Accessed July 2016.
13. Brunner HI, Lovell DJ, Finck BKGE. Preliminary definition of disease flare in juvenile rheumatoid arthritis. J Rheumatol. 2002;29(5):1058–64.
14. Perez-Romero P, Bulnes-Ramos A, Torre-Cisneros J, Gavaldá J, Aydillo TA, Moreno A, et al. Influenza vaccination during the first 6 months after solid organ transplantation is efficacious and safe. Clin Microbiol Infect. 2015;21(11): 1040.e11–8.
15. The European Agency for the Evaluation of Medicinal Products (EMEA). Comitte for Proprietary Medicinal Products (CPMP). Note for guidence on harmonisation of requirements for influenza vaccines. WwwEudraOrg/

EmeaHtml [Internet]. 1997;19. Available from: http://www.ema.europa.eu/docs/en_GB/document_library/Scientific_guideline/2009/09/WC500003945.pdf. Accessed July 2016.
16. Trombetta C, Perini D, Mather S, Temperton N, Montomoli E. Overview of Serological Techniques for Influenza Vaccine Evaluation: Past, Present and Future. Vaccine. 2014;2(4):707–34. Available from: http://www.mdpi.com/2076-393X/2/4/707/
17. Consolaro A, Giancane G, Schiappapietra B, Davì S, Calandra S, Lanni S, et al. Clinical outcome measures in juvenile idiopathic arthritis. Pediatr Rheumatol Online J. 2016;14(1):23. Available from: http://www.ncbi.nlm.nih.gov/pubmed/27089922%5Cn, http://www.pubmedcentral.nih.gov/articlerender.fcgi?artid=PMC4836071
18. Toplak N, Šubelj V, Kveder T, Čučnik S, Prosenc K, Trampuš-Bakija A, et al. Paediatric rheumatology Safety and efficacy of influenza vaccination in a prospective longitudinal study of 31 children with juvenile idiopathic arthritis. Clin Exp Rheumatol. 2012;30:436–44.
19. Verschoor CP, Singh P, Russell ML, Bowdish DME, Brewer A, Cyr L, et al. Microneutralization assay titres correlate with protection against seasonal influenza H1N1 and H3N2 in children. PLoS One. 2015;10(6):7–13.
20. Black S, Nicolay U, Vesikari T, Knuf M, Del Giudice G, Della Cioppa G, et al. Hemagglutination Inhibition Antibody Titers as a Correlate of Protection for Inactivated Influenza Vaccines in Children. Pediatr Infect Dis J. 2012;30(12):1081–5.
21. Cagigi A, Cotugno N, Rinaldi S, Santilli V, Rossi P, Palma P. Downfall of the current antibody correlates of influenza vaccine response in yearly vaccinated subjects: Toward qualitative rather than quantitative assays. Pediatr Allergy Immunol 2016;27(1):22–7.
22. Shirota Y, Yarboro C, Fischer R, Pham T, Lipsky P, Illei GG. Impact of anti-interleukin-6 receptor blockade on circulating T and B cell subsets in patients with systemic lupus erythematosus. Ann Rheum Dis. 2013;72(1):118–28.
23. Chioato A, Noseda E, Felix SD, Stevens M, Del Giudice G, Fitoussi S, et al. Influenza and meningococcal vaccinations are effective in healthy subjects treated with the interleukin-1-blocking antibody canakinumab: Results of an open-label, parallel group, randomized, single-center study. Clin Vaccine Immunol. 2010;17(12):1952–7.
24. Kobie JJ, Zheng B, Bryk P, Barnes M, Ritchlin CT, Tabechian DA, et al. Decreased influenza-specific B cell responses in rheumatoid arthritis patients treated with anti-tumor necrosis factor. Arthritis Res Ther. 2011;13(6):R209. Available from: http://www.ncbi.nlm.nih.gov/pubmed/22177419.
25. Dell'Era L, Corona F, Daleno C, Scala A, Principi N, Esposito S. Immunogenicity, safety and tolerability of MF59-adjuvanted seasonal influenza vaccine in children with juvenile idiopathic arthritis. Vaccine. 2012;20;30(5):936–40.
26. Aikawa NE, Campos LMA, Goldenstein-Schainberg C, Saad CGS, Ribeiro AC, Bueno C, et al. Effective seroconversion and safety following the pandemic influenza vaccination (anti-H1N1) in patients with juvenile idiopathic arthritis. Scand J Rheumatol [Internet]. 2013;42(1):34–40. Available from: http://www.ncbi.nlm.nih.gov/pubmed/22992045.
27. Woerner A, Sauvain M-J, Aebi C, Otth M, Bolt IB. Immune response to influenza vaccination in children treated with methotrexate or/and tumor necrosis factor-alpha inhibitors. Hum Vaccin. 2011;7(12):1293–8.
28. Sengler C, Niewerth M, Kallinich T, Nimtz-Talaska A, Haller M, Huppertz HI, et al. Survey about tolerance of the AS03-adjuvanted H1N1 influenza vaccine in children with rheumatic diseases. Clin Rheumatol. 2014;33(1):137–9.
29. Aikawa NE, França ILA, Ribeiro AC, Sallum AME, Bonfa E, Silva CA. Short and long-term immunogenicity and safety following the 23-valent polysaccharide pneumococcal vaccine in juvenile idiopathic arthritis patients under conventional DMARDs with or without anti-TNF therapy. Vaccine. 2015;33(5):604–9.
30. Campos LMA, Silva CA, Aikawa NE, Jesus AA, Moraes JCB, Miraglia J, et al. High disease activity: An independent factor for reduced immunogenicity of the pandemic influenza a vaccine in patients with juvenile systemic lupus erythematosus. Arthritis Care Res. 2013;65(7):1121–7.
31. Trzonkowski P, Myśliwska J, Szmit E, Więckiewicz J, Łukaszuk K, Brydak LB, et al. Association between cytomegalovirus infection, enhanced proinflammatory response and low level of anti-hemagglutinins during the anti-influenza vaccination - An impact of immunosenescence. Vaccine. 2003;21(25–26):3826–36.
32. Cordero E, Aydillo TA, Perez-Ordoñez A, Torre-Cisneros J, Lara R, Segura C, et al. Deficient long-term response to pandemic vaccine results in an insufficient antibody response to seasonal influenza vaccination in solid organ transplant recipients. Transplantation [Internet]. 2012;93(8):847–854. Available from: http://www.ncbi.nlm.nih.gov/pubmed/22377789

Joint cartilage thickness and automated determination of bone age and bone health in juvenile idiopathic arthritis

Marinka Twilt[1,2], Dan Pradsgaard[2], Anne Helene Spannow[2], Arne Horlyck[3], Carsten Heuck[2] and Troels Herlin[2,4*]

Abstract

Background: BoneXpert is an automated method to calculate bone maturation and bone health index (BHI) in children with juvenile idiopathic arthritis (JIA). Cartilage thickness can also be seen as an indicator for bone health and arthritis damage. The objective of this study was to evaluate the relation between cartilage thickness, bone maturation and bone health in patients with JIA.

Methods: Patients with JIA diagnosed according ILAR criteria included in a previous ultrasonography (US) study were eligible if hand radiographs were taken at the same time as the US examination. Of the 95 patients 67 met the inclusion criteria.

Results: Decreased cartilage thickness was seen in 27% of the examined joints. Decreased BHI was seen in half of the JIA patient, and delayed bone maturation was seen in 33% of patients. A combination of decreased BHI and bone age was seen in 1 out of 5 JIA patients. Decreased cartilage thickness in the knee, wrist and MCP joint was negatively correlated with delayed bone maturation but not with bone health index.

Conclusion: Delayed bone maturation and decreased BHI were not related to a thinner cartilage, but a thicker cartilage. No relation with JADAS 10 was found. The rheumatologist should remain aware of delayed bone maturation and BHI in JIA patients with cartilage changes, even in the biologic era.

Keywords: Juvenile idiopathic arthritis, Joint cartilage, Bone age, Bone health index, Musculoskeletal ultrasonography

Background

Juvenile Idiopathic Arthritis (JIA) is the most common rheumatic disease in childhood. It can result in musculoskeletal pain, joint stiffness and swelling and decreased range of motion. If left untreated JIA will lead to disability of the affected joints. If kept untreated, chronically inflamed synovium and involvement of associated muscle and soft tissues, eventually leading to degeneration of the osteocartilaginous structures, are the primary cause for functional disability in JIA [1]. In pediatric rheumatology it is of great importance to follow osteocartilaginous degeneration [2]. The imaging modalities frequently used to visualize this process are conventional radiography, magnetic resonance imaging (MRI), and within the last decade ultrasonography (US). US is of particular benefit in the assessment of early signs of arthritis, such as joint effusion and synovial thickening [3]. Unlike with the MRI, without using any contrast, hyperemia in the synovial microcirculation as part of the inflammatory process can be detected using the color Doppler or the power Doppler technique [4]. US is relatively inexpensive and does not require any radiation. US is well tolerated, even in the very young patients, can be used to view different joints in one session, and can be viewed at the bedside or in the clinic room.

High frequency US can be used to easily view the joint cartilage as an anechoic structure, as cartilage has a high water content. In previous studies, we validated the assessment of cartilage thickness by US in a pediatric setting [5, 6]. We found a low intra- and inter-observer variability and a good level of agreement, with no

* Correspondence: troeherl@rm.dk
[2]Department of Paediatrics, Division of Rheumatology, Aarhus University Hospital, Aarhus, Denmark
[4]Pediatric Rheumatology Clinic, Department of Pediatrics, Aarhus University Hospital, Palle Juul-Jensens Boulevard 99, DK-8200 Århus N, Denmark

significant systematic joint size-related differences in cartilage thickness measurements between MRI and US [7, 8]. Based on a large cohort of healthy children we established age- and sex-related normal reference values for cartilage thickness of the knee, ankle, wrist, second metacarpophalangeal (MCP) and second proximal interphalangeal (PIP) joints [5]. In a subsequent study we measured cartilage thickness of those joints in JIA patients and found reduced cartilage thickness in children with JIA compared to healthy controls [2, 8]. Children with polyarticular or systemic JIA had thinner cartilage than children with oligoarticular JIA [2].

Continuous exposure to inflammatory cytokines, together with glucocorticoid therapy, affects bone formation [9–11]. This, combined with decreased physical activity and pubertal delay puts JIA patients at increased risk of impaired growth and reduced bone mineral density (BMD) [12]. The assessment of bone age is usually made using the Greulich and Pyle atlas [13]. Dual-energy X-ray densitometry (DXA) is the most commonly used method to assess BMD [14]. Recently, BoneXpert was developed bringing back the use of radiogrammetry, one of the oldest methods to assess BMD. This new digital X-ray radiogrammetry (DXR) method combines the assessment of bone-age with radiogrammetric assessment of (cortical) BMD) of the second to the fourth metacarpal joints [15, 16]. BoneXpert expresses the cortical BMD as a Bone Health Index (BHI), in which cortical BMD is corrected for size. The BoneXpert method makes use of conventional radiography of the hand, thereby making it attractive due to relatively low costs, and lower effective radiation dose compared to other effective methods [16]. The application has been tested in healthy pediatric populations and in the JIA population and showed to be a reliable method for assessing bone age and cortical BMD [17–19]. BoneXpert method is an easy-to-use method provided that radiographs are of reasonable quality and the patients' bone age lies within the age ranges of the program [17, 18]. The JIA population, derived from a biologic registry (Dutch) ABC register showed a delayed bone maturation and lower cortical BMD than healthy patients [19].

In the literature no reports are recorded to look at the relationship between cartilage thickness and bone health in JIA.

Therefore, the aim of our study was to evaluate bone maturation and bone density by using BoneXpert in a cross-sectional JIA population and correlate these findings to the cartilage thickness assessed by US.

Methods

Patients

Children diagnosed with JIA according to the 2001 revised International League of Associations for Rheumatology (ILAR) classification aged 5–15 years and followed at the pediatric rheumatology department of Aarhus University Hospital, Denmark, were invited to participate [20]. Inclusion criteria were; systemic JIA, persistent and extended oligoarticular JIA, and rheumatoid factor (RF)- positive or RF-negative polyarticular JIA. Informed consent was received from the parents. Patients were excluded if they had received an intra articular corticosteroid injection (IACI) within 1 month prior to examination or had a history of previous joint surgery.

Demographic information was retrieved from the medical records and included; disease subtype, age at onset, disease duration. The history of affected joints during the disease course was recorded.

Joint activity was assessed by an experienced pediatric rheumatologist on the same day as the US and BoneXpert x-ray. Joint activity was defined as swelling within a joint, or limitation in the range of joint movement with joint pain or tenderness. The Juvenile Arthritis Diseases Activity Score (JADAS) was established for every patient, consisting of the active joint count of the 10 joints that were scanned by US, ESR, parents' global assessment, and physician's global assessment.

US examination

A Hitachi EUB 7500 scanner with a 6–14 MHz linear transducer (EUP-L65) was used for the US measurements. All US examinations were performed by the same observer throughout the study (DOP). The patients were examined as described, using the same US settings (European League Against Rheumatism (EULAR) standards) described in a healthy age- and sex-matched cohort [5–7]. This ensured consensus with respect to cartilage thickness measurements. The US scans were performed with the observer blinded to the clinical information regarding JIA subtype, joint status, disease duration, and treatment. The images were saved and stored anonymously on a hard drive using 9-digit code. The pressure of the probe was adjusted to a level just below visible deformation on the anatomical structure. Greyscale examinations of distal femoral cartilage (knee joint), anterior talar cartilage (ankle joint), proximal dorsal scaphoid bone cartilage (wrist joint), distal second metacarpal cartilage (second MCP joint), and distal cartilage of the second proximal interphalangeal bone (second PIP joint). Cartilage thickness was measured in mm. Standard scans of hyaline cartilage thickness are based on the guideline recommendations by EULAR [21].

BoneXpert

The stand-alone Windows product of BoneXpert (BoneXpert Version 2.1.0.12;Visiana, Holte, Denmark) was used to analyze the hand radiographs. BoneXpert automatically generates the following outcome variables: (calendar) age, bone age based on Tanner and Whitehouse (TW) method [22] and Greulich and Pyle (GP) method [13], Z-scores of GP bone age (compared with a healthy reference population: girls <15 years, boys <17 years) [23], BHI and Z-score of BHI [15]. BHI is based on cortical thickness (T) of the three middle metacarpal bones. To compensate for the high variation in stature of growing children BoneXpert incorporated the metacarpal width (W) and length (L) in the construction of BHI [16]:

$$\text{BHI} = \pi T(1-T/W)/(LW)^{0.33}$$

The complete hand and wrist joint of both the left and right sides were included in the radiographs (Fig. 1).

Statistics

Descriptive statistics are reported in terms of absolute numbers, median and interquartile range (IQR). To determine whether the Z-score of cartilage thickness or bone age and BHI were different from those in the healthy population, a one sample t-test was used. Correlation coefficient (Spearman's Rho) was used to determine the correlation between Z-score of cartilage thickness and bone age and BHI. IBM SPSS Statistics, version 24 (IBM Corp, Armonk, NY, USA) was used for all analyses.

Results

This study was performed within a larger study on the use of US in JIA. In this study 155 patients with JIA aged between 5 and 15 years were invited to participate, 52 patients declined, 4 had unclassified arthritis, and 5 canceled their scheduled appointment due to illness. As a result, 94 patients were included in the initial study. In 27 patients digital radiogrammetry of the hand was not performed. Therefore, a total of 67 patients were evaluated by US and BoneXpert and included in the current study. The study included 16 boys and 51 girls, with a median age at investigation of 10.9 years (range 7.8–14.4 years), and a median disease duration of 41 months. Patient demographics, including distribution of JIA subcategories, are described in Table 1.

A total of 680 joints were assessed by US for cartilage thickness. Decreased cartilage thickness compared to healthy age-matched controls [5–7] < −1 SD) was present in 27% of the examined joints (181 joints). The most common joint with decreased cartilage thickness was the second PIP joint, followed by the wrist. Decreased cartilage thickness was uncommon in the ankle joint (Table 2). If controlling for age and gender a significant decreased cartilage thickness was seen in the knees, wrists and second PIP joints, but not in the ankles or second MCP joints (Table 2). We found a highly

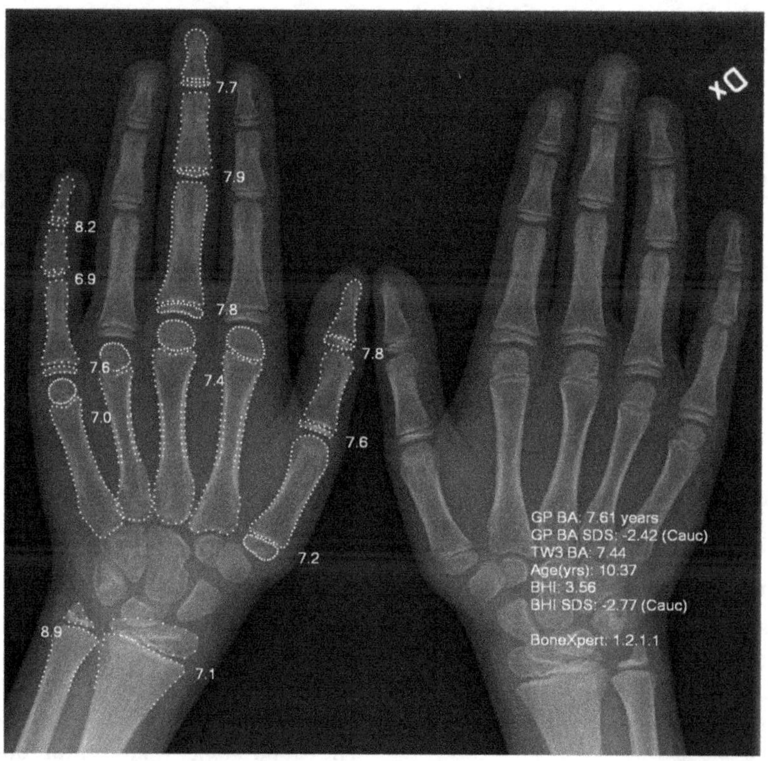

Fig. 1 Digital X-ray radiogrammetry of the left and right hand of a patient with JIA. BoneXpert® software was used to perform automated determination of bone age based on the radius, ulna and the bones in ray 1, 3 and 5 (marked with *white dots*). Bone health index (BHI) is based on the measurements of cortical thickness in the three middle metacarpals

Table 1 Demographic data for study patients (n = 67)

	Number	Age (months)	Disease duration (months)
All	67 (16 boys, 51 girls)	131 (94–168)	41 (15–80)
Oligo-persistent	25	107 (92–144)	15.5 (6.5–47.5)
Oligo-extended	13	157 (118.5–176)	83 (54.5–133.5)
Polyarticular RF-neg	17	128 (120–173.5)	51 (23.5–87)
Polyarticular RF-pos	4	167 (149–183)	20.5 (7–26.5)
Systemic	8	107.5 (85–172.5)	48 (29–117.5)

Values are expressed as median (interquartile range)

significant correlation between the cartilage thickness measured in either the right- or left knee, right or left ankle, right or left wrist and right or left finger joints (r = 0.561–0.884, p < 0.001).

The automated bone age, using either the Greulich-Pyle or Tanner-Whitehouse method, correlated closely (r = 0.992, p < 0.001) and showed significantly lower bone age in JIA patients compared to healthy controls, when controlled for age and gender (Table 3). Delayed bone maturation was found in 22 (33%) patients (bone age < −1SD) of which 10 patients had a bone age < −2SD. BHI was decreased in children with JIA (Table 3). Thirty-four (50.7%) of the patients showed a decreased BHI below −1 SD of which 9/66 had a BHI < −2SD. Fourteen patients demonstrated a combination of a decreased BHI and a decreased bone age.

The decreased bone age was significantly correlated with a longer disease duration. This was not seen for the BHI. Both the bone age and BHI were not correlated to JADAS 10 (r = 0.056, p = 0.67 and r = 0.082, p = 0.52, respectively.

Decreased cartilage thickness measured by US in the knee, wrist and second MCPs was significantly negatively correlated with standardized bone age but this was not found for the ankle and 2nd PIP joints (Table 4). There is no difference in cartilage thickness and BHI, regardless whether BHI was < − 1 SD or < − 2 SD. Thus, no correlation was observed between cartilage thickness and BHI (table 4). Children with a bone age < −1 SD (n = 22) showed a significantly increased cartilage thickness in the right knee, both wrists, and both second MCPs, compared to children with a bone age > −1 SD (not shown). Decreased bone health and bone age were more pronounced in Tanner stage 1–3 (Table 5).

Table 2 US measurement of joint cartilage thickness in children with JIA

Joint	Median (IQR)	t	p
Knee R	- 1.927 (– 2.50 – (– 1.06))	- 10.465	< 0.001
Knee L	- 1.63 (−2.31 – (−0.71))	- 9.203	< 0.001
Ankle R	0.13 (– 0.7–1.25)	0.933	0.458
Ankle L	0.20 (– 0.96 – (1.19))	1.234	0.325
Wrist R	- 0.81 (– 1.45 – (– 0.10))	- 6.513	< 0.001
Wrist L	- 0.89 (– 1.63 – (– 0.22))	- 8.277	< 0.001
MCP R	0.02 (– 1.01–1.15)	0.508	0.705
MCP L	0.02 (– 0.89–1.16)	1.482	0.142
PIP R	- 2.24 (– 3.27 – (– 1.39))	- 13.254	< 0.001
PIP L	- 2.19 (– 3.50 – (−1.27))	- 11.969	< 0.001

One sample t-test. US assessed joint cartilage thickness when controlled for age and gender expressed as median Z-score (interquartile range). N = 67

Table 3 Automated bone age and bone health index as assessed by digital radiogrammetry. N = 67

		Median (IQR)	t	p
Age (years)	67	10.9 (7.8–14.4)		
Bone age GP	67	9.98 (7.28–13.86)		
Bone age GP (SDS)	63	- 0.49 (– 1.32–0.25)	- 2.875	0.006
Bone age TW	67	9.65 (7.03–13.5)		
Bone health Index	66	4.35 (4.06–4.70)		
Bone health Index (SDS)	66	- 1.02 (– 1.60 – (– 0.30)	- 7.199	< 0.001
Disease duration (months)	67	41 (15–80)		

GP Automated digital Greulich-Pyle bone age method. *TW* Automated digital Tanner-Whitehouse bone age method. *SDS* standard deviation score. SDS for the Tanner Whitehouse bone age method is not available. One sample t-test

Discussion

This is the first paper to investigate the relation between cartilage thickness measured by US and automated bone maturation and bone health index. JIA patients show a thinner cartilage than healthy controls. One in two patients showed a decreased BHI (<= −1SD), indicating the heavy burden of JIA on the bone health of these patients. Notably they have a lower cartilage thickness in their second MCP joint, this is one of the MCP joints that are used to to calculate the BHI. Interestingly, there is no correlation between cartilage thickness and BHI. This might be explained by the 3rd and 4th metacarpal joint,

Table 4 Correlation between US-assessed joint cartilage thicknesses measured as Z-score and Bone age and bone health index assessed by digital radiogrammetry. N = 67

US mean Z score	Bone age GP SDS		BHI SDS	
	r	p	r	p
Knee	- 0.288	0.023*	- 0.069	0.587
Ankle	- 0.172	0.177	- 0.222	0.073
Wrist	- 0.298	0.018*	- 0.121	0.331
2nd MCP	- 0.500	<0.001*	0.019	0.880
2nd PIP	- 0.058	0.649	−0.009	0.945

US mean Z score: mean of the Z score of joint cartilage thickness assessed by ultrasonography of the left and right joint. *GP* Greulich-Pyle, *BHI* Bone health index, *SDS* standard deviation score. *: significant correlation p < 0.05

Table 5 Tanner stage and automated bone age and bone health index determined by digital radiogrammetry in juvenile idiopathic arthritis

Tanner stage	Number	Bone age GP	Bone age GP (SDS)	BHI SDS	BMI
1	33	7.3 (5.8–8.2)	−0.83 (−1.57-(−0.08))	−0.75 (−1.57-(−0.33))	15.9 (14.8–16.4)
2	12	11.0 (10–11.7)	−0.41 (−1.1–0.17)	−1.28 (−2.13-(−0.83))	17.8 (16.1–20.2)
3	7	13.9 (12.1–14.9)	−0.88 (−1.36-(−0.28))	−1.48 (−1.58–0.30)	19.2 (16.9–19.7)
4	9	15.5 (13.8–16.7)	0.26 (−0.76–1.12)	0.94 (−1.52–0.05)	18.4 (16.2–19.3)
5	6	16.8 (16–18)	2.33 (1.08–2.54)	−1.47 (−2.15–0.28)	25.1 (20.4–29.5)

GP Greulich-Pyle, *BHI* Bone health index, *SDS* standard deviation score, *BMI* body mass index

which are taken into account while calculating the BHI, but were not assessed by US.

Previous studies have shown that patients with JIA are known to have a delayed bone maturation [9–12]. This was, however, not studied in relation to the cartilage thickness. Surprisingly, in the knee, wrist and MCP there is a significant correlation between a thicker cartilage and a delayed bone maturation, which is in contrast with one would have expected. However, in JIA, enhanced focal bone maturation is a well-known phenomenon as a result of joint inflammation, which may lead to accelerated thinning of the cartilage. One in five JIA patients showed both a decreased bone age and a decreased BHI.

The BoneXpert method used to measure bone maturation and BHI is an easy to use, high precision method. This study is one of the first research studies to demonstrate the use of the BoneXpert method in JIA. Nusman et al. reported on the feasibility of this method in JIA and the small difference between left- and right-hand radiographs [19].

The ongoing delayed bone maturation and decreased BHI in JIA patients with relatively mild disease, and no correlation with JADAS 10 score, shows the need for ongoing bone health strategies in JIA. Early on, corticosteroids were blamed for the bone health issues in JIA, however with the new treatments available and the continuing decreased usage of corticosteroids, bone health in JIA is still under threat.

This study is limited by the very specific population studied within an US cohort as previously described [2, 8]. These factors introduce a selection bias, which limits the generalizability to the full JIA population. However, patients included in this cohort were recruited consecutively in clinic and the subgroup evaluated in this study is a representation of that group. This group, however is a group of patients with longer standing diseases and may not represent the new JIA patient. Another limitation is that degradation of the cartilage may not appear uniformly. The degradation might affect the joint more severely on either side of the scanned area. Unlike the MRI, US cannot visualize the entire cartilage surface, which was a limitation of the study.

Conclusion

This first study on cartilage thickness, bone maturation and bone health shows the ongoing delayed bone maturation and decreased BHI in JIA patients. The delayed bone age is not related to a thinner cartilage, but a thicker cartilage assessed by US. Rheumatologist need to be aware of the ongoing issue with bone health in JIA patients, even in the biologic era.

Abbreviations

BA: Bone age; BHI: Bone health index; BMD: Bone mineral density; DXA: Dual energy X-ray densitometry; DXR: Digital X-ray radiogrammetry; ESR: Erythrocyte sedimentation rate; EULAR: European League Against Rheumatism; GP: Greulich-Pyle; IACI: Intraarticular corticosteroid injection; ILAR: International League of Associations for Rheumatology; IQR: Interquartile range; JADAS: Juvenile arthritis disease activity score; JIA: Juvenile idiopathic arthritis; MCP: Metacarpophalangeal joint; MRI: Magnetic resonance imaging; PIP: Proximal interphalangeal joint; RF: Rheumatoid factor; SD: Standard deviation; TW: Tanner-Whitehouse; US: Ultrasonography

Acknowledgements

The Danish Rheumatism Association is thanked for its financial support.

Author's contribution

DP, AHS, CH and TH accompanied in designing the study. MT and TH supervised data collection, analyzed and interpreted the data, drafted the initial manuscript, and approved the final manuscript as submitted. DP collected the ultrasound data, and AH collected the radiology data. All authors critically reviewed and revised the manuscript, and approved the final manuscript as submitted.

Funding

Study was supported by a grant from the Danish Rheumatism Association (R97-A2820).

Consent for publication

Not applicable.

Competing interests

The authors declare that they have no competing interests.

Author details
[1]Department of Paediatrics, Section of Rheumatology, Alberta Children's Hospital, University of Calgary, Calgary, AB, Canada. [2]Department of Paediatrics, Division of Rheumatology, Aarhus University Hospital, Aarhus, Denmark. [3]Department of Radiology, Aarhus University Hospital, Aarhus, Denmark. [4]Pediatric Rheumatology Clinic, Department of Pediatrics, Aarhus University Hospital, Palle Juul-Jensens Boulevard 99, DK-8200 Århus N, Denmark.

References

1. Oen K, Reed M, Malleson PN, Cabral DA, Petty RE, Rosenberg AM, et al. Radiologic outcome and its relationship to functional disability in juvenile rheumatoid arthritis. J Rheumatol. 2003;30:832–40.
2. Pradsgaard DO, Spannow AH, Heuck C, Herlin T. Decreased cartilage thickness in juvenile idiopathic arthritis assessed by ultrasonography. J Rheumatol. 2013;40:1596–603.
3. Kane D, Balint PV, Sturrock RD. Ultrasonography is superior to clinical examination in the detection and localization of knee joint effusion in rheumatoid arthritis. J Rheumatol. 2003;30:966–71.
4. Roth J, Ravagnani V, Backhaus M, Balint P, Bruns A, Bruyn GA, et al. Preliminary definitions for the sonographic features of synovitis in children. Arthritis Care Res (Hoboken). 2017;69:1217-23.
5. Spannow AH, Pfeiffer-Jensen M, Andersen NT, Herlin T, Stenbog E. Ultrasonographic measurements of joint cartilage thickness in healthy children: age- and sex-related standard reference values. J Rheumatol. 2010;37:2595–601.
6. Spannow AH, Pfeiffer-Jensen M, Andersen NT, Stenbog E, Herlin T. Inter -and intraobserver variation of ultrasonographic cartilage thickness assessments in small and large joints in healthy children. Pediatr Rheumatol Online J. 2009;7:12.
7. Spannow AH, Stenboeg E, Pfeiffer-Jensen M, Fiirgaard B, Haislund M, Ostergaard M, et al. Ultrasound and MRI measurements of joint cartilage in healthy children: a validation study. Ultraschall Med. 2011;32(Suppl 1):S110–6.
8. Pradsgaard DO, Fiirgaard B, Spannow AH, Heuck C, Herlin T. Cartilage thickness of the knee joint in juvenile idiopathic arthritis: comparative assessment by ultrasonography and magnetic resonance imaging. J Rheumatol. 2015;42:534–40.
9. Thornton J, Pye SR, O'Neill TW, Rawlings D, Francis RM, Symmons DP, et al. Bone health in adult men and women with a history of juvenile idiopathic arthritis. J Rheumatol. 2011;38:1689–93.
10. Burnham JM. Inflammatory diseases and bone health in children. Curr Opin Rheumatol. 2012;24:548–53.
11. Stagi S, Cavalli L, Signorini C, Bertini F, Cerinic MM, Brandi ML, et al. Bone mass and quality in patients with juvenile idiopathic arthritis: longitudinal evaluation of bone-mass determinants by using dual-energy x-ray absorptiometry, peripheral quantitative computed tomography, and quantitative ultrasonography. Arthritis Res Ther. 2014;16:R83.
12. Sandstedt E, Fasth A, Fors H, Beckung E. Bone health in children and adolescents with juvenile idiopathic arthritis and the influence of short-term physical exercise. Pediatr Phys Ther. 2012;24:155–61.
13. Greulich WW, Pyle SI. Radiographic atlas of the skeletal development of the hand and wrist. 2nd ed. Stanford: Stanford University Press; 1959.
14. van Rijn RR, Van Kuijk C. Of small bones and big mistakes; bone densitometry in children revisited. Eur J Radiol. 2009;71:432–9.
15. Thodberg HH, van Rijn RR, Tanaka T, Martin DD, Kreiborg S. A paediatric bone index derived by automated radiogrammetry. Osteoporos Int. 2010; 21:1391–400.
16. BoneXpert. Available from: http://www.bonexpert.com/.
17. Thodberg HH, Savendahl L. Validation and reference values of automated bone age determination for four ethnicities. Acad Radiol. 2010;17:1425–32.
18. van Rijn RR, Lequin MH, Thodberg HH. Automatic determination of Greulich and Pyle bone age in healthy Dutch children. Pediatr Radiol. 2009;39:591–7.
19. Anink J, Nusman CM, van Suijlekom-Smit LW, van Rijn RR, Maas M, van Rossum MA. Automated determination of bone age and bone mineral density in patients with juvenile idiopathic arthritis: a feasibility study. Arthritis Res Ther. 2014;16:424.
20. Petty RE, Southwood TR, Manners P, Baum J, Glass DN, Goldenberg J, et al. International League of Associations for Rheumatology classification of juvenile idiopathic arthritis: second revision, Edmonton, 2001. J Rheumatol. 2004;31:390–2.
21. Backhaus M, Burmester GR, Gerber T, Grassi W, Machold KP, Swen WA, et al. Guidelines for musculoskeletal ultrasound in rheumatology. Ann Rheum Dis. 2001;60:641–9.
22. Thodberg HH, Jenni OG, Ranke MB, Martin DD. Standardization of the Tanner-Whitehouse bone age method in the context of automated image analysis. Ann Hum Biol. 2012;39:68–75.
23. Thodberg HH, Kreiborg S, Juul A, Pedersen KD. The BoneXpert method for automated determination of skeletal maturity. IEEE Trans Med Imaging. 2009;28:52–66.

7

Incidence and predictors of Uveitis in juvenile idiopathic arthritis in a Nordic long-term cohort study

Ellen Nordal[1*], Veronika Rypdal[1], Terje Christoffersen[2], Kristiina Aalto[3], Lillemor Berntson[4], Anders Fasth[5], Troels Herlin[6], Susan Nielsen[7], Suvi Peltoniemi[3], Bjørn Straume[8], Marek Zak[7], Marite Rygg[9] and for the Nordic Study Group of Pediatric Rheumatology (NoSPeR)

Abstract

Background: The incidence of uveitis associated with juvenile idiopathic arthritis (JIA) varies around the world. Our aim was to investigate the incidence and predictors of uveitis in a Nordic population-based cohort.

Methods: Consecutive JIA cases from defined geographical areas in Denmark, Finland, Sweden and Norway with disease onset between January 1997 to June 2000 were followed for median 98 months in this prospective longitudinal cohort study. Potential clinical and immunological predictors of uveitis were identified with logistic regression analysis.

Results: Uveitis occurred in 89 (20.5%) of the 435 children with regular ophtalmologic follow-up among the 500 included. Chronic asymptomatic uveitis developed in 80 and acute symptomatic uveitis in 9 children. Uveitis developed at a median interval of 0.8 (range − 4.7 to 9.4) years after onset of arthritis. Predictors of uveitis were age < 7 years at JIA onset (Odds ratio (OR) 2.1, 95% confidence interval (CI) 1.3 to 3.5), presence of antihistone antibodies (AHA) > 15 U/ml (OR 4.8 (1.8 to 13.4)) and antinuclear antibodies (ANA) (OR 2.4 (1.5 to 4.0)). Mean combined IgM/IgG AHA was significantly higher in the uveitis group (19.2 U/ml) than in the non-uveitis group (10.2 U/ml) ($p = 0.002$). Young age at JIA onset predicted uveitis in girls ($p < 0.001$), but not in boys ($p = 0.390$).

Conclusion: Early-onset arthritis and presence of AHA in girls, as well as presence of ANA in both genders, were significant predictors of chronic uveitis. The high incidence of uveitis in this long-term Nordic JIA cohort may have severe implications in a lifelong perspective.

Keywords: Juvenile idiopathic arthritis, Uveitis, Epidemiology, Biomarkers, Histones, Antinuclear antibody

Background

Uveitis is the most common extra-articular manifestation of juvenile idiopathic arthritis (JIA). This sight-threatening condition contributes significantly to the disease burden of JIA [1, 2]. Chronic insidious uveitis in JIA is often asymptomatic, and it is a major challenge to diagnose the condition as early as possible for prompt and adequate treatment [3, 4]. The diagnosis may be obvious in cases with acute uveitis [5], but the challenge remains to provide optimal screening programs and treatment to minimize long-term complications in all forms of JIA-associated uveitis. The reported prevalence of uveitis in JIA varies highly, and ethnic and geographic differences seem to exist. Recent publications show a prevalence of 8–25% in most Caucasian populations [6, 7], while some studies from other continents show lower percentage of uveitis, 1 to 7% [8, 9]. Young age at onset of arthritis and presence of ANA were predictors of uveitis in most studies [3, 10–12]. In some larger cohort studies and registries, oligoarticular onset category and female gender were also statistically significant predictors of uveitis, but with less clinical impact [3, 13].

* Correspondence: ellen.nordal@icloud.com
[1]Department of Pediatrics, University Hospital of North Norway, and Department of Clinical Medicine, UiT the Arctic University of Norway, Tromsø, Norway

Histones are subcomponents of chromatin where these basic DNA-binding proteins are found in highly organized nucleosomal particles [14]. Antihistone antibodies (AHA) are among the ANA subtypes identified in subsets of children with JIA, while other subtypes associated with connective tissue diseases such as anti-DNA, anti-RNP, anti-SSA and anti-SSB antibodies are rarely found [15, 16]. AHA were reported to be associated with early-onset JIA, oligoarthritis and uveitis [17]. We showed previously that AHA is a significant predictor of chronic uveitis in a Norwegian JIA cohort [11]. Whether this association is merely an epiphenomenon is not yet known, although new interest for histones in autoimmune diseases has emerged through recent epigenetic findings [18, 19].

A longitudinal cohort study of JIA in a population-based setting in the Nordic countries started in 1997 and is still ongoing [20, 21]. The ophthalmologic data of a follow-up 8 years after disease onset of this Nordic JIA cohort were analyzed in the present study. The main objective was to describe the incidence and the predictors of uveitis in JIA during the first decade after disease onset. We also wanted to extend the previous Norwegian pilot study to the Nordic JIA cohort regarding the presence of histone antibodies in patients with JIA with and without uveitis, respectively.

Methods

Patients

In this longitudinal study, children with long-term ophthalmologic follow-up were selected from a prospective multicentre Nordic JIA cohort. The original multicentre cohort consisted of consecutive children with newly diagnosed JIA and disease onset between January 1, 1997 to June 30, 2000 from defined geographical areas of Denmark, Finland, Norway and Sweden aiming for the cohort to be population-based [20]. Clinical information including family history, assessment of disease activity, self-reported questionnaires and information from ophthalmology visits was registered per protocol at baseline and at 1 to 3 year intervals. Detailed description of the methods of patient accrual and data collection has been published previously [21].

At the final study visit, at least 7.0 years (median 98 months, range 84–147 months) after disease onset, extended data including information from the most recent ophthalmologic visit was collected. The interval of ophthalmologic visits was every 2–3 months the first 2 years, then longer intervals according to time after disease onset and JIA category. The intervals were in line with the guidelines for uveitis screening at each center, based on international uveitis screening guidelines. Uveitis was registered as present and active, when the ophthalmologist prescribed treatment for inflammation in the uvea. Uveitis was classified according to the recommendations by the Standardization of Uveitis Nomenclature (SUN) working group [22]. Uveitis was classified as "acute"; symptomatic with acute onset, sometimes recurrent course but of limited duration, or "chronic"; insidious onset, mainly asymptomatic with chronic recurrent or persistent course. Collected data also included locally analyzed HLA-B27, antinuclear antibodies (ANA) and rheumatoid factor (RF), and a positive result of the latter two had to be confirmed, at least 3 months apart. Each physician interpreted the results of ANA and RF analysis as positive or negative according to the reference values of their local laboratory; the cut-off value for a positive test was ≥ 1/80 in Tromsø, Trondheim and parts of Sweden, ≥ 1/320 in Finland, and ≥ 1/160 in Copenhagen, Århus and some parts of Sweden. ANA was measured using immunofluorescence on HEp-2 cells. Serum was taken at a median of 4 (1st quartile of 2, 3rd quartile of 7) months after the disease was diagnosed, frozen and stored at −70 °C in aliquots to avoid repeated freeze-thaw cycles. AHA were detected with Varelisa Histone Antibodies Enzyme Induced Assay (EIA) kit for anti-histone IgM/IgG antibodies using a combined IgM/IgG conjugate (Phadia Diagnostics, Freiburg, Germany) at UIT The Arctic University of Norway, Tromsø, Norway. Tests were run according to the manufacturer's instructions [23]. According to the kit instructions a level ≥ 30 U/ml is considered positive, 15–29 U/ml borderline, and < 15 U/ml negative, based on a test population of 432 healthy adults, normative values are not given for children. In the present study, we investigated ≥ 15 U/ml as a positive threshold based on our previous study reporting a mean concentration of 4.3 U/ml in 58 healthy children utilizing the same Varelisa Histone EIA-kit [11]. The presence of AHA in a Norwegian JIA cohort, also including the Norwegian subsets of this Nordic JIA cohort, has previously been reported and was therefore not included here [11]. No sera were available from the Finnish participants, and subsequently analyses of the AHA were performed only in the Swedish and Danish sera.

Approval from medical research ethical committees and data protection authorities was granted according to the regulations of each participating country, in Norway from Regional Committee for Medical and Health Research Ethics NORD, number 53/96. Oral informed assent was obtained from all children. Written informed consent was obtained from parents of children aged < 16 years and from the children if aged ≥ 16 years.

Statistical analyses

The study report followed the STROBE guidelines [24]. Statistical analyses were performed using the STATA version 14 software (STATA Corp., College Station, TX, USA). Descriptive statistics were used to summarize clinical characteristics of the population and disease activity measures. The chi-square test was used as appropriate for comparison of categorical variables. The Student's *t*-test was used to compare means in continuous outcomes between groups, and Mann-Whitney rank sum test for comparison of medians for skewed data. A logistic regression analysis of baseline characteristics was performed to calculate odds ratio for developing uveitis. The *p*-value <0.05 was considered significant.

Results

Regular ophthalmologic follow-up for more than 7 years was available in 435 (87.0%) of the 500 children included in the prospective multi-centre Nordic JIA-cohort; 60 children were lost to follow-up, and in 5 children long-term ophthalmological data were missing. Baseline clinical characteristics of the group with or without long-term follow-up were mostly similar and have previously been published [21].

Incidence

Uveitis developed in 89 (20.5%) of the 435 children. Clinical characteristics at baseline according to the presence of acute and chronic uveitis is shown in Table 1. Among the 9 children with acute uveitis, 8 had enthesitis-related arthritis (ERA), and 7 were HLA-B27 positive. Chronic insidious uveitis developed in 80 (18.4%) children. The cumulative incidence of uveitis according to the International League of Associations for Rheumatology (ILAR) categories is shown in Table 2. There were no uveitis in the systemic nor in the polyarticular RF positive categories, and highest incidence was noted in the juvenile psoriatic arthritis (35.7%) and enthesitis-related arthritis (25.0%) categories. The incidence of uveitis was significantly higher in Finland than in the other Nordic countries (Table 3). Finland also had the highest proportion of children with young age at onset of JIA, but neither gender, oligoarticular onset nor the prevalence of HLA-B27, ANA, or AHA showed any corresponding difference between countries.

Time from onset of arthritis to onset of uveitis is shown in Fig. 1, including 5 children in which uveitis was diagnosed before the arthritis, one of these had acute uveitis. Uveitis developed within the first year after onset of arthritis in 48 (53.9%), within 4 years in 73 (82.0%) of the children, and 4 children (4.5%) had onset of uveitis more than 8 years after onset of arthritis, 2 of these had chronic asymptomatic uveitis. The number of children developing uveitis within the first year after onset of arthritis is 6 times the number developing uveitis during the second year, and 16 times the number during the fifth year. All together uveitis developed with an interval of median 0.8 (range − 4.7 to 9.4) years after onset of arthritis, while chronic uveitis developed with a median interval of 0.7 (range − 3.0 to 8.6) years after onset of arthritis.

Table 1 Clinical characteristics at the first study visit in 435 children in the Nordic juvenile idiopathic arthritis (JIA) cohort according to the presence of acute or chronic uveitis during > 7 years of follow-up

	All children		No uveitis		Acute uveitis		Chronic uveitis	
	N		N		N		N	
Female gender	435	286 (65.8)	346	227 (65.6)	9	4 (44.4)	80	55 (68.8)
Age at onset, median (1st, 3rd q)	435	5.5 (2.4, 9.5)	346	6.2 (2.8, 10)	9	10.8 (9.3, 12.9)	80	3.2 (1.8, 5.9)
Oligoarticular onset[a]	435	224 (51.5)	346	180 (52.0)	9	1 (11.1)	80	43 (53.8)
ANA positive	427	116 (27.2)	340	79 (23.2)	9	0 (0)	78	37 (47.4)
AHA >15 U/ml	134	23 (17.2)	112	14 (12.5)	3	1 (33.3)	19	8 (42.1)
RF positive	424	10 (2.4)	336	9 (2.7)	9	1 (11.1)	79	0 (0.0)
HLA-B27 positive	413	87 (21.1)	325	62 (19.1)	9	7 (77.8)	79	18 (22.8)
ESR, median (1st, 3rd q)	354	14 (8, 28)	276	14 (8, 26)	8	23 (10, 41)	70	16 (9, 36)
CRP, median (1st, 3rd q)	350	0 (0, 10)	276	0 (0, 10)	9	0 (0, 16)	65	0 (0, 14)
JADAS27, median (1st, 3rd q)	194	5.1 (2.0, 11.0)	157	5.0 (2.0, 9.8)	7	10.4 (5.6, 14.9)	30	3.8 (1.6, 12.5)
CHAQ, median (1st, 3rd q))	273	0.3 (0.0, 1.0)	222	0.4 (0.0, 1.0)	8	0.4 (0.1, 1.2)	43	0.3 (0.0, 1.0)
DMARD use 2nd visit[b]	350	125 (35.6)	316	111 (35.1)	7	3 (37.5)	27	11 (42.3)

Data are presented as numbers (%), unless otherwise noted

ANA antinuclear antibodies measured by immunofluorescence on Hep-2 cells, and *RF* rheumatoid factor; two positive tests taken > 3 months apart in participants with one or more tests taken, *AHA > 15 U/ml* antihistone antibodies IgM/IgG >15 U/ml, *HLA-B27* human leucocyte antigen B27, *Age at onset* age at onset of arthritis in years, *ESR* erythrocyte sedimentation rate, *CRP* C-reactive protein *JADAS27* Juvenile arthritis disease activity score based on 27 joint count, *CHAQ* Child health assessment questionnaire

[a]Oligoarticular JIA 6 months after disease onset, according to the International League of Associations for Rheumatology (ILAR) classification criteria. [25]

[b]Percentage of DMARD = Disease modifying anti-rheumatic drugs including biological agents used within the 2nd visit (median 13 months (IQR 12–14)) in 350 children without uveitis at the time of the 2nd study visit, differentiating into no uveitis, acute, or chronic uveitis during further follow-up

Table 2 Presence of acute or chronic uveitis in the different JIA categories according to the International League of Associations for Rheumatology (ILAR) classification criteria at the final study visit in 435 children in the Nordic juvenile idiopathic arthritis (JIA) cohort

JIA category	All children $n = 435$ (% of all)	No uveitis $n = 346$ (%)	Acute uveitis $n = 9$ (%)	Chronic uveitis $n = 80$ (%)	Cumulative total uveitis incidence (95% CI)[a]
Systemic	18 (4.1)	18 (100.0)	0 (0)	0 (0)	0 (0, 18.5)
Oligoarticular persistent	131 (30.1)	106 (80.9)	0 (0)	25 (19.1)	19.1 (12.7, 26.9)
Oligoarticular extended	78 (17.9)	62 (79.5)	0 (0)	16 (20.5)	20.5 (12.2, 31.2)
Polyarticular RF negative	80 (18.4)	62 (77.5)	0 (0)	18 (22.5)	22.5 (13.9, 33.2)
Polyarticular RF positive	3 (0.7)	3 (100.0)	0 (0.0)	0 (0.0)	0 (0, 70.8)
Juvenile psoriatic arthritis	14 (3.2)	9 (64.3)	0 (0.0)	5 (35.7)	35.7 (12.8, 64.9)
Enthesitis-related arthritis	48 (11.0)	36 (75.0)	8 (16.7)	4 (8.3)	25.0 (13.6, 39.6)
Undifferentiated arthritis	63 (14.5)	50 (79.4)	1 (1.6)	12 (19.0)	20.6 (11.5, 32.7)

[a]CI, confidence interval

Predictors of uveitis

Young age at onset of JIA and ANA were significant predictors of uveitis (Tables 4 and 5). AHA ≥ 15 U/ml was found in 23 (17.2%) and AHA ≥ 30 U/ml in 10 (7.5%) of the 134 participants with AHA analyses. AHA ≥ 30 U/ml was found in 3 of the 5 females with uveitis and AHA analyses. The presence of AHA ≥ 15 U/ml was significantly higher in children with uveitis than in children without (OR 4.8 (1.8 to 13.4)) (Table 4). Serum concentration of AHA IgM/IgG antibodies was significantly higher in the group with uveitis (mean 19.2 U/ml) than in children without uveitis (mean 10.2 U/ml) in the Swedish and Danish cohort with available sera for antihistone analyses ($p = 0.002$; chi-square, data not shown).

Neither gender, oligoarticular onset nor other ILAR categories predicted uveitis. Presence of HLA-B27 was borderline significant as a predictor of uveitis, primarily because there was a high presence of HLA-B27 among children with acute uveitis (Tables 1 and 4). There was no significantly reduced risk of developing uveitis in children that had started disease-modyfing antirheumatic drug (DMARD) treatment, including biologics, neither at the first (data not shown) nor at the second study visit (Tables 1 and 4), taking into account the start date of DMARDs and the date of diagnosis of uveitis. At the final study visit the percentage of children ever using DMARDs was higher in the uveitis group (78.7%) compared to the group without uveitis (53.2%) (data not shown), but the number of children receiving DMARDs to treat primarily their uveitis is not known. These analyses on DMARDs were also performed for methotrexate, showing the same result. There were no significant difference in incidence of uveitis in children that had used etanercept (18.5%) during the disease course versus those that never used etanercept (20.7%), $p = 0.706$. Also the incidence of uveitis was similar in children that had used sulfasalazine (16.1%) versus those that never used sulfasalazine (21.2%), $p = 0.361$. During the disease course, 14.3% of the cohort used sulfasalazine, while 12.4% used etanercept. The main predictors of uveitis in Table 4 were stratified for gender (Table 5). This analysis showed that girls with uveitis had a lower median age at onset of arthritis of 3.4 versus 6.8 in girls without uveitis ($p < 0.001$). The difference in age at onset was highly significant in girls, but not in boys ($p = 0.390$) (Tables 4 and 5). ANA was a significant predictor, both in girls and in boys (Table 4). Analysis stratified for gender showed that median median AHA was significantly higher in girls ($p = 0.003$), but not in boys ($p = 0.794$) (Table 5).

Table 3 Presence of uveitis, antinuclear antibodies, antihistone antibody levels and HLA-B27 according to country of origin in 435 children in the Nordic juvenile idiopathic arthritis (JIA) cohort

	Denmark $n = 91$	Norway $n = 105$	Sweden $n = 101$	Finland $n = 138$
No uveitis	73 (80.2)	86 (81.9)	87 (86.1)	100 (72.5)
Acute uveitis	3 (3.3)	4 (3.8)	1 (1.1)	1 (0.7)
Chronic uveitis	15 (16.5)	15 (14.3)	13 (12.9)	37 (26.8)
Female gender	62 (68.1)	67 (70.5)	67 (66.3)	83 (60.1)
Oligoarticular onset	45 (49.5)	51 (48.6)	55 (54.5)	73 (52.9)
Age at onset	4.8 (2.2, 9.3)	5.9 (2.8, 9.9)	6.9 (3.2, 11.3)	5.1 (2.3, 8.7)
ANA positive	28 (30.8)	32 (32.0)	23 (22.8)	33 (24.4)
HLA-B27 positive	14 (15.6)	29 (27.6)	20 (21.5)	24 (19.2)

Data are numbers (percent) except median (1st and 3rd quartile) for Age at onset; age at onset of arthritis, *ANA* antinuclear antibodies measured by immunofluorescence on Hep-2 cells, two positive tests taken more than 3 months apart in participants with one or more tests takenm *HLA-B27* human leucocyte antigen B27

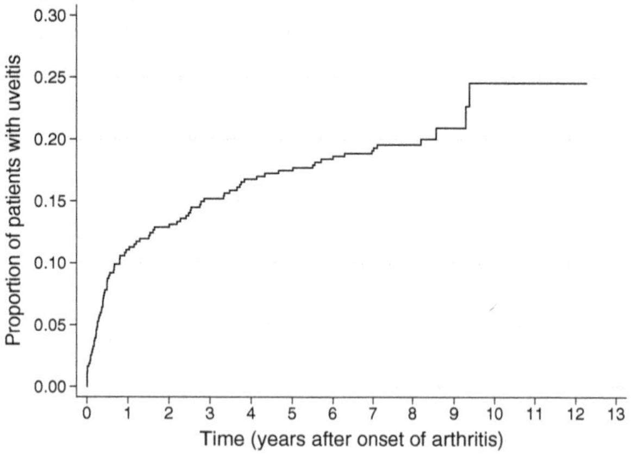

Fig. 1 Onset of uveitis in years after onset of arthritis in 435 children in the Nordic JIA cohort, including 5 children developing uveitis before onset of arthritis (time 0)

Discussion

In this Nordic multicenter JIA study, we found a high cumulative incidence of uveitis, and a geographic difference with a higher incidence in Finland compared to Norway, Sweden and Denmark. Young age at onset of arthritis, ANA and AHA were significant predictors of uveitis, but stratified for gender both young age at onset and AHA were significant predictors only in girls. Mean serum levels of AHA were higher in the uveitis group than in the children with no uveitis.

The prospective, longitudinal design and population-based context are the strengths of this multi-center study. The proportion of children lost to follow-up was small compared to other longitudinal studies [26–29]. A weakness is the few patients in each JIA category that made analyses of uveitis and its predictors in some of the categories less reliable. Another weakness is that information on uveitis such as differentiation between acute and chronic uveitis were registered from available ophthalmologic records by the pediatric rheumatologists and not by the ophthalmologists themselves.

Table 4 Baseline clinical and demographic predictors of uveitis in 435 participants in the Nordic juvenile idiopathic arthritis (JIA) cohort

	No uveitis		Uveitis		OR (95% CI)
	N	n (%)	N	n (%)	
Female gender	346	227 (65.6)	89	59 (66.3)	1.0 (0.6, 1.6)
Oligoarticular onset	346	168 (48.6)	89	41 (46.1)	0.9 (0.6, 1.4)
Age at onset (< 7 years)	346	189 (54.6)	89	64 (71.9)	2.1 (1.3, 3.5)
ANA positive	340	79 (23.2)	87	37 (42.5)	2.4 (1.5, 4.0)
AHA > 15 U	112	14 (12.5)	22	9 (40.9)	4.8 (1.8, 13.4)
HLA-B27 positive	325	62 (19.1)	87	25 (28.7)	1.7 (1.0, 2.9)
ESR > 20 mm/H	276	95 (34.4)	78	34 (43.6)	1.5 (0.9, 2.5)
CRP > 10 mg/L	276	77 (27.9)	74	27 (36.5)	1.5 (0.9, 2.6)
DMARD use ≤ 2nd visit[a]	316	111 (35.1)	34	14 (41.2)	1.3 (0.6, 2.7)

[a]In 350 children with no uveitis at the time of 2nd study visit, percentage of DMARD used within 2nd visit (median 13 (1st q 12, 3rd q 14) months) in children with no uveitis versus children with uveitis during further follow-up.
Odds ratio (OR) of developing uveitis calculated with logistic regression. Oligoarticular onset, oligoarticular category 6 months after onset of disease, according to the International League of Associations for Rheumatology (ILAR) classification criteria (5); *ANA* antinuclear antibodies measured by immunofluorescence on *Hep-2 cells* two positive tests taken > 3 months apart in participants with one or more tests taken

The high rate of uveitis in our population is in line with previous findings in the Nordic countries [6, 11, 30, 31]. A prevalence of 8–15% was reported from Sweden [30, 32], 14–18% in northern Norway [11, 31], 9–19% in Denmark [33, 34], while higher rates were previously reported from Finland (24%) [6, 35]. Even though the background rate of HLA-B27 is reported to be higher in northern areas such as Finland and northern Norway [36, 37], we did not find this in our cohort from the Helsinki area in the southern part of Finland. There were also no differences in the presence of ANA between countries. The higher incidence of uveitis during the first 8 years of disease in Finland compared to the other Nordic countries in the present study may be explained by the trend of younger age at onset of arthritis in Finland and/or genetic differences. This finding is in line with the striking worldwide ethnic and genetic differences in uveitis incidence, differences beyond what can be expected by variations in patient accrual and study design. In two large studies from North America of multiethnic populations both Saurenmann et al. and Angeles-Han et al. found that uveitis was more common among Caucasians than among children of black American, Arab and Indian origin [12, 13]. Our cohort was of mostly Caucasian origin.

In line with other studies we found that the risk of developing uveitis during the first year was more than 6 times the risk during the second year, and almost 16-fold the risk during the fifth year after onset of arthritis. This underlines the need for immediate eye examination in children with onset of non-septic or non-specific arthritis even before the diagnosis of JIA is confirmed, and frequent early follow-up when a diagnosis of JIA has been established. Even though a clear majority of 82% developed uveitis within the first 4 years, our data show that uveitis may develop late in the JIA disease course. An important finding was that 4 cases of uveitis developed more than 8 years after onset of arthritis. Of these cases 2 were asymptomatic uveitis, which may not have been diagnosed without long-term screening. Zak et al. found in their 26-years follow-up of a Danish JIA cohort that both new onset of uveitis and complications may develop late [26]. Based on these data long-term ophthalmologic follow-up into adulthood must be considered.

Robust predictors of uveitis will help selecting high-risk children for frequent eye examinations to ensure early diagnosis and treatment. In acute uveitis with

Table 5 Age at onset of arthritis, antihistone antibody levels and presence of antinuclear antibodies according to gender and presence of uveitis in 435 participants in the Nordic juvenile idiopathic arthritis (JIA) cohort

	No uveitis		Uveitis		p
	n	Age at onset of arthritis	n	Age at onset of arthritis	
Female	227	6.8 (2.5, 10.4)	59	3.4 (1.7, 7.5)	< 0.001
Male	121	5.9 (3.2, 9.2)	27	3.9 (2.3, 7.9)	0.390
	n	Presence of ANA	n	Presence of ANA[a]	
Female	222	65 (29.3)	59	27 (45.8)	0.016
Male	118	14 (11.9)	28	10 (35.7)	0.002
	n	AHA IgM/IgG U/ml	n	AHA IgM/IgG U/ml	
Female	72	6.9 (5.2, 11.4)	16	14.2 (7.2, 27.9)	0.003
Male	40	7.1 (4.7, 11.0)	6	8.2 (4.5, 11.4)	0.794

ANA antinuclear antibodies measured by immunofluorescence on Hep-2 cells, two positive tests taken >3 months apart in participants with one or more tests taken. *AHA* antihistone IgM/IgG antibodies U/ml, analyzed only in the Swedish and Danish cohort
[a]numbers (percent), analysed by Chi-square test, otherwise median (1st, 3rd quartile), analyzed with Mann-Whitney rank sum test

symptoms, the diagnosis is easy and predictors not that important, but the differentiation between acute and chronic uveitis is not always clear, and young children may have difficulties expressing complaints of a painful acute uveitis. In line with most publications we have therefore chosen to analyze predictors of all forms of JIA-associated uveitis and compared with children without uveitis [3, 12, 13]. The most consistently reported predictor of uveitis is young age at onset of arthritis. In line with Saurenmann et al. our data confirms that young age at arthritis onset implies high risk of uveitis in girls, but not in boys [38]. The predictors of uveitis are different in girls and boys, even though the rate of uveitis did not differ. This may reflect that different categories of JIA have different types of uveitis with different predicting factors. ANA is another well-documented predictor of uveitis, but this applies only to the immunofluorescence method, and not to the more automatized high-throughput method of ANA ELISA. We were not able to find the gender-specific differences of ANA that Saurenmann et al. found in their Canadian study [38], but there were few ANA positive boys with uveitis in our study.

We found increased risk of uveitis in children with high levels of antihistone antibodies. Previous findings in the Norwegian JIA cohort were now confirmed in 134 Swedish and Danish children, in whom significantly higher baseline serum levels of histone antibodies were found among those who developed uveitis compared to those who did not develop uveitis [11]. In these studies, the histone antibody levels were either borderline positive (≥ 15 U/ml) or positive (≥ 30 U/ml) according to the commercial test, however, the test and the cut-offs are established to detect drug-induced or other types of systemic lupus erythematosus in adults [23]. While the mean serum concentration of combined antihistone IgM and IgG antibodies was 19.2 U/ml in children with uveitis, and 10.2 U/ml in children without uveitis, a mean concentration of 4.3 U/ml was found in healthy children in our previous report utilizing the identical type of AHA EIA kit [11]. The reproducibility of this finding should be tested in other cohorts. Epigenetic modifications of histone such as acetylation and methylation are suggested to be involved in the pathological processes of autoimmunity [18], and may also play a role in the etiology of uveitis [39]. However, no specific intra-ocular antigen has been identified as the target of neither ANA nor AHA, and therefore their potential role in pathophysiology and etiology remains unclear. The presence of ANA immunofluorescence and AHA had similar test properties as predictors of uveitis, but with less predictive ability as the simple measure of young age at onset of arthritis. There is an ongoing discussion on classification in JIA. ANA positive young children are a quite homogeneous group regarding disease characteristics including high risk of uveitis the first 2 years after onset [40, 41]. It is interesting that the higher risk of uveitis in girls with young age at onset, was shown also for girls with higher levels of histone antibodies in our study. Whether young girls with uveitis, presence of ANA and AHA constitutes a biological subset among children with JIA remains to be shown.

We analyzed the onset of uveitis in relation to early DMARD treatment, and found that early DMARD or methotrexate treatment did not seem to prevent later development of uveitis. The inclusion period in our cohort was too short for analyses of prevalence in different time periods, the onset of disease was in the very beginning of the era of biologic agents, and our data are therefore of limited value in clarifying any uveitis-protective potential of specific drugs or modern DMARD treatment in general. Tappeiner et al. have compared prevalence of uveitis in German children with JIA in two time periods up to 2013, and found a lower prevalence in the latest period when DMARDs including biologic agents were more commonly used [42]. Whether DMARDs can prevent or only postpone development of uveitis in JIA is not known.

Conclusion

We found a high prevalence of uveitis in this Nordic JIA population-based cohort. Significant predictors of uveitis were young age at onset of arthritis and presence of AHA in girls, and presence of ANA in both genders. Further long-term follow-up are needed to focus on prevalence of late-onset uveitis, presence of complications, and impact on quality of life in young adults with JIA-associated uveitis.

Abbreviations

AHA: Antihistone antibodies; ANA: Antinuclear antibodies; CHAQ: Childhood Health Assessment Questionnaire; CI: Confidence interval; CRP: C-reactive protein; DMARD: Disease-modyfing antirheumatic drugs; EIA: Enzyme Induced Assay; ERA: enthesitis-related arthritis; ESR: Erythrocyte sedimentation rate; HLA-B27: Human leucocyte antigen B27; ILAR: International League of Associations for Rheumatology; IQR: Interquartile range; JADAS27: Juvenile Arthritis Disease Activity Score; JIA: Juvenile idiopathic arthritis; OR: Odds ratio; RF: Rheumatoid factor; SUN: Standardization of Uveitis Nomenclature

Acknowledgements

First, we thank the children and parents participating in the study. We also thank the other members of the Nordic Study group of Pediatric Rheumatology (NoSPeR); Gudmund Marhaug in Trondheim, Freddy Karup Pedersen in Copenhagen, Pekka Lahdenne in Helsinki, Boel Anderson-Gäre in Jönköping for inspiring cooperation. Finally, we thank participating physicians contributing by collecting data; Nils Thomas Songstad, Astri Lang and Anne Elisabeth Ross in Tromsø, Kjell Berntzen and Nina Moe in Trondheim, Mikael Damgaard, Maria Ekelund and Nils Olof Jonsson, Jönköping, Anders Berner and Hans Ekström, Karlstad, Eric Ronge, Skövde, Agne Lind and Lars Hammarén, Borås, Johan Robinsson, Trollhättan and Anna-Lena Nilsson, Östersund.

Funding

This work was supported by grants from the Helse Nord Research Program, and the Grete Harbitz foundation. UiT the Arctic University of Norway funded the publication costs.

Authors' contributions

EN, LB, AF, TH, TC, SN, and MR were involved in the conception and design of the study, and/or analysis and interpretation of data, drafting of the manuscript and revising it critically for important intellectual content. VR, KA, MZ, SP, BS were involved in the acquisition of data, drafting of the manuscript and revising it critically for important intellectual content. All authors read and approved the final manuscript.

Consent for publication

Not applicable.

Competing interests

The authors declare that they have no financial interests that may conflict with this manuscript.

Author details

[1]Department of Pediatrics, University Hospital of North Norway, and Department of Clinical Medicine, UiT the Arctic University of Norway, Tromsø, Norway. [2]Department of Ophtalmology, University Hospital of North Norway, and Department of Clinical Medicine, UiT the Arctic University of Norway, Tromsø, Norway. [3]Pediatric Rheumatology Clinic, Hospital for Children and Adolescents, University of Helsinki, Helsinki, Finland. [4]Department of Women's and Children's Health, Uppsala University, Uppsala, Sweden. [5]Department of Pediatrics, Institute of Clinical Sciences, Sahlgrenska Academy, University of Gothenburg, Gothenburg, Sweden. [6]Department of Pediatrics, Aarhus University Hospital, Aarhus, Denmark. [7]Pediatric Rheumatology Clinic, Rigshospitalet Copenhagen University Hospital, Copenhagen, Denmark. [8]Department of Community Medicine, UiT the Arctic University of Norway, Tromsø, Norway. [9]Department of Clinical and Molecular Medicine, NTNU - Norwegian University of Science and Technology, and Department of Pediatrics, St. Olavs Hospital, Trondheim, Norway.

References

1. Skarin A, Elborgh R, Edlund E, Bengtsson-Stigmar E. Long-term follow-up of patients with uveitis associated with juvenile idiopathic arthritis: a cohort study. Ocul Immunol Inflamm. 2009;17:104–8.
2. Paroli MP, Abbouda A, Restivo L, Sapia A, Abicca I, Pivetti PP. Juvenile idiopathic arthritis-associated uveitis at an Italian tertiary referral center: clinical features and complications. Ocul Immunol Inflamm. 2015;23:74–81.
3. Heiligenhaus A, Niewerth M, Ganser G, Heinz C, Minden K. Prevalence and complications of uveitis in juvenile idiopathic arthritis in a population-based nation-wide study in Germany: suggested modification of the current screening guidelines. Rheumatology (Oxford). 2007;46:1015–9.
4. Clarke SL, Sen ES, Ramanan AV. Juvenile idiopathic arthritis-associated uveitis. Pediatr Rheumatol Online. 2016;14:27.
5. Sen ES, Dick AD, Ramanan AV. Uveitis associated with juvenile idiopathic arthritis. Nature Rev Rheumatol. 2015;11:338–48.
6. Kotaniemi K, Sihto-Kauppi K, Salomaa P, Saila H, Ristolainen L, Kauppi M. The frequency and outcome of uveitis in patients with newly diagnosed juvenile idiopathic arthritis in two 4-year cohorts from 1990-1993 and 2000-2003. Clin Exp Rheumatol. 2014;32:143–7.
7. Angeles-Han ST, McCracken C, Yeh S, Jenkins K, Stryker D, Travers C, et al. The Association of Race With Childhood Uveitis. Am J Ophthalmol. 2015;160:919–28.
8. Shen CC, Yeh KW, Ou LS, Yao TC, Chen LC, Huang JL. Clinical features of children with juvenile idiopathic arthritis using the ILAR classification criteria: a community-based cohort study in Taiwan. J Microbiol Immunol. 2013;46:288–94.
9. Arguedas O, Fasth A, Andersson-Gare B, Porras O. Juvenile chronic arthritis in urban San Jose, Costa Rica: a 2 year prospective study. J Rheumatol. 1998;25:1844–50.
10. Berntson L, Nordal E, Aalto K, Peltoniemi S, Herlin T, Zak M, et al. HLA-B27 predicts a more chronic disease course in an 8-year followup cohort of patients with juvenile idiopathic arthritis. J Rheumatol. 2013;40:725–31.
11. Nordal EB, Songstad NT, Berntson L, Moen T, Straume B, Rygg M. Biomarkers of chronic uveitis in juvenile idiopathic arthritis: predictive value of antihistone antibodies and antinuclear antibodies. J Rheumatol. 2009;36:1737–43.
12. Saurenmann RK, Levin AV, Feldman BM, Rose JB, Laxer RM, Schneider R, et al. Prevalence, risk factors, and outcome of uveitis in juvenile idiopathic arthritis: A long-term followup study. Arthritis Rheum. 2007;56:647–57.
13. Angeles-Han ST, Pelajo CF, Vogler LB, Rouster-Stevens K, Kennedy C, Ponder L, et al. Risk markers of juvenile idiopathic arthritis-associated uveitis in the Childhood Arthritis and Rheumatology Research Alliance (CARRA) Registry. J Rheumatol. 2013;40:2088–96.

14. Rekvig OP, van der Vlag J, Seredkina N. Review: antinucleosome antibodies: a critical reflection on their specificities and diagnostic impact. Arthritis Rheumatol. 2014;66:1061–9.
15. Sparchez M, Delean D, Samasca G, Miu N, Sparchez Z. Antinuclear antibody screening by ELISA and IF techniques: discrepant results in juvenile idiopathic arthritis but consistency in childhood systemic lupus erythematous. Clin Rheumatol. 2014;33:643–7.
16. Southwood TR, Malleson PN. Antinuclear antibodies and juvenile chronic arthritis (JCA): search for a specific autoantibody associated with JCA. Ann Rheum Dis. 1991;50:595–8.
17. Monestier M, Losman JA, Fasy TM, Debbas ME, Massa M, Albani S, et al. Antihistone antibodies in antinuclear antibody-positive juvenile arthritis. Arthritis Rheum. 1990;33:1836–41.
18. Picascia A, Grimaldi V, Pignalosa O, De Pascale MR, Schiano C, Napoli C. Epigenetic control of autoimmune diseases: from bench to bedside. Clin Immunol. 2015;157:1–15.
19. Meda F, Folci M, Baccarelli A, Selmi C. The epigenetics of autoimmunity. Cell Mol Immunol. 2011;8:226–36.
20. Berntson L, Andersson GB, Fasth A, Herlin T, Kristinsson J, Lahdenne P, et al. Incidence of juvenile idiopathic arthritis in the Nordic countries. A population based study with special reference to the validity of the ILAR and EULAR criteria. J Rheumatol. 2003;30:2275–82.
21. Nordal E, Zak M, Aalto K, Berntson L, Fasth A, Herlin T, et al. Ongoing disease activity and changing categories in a long-term nordic cohort study of juvenile idiopathic arthritis. Arthritis Rheum. 2011;63:2809–18.
22. Jabs DA, Nussenblatt RB, Rosenbaum JT. Standardization of uveitis nomenclature for reporting clinical data. Results of the First International Workshop. Am J Ophthalmol. 2005;140:509–16.
23. Pharmacia Deutschland GmbH DD. Varelisa Histone Antibodies, Directions for Use. Freiburg: Phadia GmbH; 2008.
24. Vandenbroucke JP, von Elm E, Altman DG, Gotzsche PC, Mulrow CD, Pocock SJ, et al. Strengthening the Reporting of Observational Studies in Epidemiology (STROBE): explanation and elaboration. Epidemiology. 2007;18:805–35.
25. Petty RE, Southwood TR, Manners P, Baum J, Glass DN, Goldenberg J, et al. International League of Associations for Rheumatology classification of juvenile idiopathic arthritis: second revision, Edmonton, 2001. J Rheumatol. 2004;31:390–2.
26. Zak M, Pedersen FK. Juvenile chronic arthritis into adulthood: a long-term follow-up study. Rheumatology (Oxford). 2000;39:198–204.
27. Minden K, Niewerth M, Listing J, Biedermann T, Bollow M, Schontube M, et al. Long-term outcome in patients with juvenile idiopathic arthritis. Arthritis Rheum. 2002;46:2392–401.
28. Oen K, Malleson PN, Cabral DA, Rosenberg AM, Petty RE, Cheang M. Disease course and outcome of juvenile rheumatoid arthritis in a multicenter cohort. J Rheumatol. 2002;29:1989–99.
29. Bertilsson L, Andersson-Gare B, Fasth A, Petersson IF, Forsblad-D'elia H. Disease course, outcome, and predictors of outcome in a population-based juvenile chronic arthritis cohort followed for 17 years. J Rheumatol. 2013;40:715–24.
30. Bertilsson L, Andersson-Gare B, Fasth A, Forsblad-d'Elia H. A 5-year prospective population-based study of juvenile chronic arthritis: onset, disease process, and outcome. Scand J Rheumatol. 2012;41:379–82.
31. Moe N, Rygg M. Epidemiology of juvenile chronic arthritis in northern Norway: a ten-year retrospective study. Clin Exp Rheumatol. 1998;16:99–101.
32. Andersson GB, Fasth A, Andersson J, Berglund G, Ekstrom H, Eriksson M, et al. Incidence and prevalence of juvenile chronic arthritis: a population survey. Ann Rheum Dis. 1987;46:277–81.
33. Zak M, Fledelius H, Pedersen FK. Ocular complications and visual outcome in juvenile chronic arthritis: a 25-year follow-up study. Acta Ophthalmol Scand. 2003;81:211–5.
34. Glerup M, Herlin T, Twilt M. Remission rate is not dependent on the presence of antinuclear antibodies in juvenile idiopathic arthritis. Clin Rheumatol. 2017;17 doi:https://doi.org/10.1007/s10067-017-3540-x.
35. Kotaniemi K, Kautiainen H, Karma A, Aho K. Occurrence of uveitis in recently diagnosed juvenile chronic arthritis: a prospective study. Ophthalmology. 2001;108:2071–5.
36. Gran JT, Mellby AS, Husby G. The prevalence of HLA-B27 in Northern Norway. Scand J Rheumatol. 1984;13:173–6.
37. Kotaniemi K, Arkela-Kautiainen M, Haapasaari J, Leirisalo-Repo M. Uveitis in young adults with juvenile idiopathic arthritis: a clinical evaluation of 123 patients. Ann Rheum Dis. 2005;64:871–4.
38. Saurenmann RK, Levin AV, Feldman BM, Laxer RM, Schneider R, Silverman ED. Risk factors for development of uveitis differ between girls and boys with juvenile idiopathic arthritis. Arthritis Rheum. 2010;62:1824–8.
39. Yan B, Yao J, Tao ZF, Jiang Q. Epigenetics and ocular diseases: from basic biology to clinical study. J Cell Physiol. 2014;229:825–33.
40. Ravelli A, Felici E, Magni-Manzoni S, Pistorio A, Novarini C, Bozzola E, et al. Patients with antinuclear antibody-positive juvenile idiopathic arthritis constitute a homogeneous subgroup irrespective of the course of joint disease. Arthritis Rheum. 2005;52:826–32.
41. Ravelli A, Varnier GC, Oliveira S, Castell E, Arguedas O, Magnani A, et al. Antinuclear antibody-positive patients should be grouped as a separate category in the classification of juvenile idiopathic arthritis. Arthritis Rheum. 2011;63:267–75.
42. Tappeiner C, Klotsche J, Schenck S, Niewerth M, Minden K, Heiligenhaus A. Temporal change in prevalence and complications of uveitis associated with juvenile idiopathic arthritis:data from a cross-sectional analysis of a prospective nationwide study. Clin Exp Rheumatol. 2015;33:936–44.

8

Growth and weight gain in children with juvenile idiopathic arthritis: results from the ReACCh-Out cohort

Jaime Guzman[1,19*], Tristan Kerr[19], Leanne M. Ward[10], Jinhui Ma[10], Kiem Oen[6], Alan M. Rosenberg[5], Brian M. Feldman[9], Gilles Boire[14], Kristin Houghton[1], Paul Dancey[17], Rosie Scuccimarri[11], Alessandra Bruns[14], Adam M. Huber[16], Karen Watanabe Duffy[10], Natalie J. Shiff[18], Roberta A. Berard[7], Deborah M. Levy[9], Elizabeth Stringer[16], Kimberly Morishita[1], Nicole Johnson[4], David A. Cabral[1], Maggie Larché[8], Ross E. Petty[1], Ronald M. Laxer[9], Earl Silverman[9], Paivi Miettunen[4], Anne-Laure Chetaille[15], Elie Haddad[12], Lynn Spiegel[9], Stuart E. Turvey[1], Heinrike Schmeling[4], Bianca Lang[16], Janet Ellsworth[3], Suzanne E. Ramsey[16], Johannes Roth[10], Sarah Campillo[11], Susanne Benseler[4], Gaëlle Chédeville[11], Rayfel Schneider[9], Shirley M. L. Tse[9], Roxana Bolaria[2], Katherine Gross[2], Debbie Feldman[13], Bonnie Cameron[9], Roman Jurencak[10], Jean Dorval[15], Claire LeBlanc[11], Claire St. Cyr[12], Michele Gibbon[10], Rae S. M. Yeung[9], Ciarán M. Duffy[10] and Lori B. Tucker[1]

Abstract

Background: With modern treatments, the effect of juvenile idiopathic arthritis (JIA) on growth may be less than previously reported. Our objective was to describe height, weight and body mass index (BMI) development in a contemporary JIA inception cohort.

Methods: Canadian children newly-diagnosed with JIA 2005–2010 had weight and height measurements every 6 months for 2 years, then yearly up to 5 years. These measurements were used to calculate mean age- and sex-standardized Z-scores, and estimate prevalence and cumulative incidence of growth impairments, and the impact of disease activity and corticosteroids on growth.

Results: One thousand one hundred forty seven children were followed for median 35.5 months. Mean Z-scores, and the point prevalence of short stature (height < 2.5th percentile, 2.5% to 3.4%) and obesity (BMI > 95th percentile, 15.8% to 16.4%) remained unchanged in the whole cohort. Thirty-three children (2.9%) developed new-onset short stature, while 27 (2.4%) developed tall stature (>97.5th percentile). Children with systemic arthritis ($n = 77$) had an estimated 3-year cumulative incidence of 9.3% (95%CI: 4.3–19.7) for new-onset short stature and 34.4% (23–49.4) for obesity. Most children (81.7%) received no systemic corticosteroids, but 1 mg/Kg/day prednisone-equivalent maintained for 6 months corresponded to a drop of 0.64 height Z-scores (0.56–0.82) and an increase of 0.74 BMI Z-scores (0.56–0.92). An increase of 1 in the 10-cm physician global assessment of disease activity maintained for 6 months corresponded to a drop of 0.01 height Z-scores (0–0.02).

Conclusions: Most children in this modern JIA cohort grew and gained weight as children in the general population. About 1 in 10 children who had systemic arthritis, uncontrolled disease and/or prolonged corticosteroid use, had increased risk of growth impairment.

Keywords: Juvenile arthritis, Growth, Obesity, Corticosteroids

* Correspondence: jguzman@cw.bc.ca
[1]From British Columbia Children's Hospital and University of British Columbia, Vancouver, Canada
[19]Division of Pediatric Rheumatology, BC Children's Hospital, 4500 Oak St, Suite K4-122, Vancouver, BC V6H 3N1, Canada
Full list of author information is available at the end of the article

Background

Juvenile idiopathic arthritis (JIA) is the most common rheumatic disease of childhood [1], and the seven JIA categories have different characteristics and outcomes [2, 3]. Chronic inflammation in children with JIA may lead to growth delay and poor weight gain, while use of corticosteroids to control inflammation may lead to growth delay and excessive weight gain. Our knowledge about growth in children with JIA is largely based on older cross-sectional studies and retrospective cohorts from single centres [4, 5]. These studies included 20 to 200 children each and reported frequent growth impairments (a deviation from healthy growth standards in height, weight or body mass index, BMI) [5]. More recently, synthetic disease-modifying antirheumatic drugs (DMARDS) and biologic medications, which help control inflammation and reduce the need for corticosteroids, have been reported to mitigate growth impairment [6–9]. Yet, as recently as 2011, significant height growth delay was reported in oligoarthritis, a usually mild JIA category rarely treated with systemic corticosteroids [10].

In this study, we used data from a prospective multicentre inception cohort of over one thousand Canadian children to determine 1) height, weight and BMI trajectories over time in children with JIA managed with modern treatments; 2) their risk of growth impairments; and 3) the impact of disease activity and corticosteroid use on growth.

Methods

Subjects

Data from the Research in Arthritis in Canadian Children emphasizing Outcomes (ReACCh-Out) cohort were used. ReACCh-Out was designed to document disease outcomes in usual practice [3, 11]. It enrolled 1497 patients newly diagnosed with JIA between 2005 and 2010 at all 16 Canadian pediatric rheumatology centres. JIA category was assigned using accepted criteria within 6 months of enrolment [2, 3]. Study visits were scheduled at enrolment and at 6, 12, 18, 24, 36, 48, and 60 months thereafter. The study was approved by research ethics boards at each participating institution. Parents provided informed written consent, and patients provided assent where appropriate. This report includes children recruited within 6 months of diagnosis who had at least two available height and weight records as of May 30th, 2012.

Measures of growth and weight gain

Standing height and weight were measured at each study visit as per usual clinic practices. We calculated age- and sex-standardized scores (Z-scores, 0 = mean of healthy children, 1 = one standard deviation in healthy children) [12], for height, weight, and BMI for each child using standards for healthy growth endorsed by the Canadian Pediatric Endocrinology Group [13]. These are equivalent to the 2007 World Health Organization standards, except that standards for both weight and BMI are provided up to age 18 years [14].

Growth impairments were defined as follows:

Short stature: a height below the 2.5th percentile for age and sex (corresponding to a Z-score < −2.0) [15].

Tall stature: a height above the 97.5th percentile for age and sex.

Obesity: a BMI above the 95th percentile for age and sex [12].

Thinness: a BMI below the 5th percentile for age and sex.

Growth delay: a decrease of 1.0 or more in height Z-score at a given visit, relative to the Z-score of that child at enrolment.

Growth acceleration: an increase of 1.0 or more in height Z-score at a given visit, relative to the Z-score of that child at enrolment.

Excessive weight gain: an increase of 1.0 or more in BMI Z-score at a given visit, relative to the Z-score of that child at enrolment.

Poor weight gain: a decrease of 1.0 or more in BMI Z-score at a given visit, relative to the Z-score of that child at enrolment.

These definitions and cut-offs have been used in previous studies, but they are not universally accepted. The Z-score at enrolment was calculated using the first available measurements of height and weight (a median of 0.5 months after diagnosis), representing our best estimate of the child's baseline growth. A change of 1.0 Z-scores from enrolment was chosen because it roughly corresponds to the crossing of a percentile channel on growth charts [16], and it had been used in a previous study [10].

Other measures

Disease activity and medication use were recorded at each study visit, and at clinic visits in-between study visits. Disease activity was reported by the pediatric rheumatologist using a standard 10-cm horizontal visual analogue scale from 0 = inactive disease to 10 = very active disease [17]. Early treatment responders (versus non-early responders) were defined as those who attained clinically inactive disease within a year of diagnosis [3, 17].

The name and current dose of oral and intravenous corticosteroids recorded at each clinic visit were used to calculate mg/kg/day in prednisone equivalent using published conversion factors [18, 19], and the most recently recorded patient's weight. Children were categorized as non-users of systemic corticosteroids, transitory users (3 months or less) or prolonged users (>3 months of cumulative use during the study), irrespective of the doses or frequency of administration; intraarticular corticosteroid administration was not considered in this categorization.

The education level of the parent with the highest level of education was used as a proxy for socio-economic status and self-reported ethnicity was recorded using Statistics Canada standard categories.

Statistical analysis

Analyses were conducted using STATA 12 software [StataCorp LP, College Station, Texas]. Trajectories of the mean Z-score over time were charted using locally weighted scatter plot smoothing with a band width of 0.6 to produce lines reflecting observed data without imposing a particular shape. Kaplan Meier survival methods were used to estimate the cumulative incidence of new-onset growth impairments. These consider only the first occurrence of growth impairment, and do not reflect persistence or resolution of the impairment. Because the number of subjects in some JIA categories was small beyond three years, we show plots only to three years after diagnosis. The log-rank test was used to compare survival curves. Mixed effects models assessed the impact of cumulative disease activity and corticosteroid use in the previous six months on Z-scores, after adjusting for parental education, ethnicity and JIA category. Models were implemented in STATA as growth curve models [20] with random intercept, random slope and a quadratic term for time since diagnosis (see Additional file 1 for details).

Sensitivity analyses to assess the robustness of our findings included use of alternative growth charts and measures of disease activity [21], analyses in children of prepubertal age (defined as <7 years at diagnosis) and calculation of cumulative incidence of reciprocal "growth impairments" (e.g. tall stature and growth acceleration) to assess to what extent our results were due to normal variability and the choice of cut-off, rather than true impairments.

Results

A total of 1147 children were included (Table 1). The reasons for ineligibility and subject disposition are shown in Fig. 1. The median age at diagnosis was 9.5 years (25th, 75th centile: 4, 13) and 64% were female. The median time from diagnosis to enrolment was 0.5 months (0, 1.9). Height and weight measurements were available on 5909 visits for a median follow-up of 35.5 months (25th, 75th centile: 23, 49). Additional file 1: Table S1 shows subjects with data at each visit.

Height, weight and BMI trajectories

Figure 2 shows trajectories of height, weight, and BMI mean Z-scores for the whole cohort and for each JIA category. Mean height Z-scores remained unchanged for the whole cohort (Fig. 2d). Children with enthesitis-related arthritis had an estimated mean height Z-score at diagnosis of +0.2 and remained unchanged over 3 years. In contrast, children with systemic arthritis also had an estimated mean height Z-score at diagnosis of +0.2 but it decreased and did not return to baseline within 3 years. Using quadratic fit equations the corresponding 95% CI become non-overlapping by one year (Additional file 1: Fig. S1).

Mean weight and BMI Z-scores in the whole cohort and in the most frequent JIA categories (oligoarthritis, RF-negative polyarthritis, enthesitis-related, undifferentiated) remained stable over time (Fig. 2). These parameters increased during the first year after diagnosis in children with systemic JIA and RF-positive polyarthritis, but their estimates at diagnosis were different: a mean BMI Z-score of +0.6 for systemic and −0.1 for RF-positive polyarthritis. Mean values of weight and BMI Z-scores of children with psoriatic arthritis were high at enrolment and decreased over time.

Growth impairments

The point prevalence of short stature in the whole cohort remained stable during the study (2.5 to 3.4%, Fig. 3). Thirty-three children (2.9%) had new-onset short stature (<2.5th percentile), while 27 (2.4%) had new-onset tall stature (>97.5th percentile) during the study. Ninety-three children (8.1%) had growth delay, while 64 (5.6%) had growth acceleration. The estimated cumulative incidence of growth delay within 3 years of diagnosis for the whole cohort was 8.5% (95%CI: 6.8–10.6, Table 2). It varied from 5.7% to 9.9% across JIA categories, except for systemic arthritis (22.5%, 14.2–34.7).

The point prevalence of obesity in the whole cohort remained stable during the study (15.8 to 16.8%, Fig. 3). Ninety-seven children (8.5%) developed new onset obesity, while 43 (3.7%) developed new onset thinness. The estimated cumulative incidence of obesity within three years of diagnosis was 10.8% (95%CI: 8.8–13.2, Table 2); it varied from 5.9% to 14.1% across JIA categories, except for systemic arthritis (34.4%, 23.0–49.4). The estimated cumulative incidence of excessive weight gain within 3 years of diagnosis varied from 5% to 15% across JIA categories, except for systemic arthritis (28.1%, 19.0–40.3).

Impact of corticosteroids and disease activity

In adjusted mixed effects models, a dose of 1 mg/kg/day prednisone equivalents maintained for 6 months corresponded to a decrease of 0.64 in height Z-scores (95%CI: 0.56–0.82) and an increase of 0.74 in BMI Z-scores (0.56–0.92) (Table 3). Additional file 1: Fig. S2 shows trajectories of mean corticosteroid dose for each JIA category. Most children received no systemic corticosteroids during the study (n = 943, 81.7%), while 88 (7.6%) were transitory users and 123 (10.6%) were prolonged users (>3 months). The estimated cumulative incidence of short stature among prolonged corticosteroid users was 6.6% within 3 years, compared to 2.6% for non-users (p = 0.07, log-rank test for survival curves). The estimated cumulative

Table 1 Characteristics of patients by JIA category[a]

Characteristic	All (*N* = 1147)	Systemic Arthritis (*n* = 77)	Oligoarthritis (*n* = 443)	RF-negative polyarthritis (*n* = 232)	RF-positive polyarthritis (*n* = 44)	Psoriatic arthritis (*n* = 70)	Enthesitis-related Arthritis (*n* = 164)	Undifferentiated (*n* = 117)
% Female	64.0	47.4	70.2	77.6	95.5	67.1	25.0	68.4
Age at diagnosis (yrs)	9.5 (4.0, 13.1)	6.6 (3.1, 12.2)	6.4 (3.0, 11.5)	9.1 (3.4, 12.7)	12.8 (9.4, 15.2)	11.6 (5.3, 13.6)	13.1 (10.8,14.5)	9.5 (3.7, 13.1)
Disease duration (months)	5.8 (3.1, 10.9)	2.9 (1.9, 5.4)	5.3 (3.0, 8.9)	6.1 (3.4, 12.4)	5.5 (3.6, 10.6)	6.5 (3.0, 13.6)	8.9 (4.2,17.3)	5.9 (3.5, 9.0)
Follow-up (months)	35.5 (23,49)	40.7 (24,52)	35.0 (23,49)	36.7 (24,52)	33.1 (23, 49)	34.5 (18, 49)	30.9 (19, 40)	35.7 (23, 48)
Height Z-score at enrolment	0.02 (−0.70, 0.82)	0.09 (−0.69, 0.91)	0.06 (−0.65, 0.83)	−0.13 (−0.77, 0.58)	0.02 (−0.59, 0.69)	0.12 (−0.68, 0.99)	0.16 (−0.52, 0.98)	−0.19 (−0.92, 0.62)
Weight Z-score at enrolment	0.31 (−0.37, 1.06)	0.58 (0.04, 1.25)	0.25 (−0.35, 0.90)	0.17 (−0.53, 0.94)	0.16 (−0.83, 0.94)	0.66 (−0.26, 1.4)	0.61 (−0.52, 1.4)	0.29 (−0.53, 0.96)
BMI percentile at enrolment	66 (34, 89)	80.4 (62, 90)	62.6 (35, 87)	64.6 (34, 87)	55.8 (18, 88)	75.3 (46, 96)	65.8 (28, 93)	67.0 (38, 88)
Disease activity (mm)	28 (12, 50)	37 (13, 62)	19 (8, 34)	46 (27, 66)	52 (26, 71)	23 (11, 51)	30 (12, 46)	26 (12, 48)
ESR, mm/h[b]	18 (7, 36)	58 (25, 89)	17 (7, 31)	18 (8, 36)	36 (16, 53)	15 (8, 36)	10 (4, 24)	16 (5, 35)
Treatments[c]								
DMARDs (%)	55.7	71.1	33.9	84.9	97.7	50.0	58.7	53.8
Biologics (%)	11.7	34.2	3.6	15.9	40.9	7.1	12.2	10.3
Corticosteroid joint injections (%)	44.3	17.1	55.5	43.5	43.2	41.4	31.4	41.9
Systemic corticosteroids (%)	18.2	85.5	9.3	28.0	63.6	17.1	23.8	23.1
Corticosteroids >3 months (%)	10.6	65.0	0.9	10.8	29.5	2.9	9.3	11.1
Ethnicity[d]								
British (%)	50.2	41.9	44.7	54.1	44.2	60.6	54.6	53.5
French (%)	31.2	22.1	35.8	26.1	18.6	34.8	22.7	42.1
Indigenous Canadian (%)	8.1	5.8	8.9	7.7	16.3	6.1	5.5	8.8
Other (%)	25.4	26.7	21.8	31.5	34.9	16.7	30.7	16.7
Parental education[e]								
Less than high school (%)	2.01	1.6	1.9	2.9	0	1.6	2.6	1.0
High school/ some postsecondary (%)	50.24	53.1	45.8	51.7	61.9	54.1	51.6	56.4
University/ postgraduate degree (%)	47.75	45.3	51.6	46.4	38.1	44.3	45.8	42.6
Inactive disease within 1 year of diagnosis (%)	49.5	44.7	65.48	36.6	22.7	42.9	37.8	39.3

[a]Numbers are median and (25th, 75th centiles) unless otherwise specified
[b]ESR was obtained in 88% of the cohort at enrolment
[c]Treatments received at any time during the study
[d]Self-reported ethnicity was available in 96% of the cohort. Other ethnicity includes Asian, African, Latin American and other European ethnicities. The sum of ethnicities may add to more than 100% because each child could report up to 6 ethnic backgrounds
[e]The level of education of the parent who had a higher level of education. Parental education for at least one parent was obtained in 93% of the cohort at enrolment

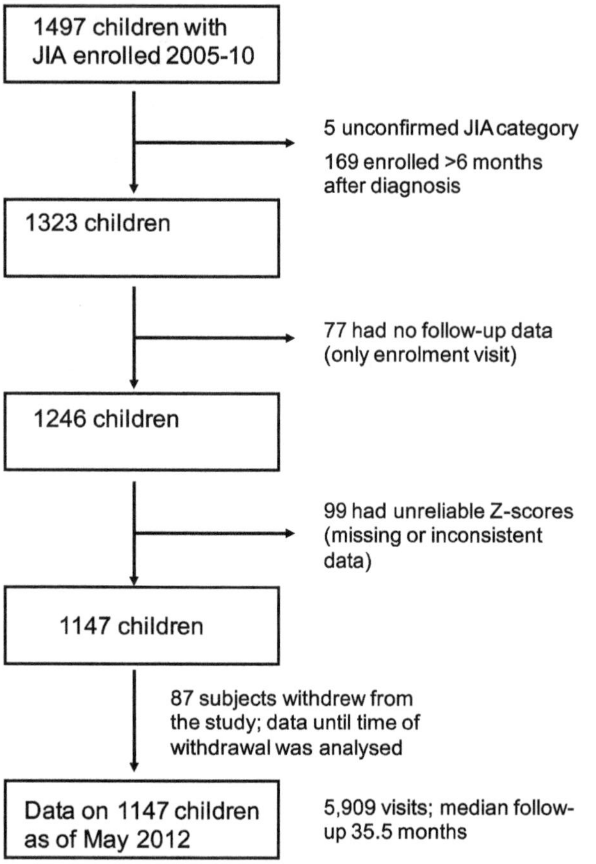

Fig. 1 Subject eligibility and disposition

incidence of obesity among prolonged corticosteroid users was 25% within 3 years, compared to 8.5% for non-users ($p < 0.0001$, log-rank test for survival curves, Additional file 1: Fig. S3).

In adjusted models, a 1 cm increase in the 10 cm physician global assessment of disease activity maintained for 6 months was associated with a decrease of 0.01 in height Z-scores (95%CI: 0.00–0.02) (Table 3). The association between disease activity and changes in BMI Z-scores was not significant. Mean disease activity decreased in all JIA categories after diagnosis (Additional file 1: Fig. S2) and 567 children (49.5%) attained inactive disease within the first year. Early treatment responders and non-early treatment responders had similar probability of growth impairments (Additional file 1: Fig. S4).

Sensitivity analyses

Using the Centers for Disease Control growth charts had minimal impact on our estimates of growth impairments, except for a lower cumulative incidence of obesity within 3 years of diagnosis of 7.5% (95%CI: 5.9–9.6) (Additional file 1: Table S2). Calculations for reciprocal "growth impairments" (growth acceleration, tall stature, poor weight gain and thinness) are shown in Additional file 1: Table S3 and suggest a substantial portion of the incidence of growth impairments reported in Table 2 is due to normal variability and our choice of cut-offs rather than to the disease; for example, the 3-year cumulative incidence of tall stature for the whole cohort was 2.3%, compared to 3.0% for short stature. Children younger than 7 years at diagnosis had higher cumulative incidence of growth impairments, relative to the whole cohort, and a different distribution of JIA categories (Additional file 1: Table S4). Use of the active joint count or the Juvenile Arthritis Disease Activity Score [21], as alternative measures of disease activity, did not substantially change our findings (Additional file 1: Table S5).

Discussion

We used data from a large prospective inception cohort of Canadian children with JIA to estimate impact of the disease and its treatment on height, weight and BMI development. For children in the most frequent JIA categories (oligoarthritis, RF-negative polyarthritis, enthesitis-related arthritis and undifferentiated arthritis, 83.5% of the cohort) the impact was negligible. On the other hand, children with systemic arthritis showed a decrease in height Z-scores and increase in BMI Z-scores, with no apparent return to baseline within 3 years. To put things in perspective, the decrease in mean height Z-scores in children with systemic JIA corresponds to approximately 2 cm for a 9 year old child. Children with RF-positive polyarthritis or psoriatic arthritis had relatively minor, but measurable, risk of growth impairments. For the whole cohort, point prevalence for short stature and obesity remained unchanged over the 3 years after diagnosis, suggesting the observed growth impairments affected too few children and/or were too short-lived to affect the overall prevalence.

Most children received no systemic corticosteroids, in those who did, larger doses of corticosteroids were clearly associated with lower height and higher BMI Z-scores. A similar impact of corticosteroids on BMI has been shown in children with a variety of rheumatic diseases [22]. In our cohort, most children with systemic JIA received high-dose corticosteroids, which likely mediated their observed growth impairments. Increased disease activity was associated with lower height Z-scores but the impact was minor, relative to that of corticosteroids.

Our original protocol considered a change of 1.0 Z-scores relative to baseline indicative of growth impairment because this roughly corresponds to crossing a percentile channel in growth charts [16], and it had been used in a previous study [10]. However, we later realized this definition may lead to apparent growth impairments even in healthy children. Growth in healthy children is complex and may have periods of relative stasis or rapid growth [23]. This may result in apparent delay or acceleration of

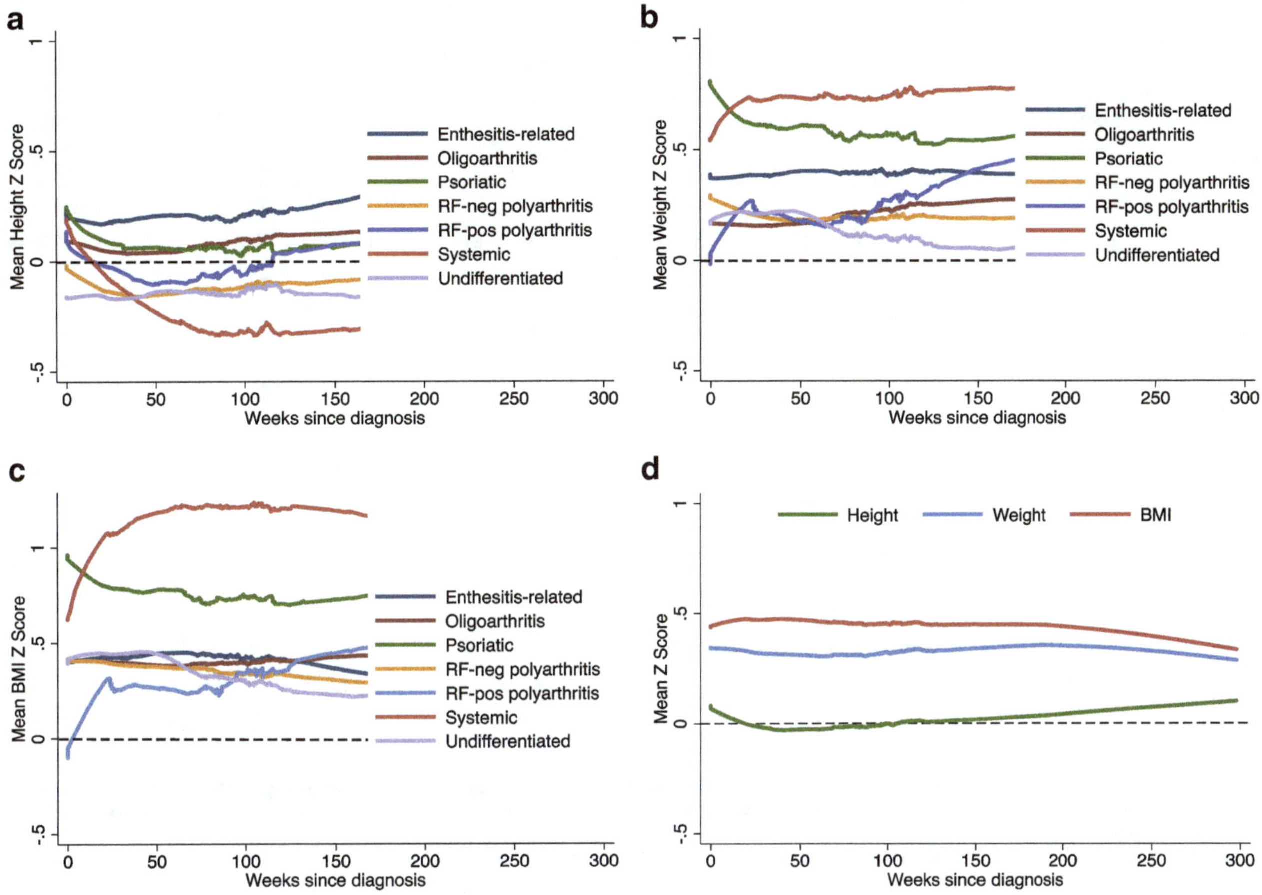

Fig. 2 Smoothed trajectories of mean Z-scores. Shown are trajectories of (**a**) height, (**b**) weight, and (**c**) BMI for each JIA category in the 3 years after diagnosis. Panel (**d**) shows Z-score trajectories for the whole cohort. Trajectories of the mean Z-score were charted using locally weighted scatter plot smoothing with a band width of 0.6. The black dashed horizontal line represents healthy growth standards

growth when comparing a child to normative growth curves [12]. For example, children with enthesitis-related arthritis in our cohort had a virtually flat trajectory of mean height Z-score (i.e. they grew at the same pace than healthy children), but over 3 years they still had a 7.2% cumulative incidence of growth delay and a 7.7% cumulative incidence of growth acceleration. We believe cumulative incidences of this level using the 1.0 Z-score cut-off likely reflect normal periods of relative stasis or rapid growth, rather than true growth impairments. This could

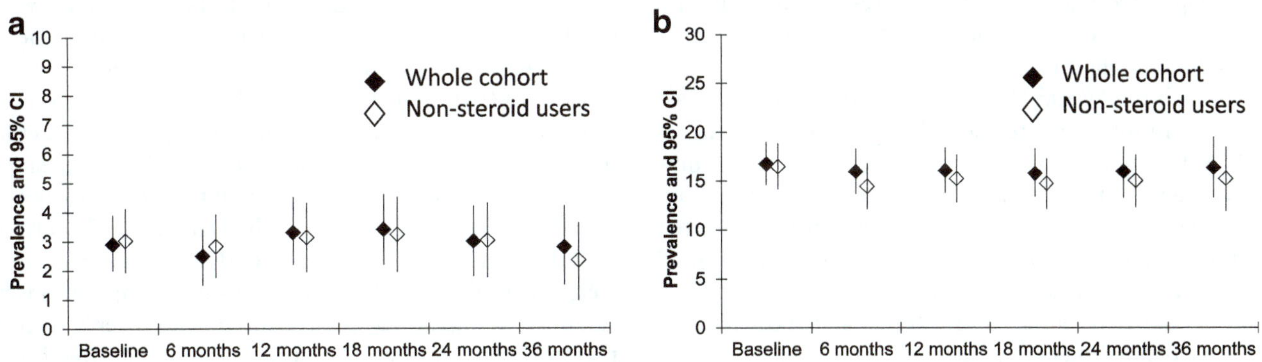

Fig. 3 Point prevalence of short stature and obesity in the whole cohort. Shown are the point prevalences of **a**) short stature and **b**) obesity in the whole cohort at every study visits for the 3 years after enrolment, and after excluding children who received corticosteroids. The vertical lines represent 95%CI

Table 2 Estimates of the cumulative incidence (%) of growth delay, short stature, excessive weight gain and obesity within 1 and 3 years after diagnosis in seven JIA categories

JIA Category	Growth delay		Short stature		Excessive weight gain		Obesity	
	1-year cumulative incidence (95% CI)	3-year cumulative incidence (95% CI)	1-year cumulative incidence (95% CI)	3-year cumulative incidence (95% CI)	1-year cumulative incidence (95% CI)	3-year cumulative incidence (95% CI)	1-year cumulative Incidence (95% CI)	3-year cumulative Incidence (95% CI)
All (*N* = 1147)	3.2 (2.4, 4.5)	8.5 (6.8, 10.6)	1.2 (0.7, 2.1)	3.0 (2.1, 4.4)	4.8 (3.7, 6.2)	10.7 (8.8, 12.9)	5.2 (4.0, 6.9)	10.8 (8.8, 13.2)
Systemic arthritis (*n* = 77)	6.8 (2.9, 15.7)	22.5 (14.2, 34.7)	1.4 (0.2, 9.8)	9.3 (4.3, 19.7)	17.2 (10.4, 27.8)	28.1 (19.0, 40.3)	22.7 (13.9, 35.9)	34.4 (23.0, 49.4)
Oligoarthritis (*n* = 443)	3.8 (2.3, 6.1)	7.8 (5.3, 11.3)	1.2 (0.5, 2.9)	2.3 (1.2, 4.4)	3.8 (2.3, 6.1)	10.5 (7.6, 14.4)	3.3 (1.9, 5.7)	8.2 (5.5, 12.1)
RF-negative polyarthritis (*n* = 232)	4.0 (2.1, 7.6)	7.4 (4.5, 12.0)	0.9 (0.2, 3.6)	0.9 (0.2, 3.6)	3.6 (1.8, 7.0)	8.9 (5.6, 14.1)	3.5 (1.7, 7.2)	8.5 (5.2, 13.8)
RF-positive polyarthritis (*n* = 44)	—	9.9 (3.1, 28.7)	—	4.3 (0.6, 27.1)	9.1 (3.5, 22.6)	15.0 (7.2, 31.9)	—	5.9 (0.8, 35.0)
Psoriatic arthritis (*n* = 70)	2.9 (0.7, 10.9)	9.5 (4.0, 21.8)	2.9 (0.7, 11.1)	9.5 (3.9, 22.0)	3.0 (0.7, 11.4)	5.0 (1.6, 14.9)	4.1 (1.0, 15.5)	11.7 (5.0, 26.0)
Enthesitis-related arthritis (*n* = 164)	1.2 (0.3, 4.7)	7.2 (3.6, 14.4)	0.6 (0.1, 4.5)	1.6 (0.4, 6.3)	3.7 (1.7, 8.1)	8.3 (4.5, 14.9)	5.4 (2.6, 10.9)	9.7 (5.4, 17.2)
Undifferentiated (*n* = 117)	1.9 (0.5, 7.2)	5.7 (2.4, 13.5)	1.9 (0.5, 7.4)	3.6 (1.1, 11.4)	3.6 (1.4, 9.3)	7.6 (3.9, 14.7)	8.4 (4.3, 16.0)	14.1 (8.4, 23.1)

Growth delay: a decrease of 1.0 or more in height Z-score relative to the z-score of that child at enrolment. Short stature: a height below the 2.5th percentile for age and sex. Excessive weight gain: an increase of 1.0 or more in BMI Z-score relative to the z-score of that child at enrolment. Obesity: a BMI above the 95th percentile for age and sex

— = Cumulative incidence could not be calculated as no child had experienced the growth impairment at this time

only be confirmed by following healthy children at the same time intervals and applying the 1.0 Z score cut-off; we are not aware of any such study.

Defining growth impairments as a change of 1.0 Z scores from baseline uses the child as his/her own control and allows identification of substantial changes in growth that may not be apparent when using the extreme limits (e.g. below 2.5th percentile or above 95th percentile). Nevertheless, some such changes may be desirable. For example, a child who is obese at baseline may drop more than 1.0 BMI Z-scores in follow-up and become closer to his/her ideal BMI (by our definition this is "poor weight gain").

Although the World Health Organization has proposed standard terminology to describe growth impairments [15], it has not been universally adopted. The recommended term for a stature <−2.0 Z-scores is 'stunting,' but we chose to use the term short stature instead, as we felt the implication that 2.5% of healthy children have stunted growth had overtly negative connotations. At the end, we chose to use neutral descriptive terms and most importantly, we defined them explicitly.

The high prevalence and cumulative incidence of obesity observed in our cohort may be a reflection of the current epidemic of obesity among North American children. An obesity point prevalence of 10.5 to 16.3% has been reported among Canadian children aged 5 to 11 years old [24], and new onset obesity has been reported in 11.9% of children in the United States between the ages of 5 and 14 years old [25]. However, children with systemic arthritis in our cohort had a three times higher incidence of obesity than these reported population values.

There were some interesting differences across JIA categories in growth parameters at enrolment (Table 1). These may reflect disease impact between symptom onset and enrolment, but they should be interpreted with caution as chance alone may explain these differences. One could postulate for example that the mean weight Z-score of 0.31 at enrolment for the whole cohort represents the current obesity epidemic among Canadian children, and that the mean z-score of 0.16 for RF-positive polyarthritis reflects weight loss during the nearly six months from symptom onset, while the mean Z-score of 0.58 for systemic JIA reflects corticosteroid-associated weight gain during the 2.9 months since symptom onset. Again, one ought to be careful not to over-interpret these differences given the large variability in growth parameters across children and small sample sizes in some JIA categories in this cohort. Of note, children with psoriatic arthritis had the highest mean weight Z-score

Table 3 Impact of corticosteroid use, disease activity and covariates on height Z-scores and BMI Z-scores

	Impact on height Z-scores				*Impact on BMI Z-scores*			
Variable	Unadjusted[a] (95% CI)	*p* value	Adjusted (95% CI)	*p* value	Unadjusted (95% CI)	*p* value	Adjusted (95% CI)	*p* value
Cumulative corticosteroids[b]	−0.69 (−0.82, −0.56)	<0.01	−0.64 (−0.77, −0.50)	<0.01	0.79 (0.63, 0.96)	<0.01	0.74 (0.56, 0.92)	<0.01
Cumulative disease activity[c]	−0.02 (−0.03, −0.01)	<0.01	−0.01 (−0.02, 0.00)	0.04	0.00 (−0.01, 0.01)	0.49	−0.01 (−0.02, 0.00)	0.17
Parental education[d]								
Less than high school	Reference		Reference		Reference		Reference	
High school/secondary	0.29 (−0.18, 0.77)	0.23	0.31 (−0.18, 0.80)	0.21	0.005 (−0.50, 0.51)	0.98	0.09 (−0.43, 0.61)	0.73
Some post-secondary	0.34 (−0.12, 0.80)	0.15	0.39 (−.08, 0.87)	0.11	−0.01 (−0.50, 0.48)	0.96	0.09 (−0.41, 0.60)	0.72
University degree	0.32 (−0.14, 0.78)	0.18	0.36 (−0.11, 0.84)	0.14	−0.17 (−0.66, 0.31)	0.49	−0.08 (−0.58, 0.43)	0.77
Postgraduate degree	0.40 (−0.08, 0.89)	0.10	0.43 (−0.07, 0.93)	0.09	−0.25 (−0.76, 0.26)	0.33	−0.11 (−0.64, 0.42)	0.68
Primary Ethnicity[e]								
British	Reference		Reference		Reference		Reference	
French	−0.09 (−0.26, 0.09)	0.32	−0.11 (−0.29, 0.07)	0.24	−0.36 (−0.55, −0.17)	<0.01	−0.33 (−0.52, −0.13)	<0.01
Indigenous Canadian	0.15 (−0.15, 0.45)	0.34	0.15 (−0.16, 0.46)	0.33	−0.05 (−0.37, 0.27)	0.76	−0.03 (−0.36, 0.30)	0.84
Other European	0.03 (−0.14, 0.19)	0.74	0.03 (−0.14, 0.20)	0.75	−0.31 (−0.49, −0.13)	<0.01	−0.23 (−0.41, −0.05)	0.01
South Asian	0.33 (0.0, 0.66)	0.05	0.34 (0.0, 0.67)	0.05	−0.13 (−0.48, 0.22)	0.47	−0.13 (−0.49, 0.23)	0.48
Other	−0.07 (−0.27, 0.13)	0.47	−0.03 (−0.24, 0.18)	0.75	−0.23 (−0.44, −0.02)	0.03	−0.13 (−0.35, 0.09)	0.25
JIA categories								
Oligoarthritis	Reference		Reference		Reference		Reference	
RF-neg polyarthritis	−0.17 (−0.34, −0.01)	0.04	−0.14 (−0.32, 0.03)	0.10	−0.01 (−0.18, 0.17)	0.96	0.00 (−0.18, 0.19)	0.99
Enthesitis-related	0.17 (−0.01, 0.36)	0.07	0.21 (0.01, 0.40)	0.04	0.08 (−0.12, 0.27)	0.45	−0.04 (−0.25, 0.18)	0.74
Systemic	−0.36 (−0.61, −0.10)	0.01	−0.23 (−0.51, 0.05)	0.10	0.68 (0.41, 0.95)	<0.01	0.44 (0.15, 0.74)	<0.01
Psoriatic	0.04 (−0.23, 0.30)	0.79	0.16 (−0.12, 0.44)	0.26	0.41 (0.13, 0.69)	<0.01	0.31 (0.01, 0.61)	0.05
RF-pos polyarthritis	−0.13 (−0.46, 0.19)	0.43	−0.03 (−0.36, 0.31)	0.88	−0.13 (−0.47, 0.21)	0.46	−0.25 (−0.60, 0.10)	0.17
Undifferentiated	−0.18 (−0.39, 0.04)	0.11	−0.11 (−0.33, 0.12)	0.37	0.03 (−0.20, 0.25)	0.82	0.02 (−0.22, 0.26)	0.86

[a]Unadjusted Beta coefficients and (95% CI) were obtained from mixed effect models including only one independent variable at a time. Adjusted beta coefficients are from a mixed effects model where cumulative corticosteroids in previous 6 months, cumulative disease activity in previous 6 months, parental education, ethnicity and JIA category were entered together. Cumulative prednisone and disease activity were time-variant variables. All mixed effects models were run by subject and included random intercept, random slope and a quadratic term for time since diagnosis in weeks. They can be represented by: dependent variable = b1*constant + b2*time + b3*time square + b4* first independent variable + b5* second independent variable

[b]Cumulative corticosteroids were calculated as area under the curve of daily prednisone equivalents per kilogram of body weight recorded at each clinic visit, using the trapezoid method; a one unit change corresponds to an increase of 1 mg/Kg of prednisone equivalents per day sustained for 6 months. For the first study visit, corticosteroids were assumed to start at diagnosis

[c]Cumulative disease activity was calculated as area under the curve of the physician global assessment of disease activity recorded at each clinic visit, using the trapezoid method; a one unit change corresponds to an increase of 1 cm in the physician global assessment sustained for 6 months. For the first study visit the physician global assessment was assumed to be zero the day before disease onset

[d]The level of education of the parent who had a higher level of education

[e]The ethnic group listed first; up to six ethnic groups could be listed for each child as defined by Statistics Canada

of 0.66 at enrolment and they rarely, if ever, used corticosteroids.

Two published retrospective cohorts are of particular relevance to our study. In a study of 67 Canadian children with JIA, Liem and Rosenberg reported that relative to children with oligoarthritis, a lower height Z-score was apparent in the second year after diagnosis for children with systemic arthritis [26]. A similar change was apparent from the first year in our study. Children with RF-positive polyarthritis tended to have negative Z-scores, while children with RF-negative polyarthritis tended to have positive Z-scores [26]. In our study, children with RF-negative polyarthritis had practically normal growth while those with RF-positive polyarthritis had measurable, but mild growth impairments.

In the second study, Padeh et al. reported on 95 children with oligoarticular JIA in a single centre in Israel. After a mean follow-up of 6 years they reported "severe growth retardation" (a decrease in height Z-score of 1.0 or more relative to baseline) in 11.6% of children [10]. This estimate is compatible with our 3-year cumulative incidence of growth delay of 7.8% using the same cut-off, but as stated above, we suspect this level of apparent growth impairment reflects normal periods of relative stasis and not true impairment.

Recent studies suggest DMARDs and biologic agents mitigate growth impairments in children with JIA [6, 7]. It is not clear whether this is due to better control of the disease, reduced doses of corticosteroids, or both. One non-controlled trial of anakinra monotherapy in systemic arthritis avoided use of corticosteroids in 13 of 20 children [27]. The 2013 update of the American College of Rheumatology juvenile arthritis treatment recommendations includes initial monotherapy with biologics as an option in children with systemic arthritis [28]. It will be important to ascertain if early monotherapy with biologics prevents the growth impairments observed in patients with systemic JIA in our cohort.

Study strengths and limitations

To our knowledge, this is the largest prospective study of growth in children with JIA published to date. It reflects more recent treatment practices than previous studies and we analysed growth in multiple ways to ensure our findings were robust. Nonetheless, our data should be interpreted in light of five limitations. First, although Z-scores are age- and sex-standardized this may not fully adjust for the effect of age and pubertal status on the child's susceptibility to growth impairment, and we did not collect data on pubertal status in this cohort. Second, because procedures to measure height and weight were not standardized and the stadiometers and balances were not cross-calibrated, some differences in Z-scores may be due to measurement variability. Third, cumulative corticosteroids and cumulative disease activity in the previous 6 months were based on few measurements, since we did not use corticosteroid diaries and disease activity was only assessed at clinic visits. Fourth, we did not report on localized growth impairments such as leg length discrepancy or jaw asymmetry, which may occur in juvenile arthritis. Finally, our estimates refer to 3 years after diagnosis, and the risk of growth impairments may change with longer follow-up. It is important to emphasize that the reported growth impairments may be transitory and that final height and weight may be normal due to catch up growth and delayed puberty. Most children in this cohort had not completed their growth at the last assessment, and we had no parental height data to allow calculation of genetic growth potential.

Implications for practice

Families of children with JIA should know that with modern treatments, their child's disease will not substantially affect growth and weight gain, unless the child has systemic JIA, requires prolonged corticosteroid use (>3 months) and/or has uncontrolled disease. Families of children with systemic arthritis should know that systemic corticosteroids may control the disease, but at the cost of potential growth impairment; a 1 in 10 risk of short stature and a 1 in 3 risk of obesity within 3 years of diagnosis. Practitioners should be wary of prolonged corticosteroid use and our results quantify their effect on growth.

Conclusions

Most children with JIA in this cohort grew and gained weight at a pace similar to modern North American populations. Children in the most frequent JIA categories grew well, but about 1 in 10 children who had systemic arthritis, uncontrolled disease activity, and/or required prolonged use of systemic corticosteroids were at risk of growth impairment. These children may benefit from earlier aggressive therapy to help prevent growth impairment, or early consultation with a pediatric endocrinologist to mitigate growth impairment by other means.

Abbreviations

BMI: Body Mass Index; DMARDs: Disease modifying Antirheumatic drugs; JIA: Juvenile idiopathic arthritis; ReACCh-Out: The Research in Arthritis in Canadian Children Emphasizing Outcomes Cohort; RF: Rheumatoid factor

Acknowledgments

A heartfelt thank you to all the Canadian families who enrolled their children in the Research in Arthritis in Canadian Children emphasizing Outcomes cohort and made this study possible.

Funding

This study was funded by a New Emerging Team research grant from the Canadian Institutes of Health Research. Additional funding support for Ms. Michele Gibbon was provided by the Fast Foundation, Toronto, Canada. Mr. Tristan Kerr received a studentship from the Canadian Rheumatology Association for his work with this project. Dr. Ward was supported by the Departments of Pediatrics and Surgery, Children's Hospital of Eastern Ontario and a University of Ottawa Research Chair award. Dr. Guzman was funded by a Clinical Investigator Award from the Child and Family Research Institute, Vancouver, Canada.

Authors' contributions

JG: drafted the initial proposal for this study, conducted statistical analyses, provided substantial input on the interpretation of findings, drafted the initial manuscript and coordinated revisions to the manuscript. TK: drafted the initial proposal for this study, conducted statistical analyses, and drafted the initial manuscript. LMW: contributed substantially to the final study proposal, the interpretation of findings and drafting of the manuscript. JM: contributed substantially to the final study proposal, design of statistical analyses, interpretation of findings and the drafting of the manuscript. KO: designed the original ReACCh-Out study that provided the data, obtained the original research grant, contributed substantially to the final proposal and interpretation of findings, and to the drafting of the manuscript. AMR: contributed substantially to the final study proposal, the interpretation of findings and drafting of the manuscript. BMF: contributed substantially to the final study proposal, the interpretation of findings and drafting of the manuscript. GB: contributed substantially to the final study proposal, the interpretation of findings and drafting of the manuscript. KH, PD, RS, AB, AMH, KWD, NJS, RAB, DML, ES, KM, NJ, DAC, ML, REP, RML, ES, PM, ALC, EH, LS, SET, HS, BL, JE, SER, JR, SC, SB, GC, RS, SMLT, RB, KG, DF, BC, RJ, JD, CL and CSC participated in subject enrolment and follow-up, and in two rounds of revisions for the manuscript. MG: was the main coordinator for the ReACCh-Out cohort, oversaw data collection and data entering and participated in two rounds of revisions for the manuscript. RSMY: designed the original ReACCh-Out study that provided the data, obtained the original research grant and participated in two rounds of revisions for the manuscript. CMD: was the nominated principal investigator for the ReACCh-Out study, designed the original ReACCh-Out study that provided the data, obtained the original research grant and participated in two rounds of revisions for the manuscript. LBT: drafted the initial proposal for this study, designed the original ReACCh-Out study that provided the data, obtained the original research grant, provided substantial input on interpretation of findings and drafting of the manuscript, and supervised Mr. Kerr's involvement in this project. All authors read and approved the final manuscript.

Consent for publication
Not applicable.

Competing interests
The authors declare that they have no competing interests.

Author details
[1]From British Columbia Children's Hospital and University of British Columbia, Vancouver, Canada. [2]Department of Pediatrics University of British Columbia, Vancouver, Canada. [3]Stollery Children's Hospital and University of Alberta, Edmonton, Canada. [4]Alberta Children's Hospital and University of Calgary, Calgary, Canada. [5]Royal University Hospital and University of Saskatchewan, Saskatoon, Canada. [6]Department of Pediatrics and Child Health, University of Manitoba, Winnipeg, Canada. [7]London Health Sciences Centre and Western University, London, Canada. [8]McMaster University, Hamilton, Canada. [9]Hospital for Sick Children and University of Toronto, Toronto, Canada. [10]Children's Hospital of Eastern Ontario and University of Ottawa, Ottawa, Canada. [11]McGill University Health Centre and McGill University, Montreal, Canada. [12]Centre Hospitalier Universitaire Ste. Justine and Université de Montréal, Montréal, Canada. [13]Université de Montréal, Montréal, Canada. [14]Centre Hospitalier Universitaire de Sherbrooke and Université de Sherbrooke, Sherbrooke, Canada. [15]Centre Hospitalier Universitaire de Laval and Université Laval, Quebec, Canada. [16]IWK Health Centre and Dalhousie University, Halifax, Canada. [17]Janeway Children's Health and Rehabilitation Centre and Memorial University, Saint John 's, Canada. [18]Shands Children's Hospital and University of Florida, Gainesville, USA. [19]Division of Pediatric Rheumatology, BC Children's Hospital, 4500 Oak St, Suite K4-122, Vancouver, BC V6H 3N1, Canada.

References
1. Harrold LR, Salman C, Shoor S, Curtis JR, Asgari MM, Gelfand GM, et al. Incidence and prevalence of juvenile idiopathic arthritis among children in a managed care population, 1996-2009. J Rheumatol. 2013;40(7):1218–25.
2. Petty RE, Southwood TR, Manners P, et al. International league of associations for rheumatology classification of juvenile idiopathic arthritis: second revision, Edmonton, 2001. J Rheumatol2004;31(2):390–2.
3. Guzman J, Oen K, Tucker LB, Huber AM, Shiff N, Boire G, Scuccimarri R, Berard R, Tse SM, Morishita K, Stringer E, Johnson N, Levy DM, Duffy KW, Cabral DA, Rosenberg AM, Larché M, Dancey P, Petty RE, Laxer RM, Silverman E, Miettunen P, Chetaille AL, Haddad E, Houghton K, Spiegel L, Turvey SE, Schmeling H, Lang B, Ellsworth J, Ramsey S, Bruns A, Campillo S, Benseler S, Chédeville G, Schneider R, Yeung R, Duffy CM, for the ReACCh-Out investigators. The outcomes of juvenile idiopathic arthritis in children managed with contemporary treatments: results from the ReACCh-Out cohort. Ann Rheum Dis. 2015;74(10):1854–60.
4. Simon D. Inflammation and growth. J Pediatr Gastroenterol Nutr. 2010; 51(Suppl3):S133–4.
5. Bechtold S, Simon D. Growth abnormalities in children and adolescents with juvenile idiopathic arthritis. Rheumatol Int. 2014;34(11):1483–8.
6. Chédeville G, Quartier P, Miranda M, Brauner R, Prieur AM. Improvements in growth parameters in children with juvenile idiopathic arthritis associated with the effect of methotrexate on disease activity. Joint Bone Spine. 2005; 72(5):392–6.
7. Giannini EH, Ilowite NT, Lovell DJ, Wallace CA, Rabinovich CE, Reiff A, Higgins G, Gottlieb B, Chon Y, Zhang N, Baumgartner SW. Effects of long-term etanercept treatment on growth in children with selected categories of juvenile idiopathic arthritis. Arthritis Rheum. 2010;62(11):3259–64.
8. Tynjälä P, Lahdenne P, Vähäsalo P, Kautiainen H, Honkanen V. Impact of anti-TNF treatment on growth in severe juvenile idiopathic arthritis. Ann Rheum Dis. 2006;65(8):1044–9.
9. Uettwiller F, Perlbarg J, Pinto G, Bader-Meunier B, Mouy R, Compeyrot-Lacassagne S, Melki I, Wouters C, Prieur AM, Landais P, Polak M, Quartier P. Effect of biologic treatments on growth in children with juvenile idiopathic arthritis. J Rheumatol. 2014;41(1):128–35.
10. Padeh S, Pinhas-Hamiel O, Zimmermann-Sloutskis D, Berkun Y. Children with oligoarticular juvenile idiopathic arthritis are at considerable risk for growth retardation. J Pediatr. 2011;159(5):832–7.
11. Oen K, Tucker L, Huber AM, et al. Predictors of early inactive disease in a juvenile idiopathic arthritis cohort: results of a Canadian multicenter, prospective inception cohort study. Arthritis Rheum. 2009;61:1077–86.
12. Wang Y, Chen H-J. Chapter 2, use of percentiles and *Z* -scores in anthropometry. In: Preedy VR, editor. Handbook of anthropometry: physical measures of human form in health and disease. Springer: New York; 2012. p. 29–48.
13. Lawrence S, Cummings E, Chanoine JP, Metzger DL, Palmert M, Sharma A, Rodd C. Canadian pediatric endocrine group extension to WHO growth charts: why bother? Paediatr Child Health. 2013;18(6):295–7.
14. de Onis M, Onyango AW, Borghi E, Siyam A, Nishida C, Siekmann J. Development of a WHO growth reference for school-aged children and adolescents. Bull World Health Organ. 2007;85(9):660–7.
15. Physical status: the use and interpretation of anthropometry. Report of a WHO Expert Committee. World Health Organ Tech Rep Ser. 1995;854:1–452.
16. A Health Professional's Guide for using the WHO growth charts for Canada. https://www.dietitians.ca/Dietitians-Views/Prenatal-and-Infant/WHO-Growth-Charts/WHO-Growth-Charts-%2D-Resources-for-Health-Professio.aspx.
17. Wallace CA, Ruperto N, Giannini EH. For the CARRA, PRINTO and PRCSG. Preliminary criteria for clinical remission for select categories of juvenile idiopathic arthritis. J Rheumatol. 2004;31(11):2290–4.
18. Corticosteroid Conversion Table. Available at med.umkc.edudocsem Corticosteroid_Table.pdf. Accessed April 28th, 2016.
19. Meikle AW, Tyler FH. Potency and duration of action of glucocorticoids. Effects of hydrocortisone, prednisone and dexamethasone on human pituitary-adrenal function. Am J Med. 1977;63(2):200–7.
20. Rabe-Hesketh S, Skrondal A. Multilevel and longitudinal modeling using Stata. Second ed. College Station, Texas: Stata Press; 2008.
21. Consolaro A, Ruperto N, Bracciolini G, Frisina A, Gallo MC, Pistorio A, Verazza S, Negro G, Gerloni V, Goldenstein-Schainberg C, Sztajnbok F. WulffraatNM, martini a, Ravelli a; Paediatric rheumatology international TrialsOrganization (PRINTO). Defining criteria for high disease activity in juvenile idiopathic arthritis based on the juvenile arthritis disease activity score. Ann Rheum Dis. 2014;73(7):1380–3.
22. Shiff NJ, Brant R, Guzman J, Cabral DA, Huber AM, Miettunen P, Roth J, Scuccimarri R, Alos N, Atkinson SA, Collet JP, Couch R, Cummings EA, Dent PB, Ellsworth J, Hay J, Houghton K, Jurencak R, Lang B, Larche M, Leblanc C, Rodd C, Saint-Cyr C, Stein R, Stephure D, Taback S, Rauch F, Ward LM. Canadian Steroid-associated Osteoporosis in the Pediatric Population Consortium. Glucocorticoid-related changes in body mass index among children and adolescents with rheumatic diseases. Arthritis Care Res (Hoboken). 2013;65(1):113–21.
23. Thalange NK, Foster PJ, Gill MS, Price DA, Clayton PE. Model of normal prepubertal growth. Arch Dis Child. 1996;75(5):427–31.
24. Roberts KC, Shields M, de Groh M, Aziz A, Gilbert JA. Overweight and obesity in children and adolescents: results from the 2009 to 2011 Canadian health measures survey. Health Rep. 2012;23(3):37–41.

25. Cunningham SA, Kramer MR, Narayan KM. Incidence of childhood obesity in the United States. N Engl J Med. 2014;370(5):403–11.
26. Liem JJ, Rosenberg AM. Growth patterns in juvenile rheumatoid arthritis. Clin Exp Rheumatol. 2003;21(5):663–8.
27. Vastert SJ, de Jager W, Noordman BJ, Holzinger D, Kuis W, Prakken BJ, Wulffraat NM. Effectiveness of first-line treatment with recombinant interleukin-1 receptor antagonist in steroid-naive patients with new-onset systemic juvenile idiopathic arthritis: results of a prospective cohort study. Arthritis Rheumatol. 2014;66(4):1034–43.
28. Ringold S, Weiss PF, Beukelman T, DeWitt EM, Ilowite NT, Kimura Y, Laxer RM, Lovell DJ, Nigrovic PA, Robinson AB, Vehe RK. American College of Rheumatology. 2013 update of the 2011 American College of Rheumatology recommendations for the treatment of juvenile idiopathic arthritis: recommendations for the medical therapy of children with systemic juvenile idiopathic arthritis and tuberculosis screening among children receiving biologic medications. Arthritis Rheum. 2013;65(10):2499–512.

9

Readout-segmented multi-shot diffusion-weighted MRI of the knee joint in patients with juvenile idiopathic arthritis

Alexander Sauer[1], Mengxia Li[2], Annette Holl-Wieden[3], Thomas Pabst[1] and Henning Neubauer[1,4,5*]

Abstract

Background: Diffusion-weighted MRI has been proposed as a new technique for imaging synovitis without intravenous contrast application. We investigated diagnostic utility of multi-shot readout-segmented diffusion-weighted MRI (multi-shot DWI) for synovial imaging of the knee joint in patients with juvenile idiopathic arthritis (JIA).

Methods: Thirty-two consecutive patients with confirmed or suspected JIA (21 girls, median age 13 years) underwent routine 1.5 T MRI with contrast-enhanced T1w imaging (contrast-enhanced MRI) and with multi-shot DWI (RESOLVE, b-values 0–50 and 800 s/mm^2). Contrast-enhanced MRI, representing the diagnostic standard, and diffusion-weighted images at b = 800 s/mm^2 were separately rated by three independent blinded readers at different levels of expertise for the presence and the degree of synovitis on a modified 5-item Likert scale along with the level of subjective diagnostic confidence.

Results: Fourteen (44%) patients had active synovitis and joint effusion, nine (28%) patients showed mild synovial enhancement not qualifying for arthritis and another nine (28%) patients had no synovial signal alterations on contrast-enhanced imaging. Ratings by the 1st reader on contrast-enhanced MRI and on DWI showed substantial agreement ($\kappa = 0.74$). Inter-observer-agreement was high for diagnosing, or ruling out, active arthritis of the knee joint on contrast-enhanced MRI and on DWI, showing full agreement between 1st and 2nd reader and disagreement in one case (3%) between 1st and 3rd reader. In contrast, ratings in cases of absent vs. little synovial inflammation were markedly inconsistent on DWI. Diagnostic confidence was lower on DWI, compared to contrast-enhanced imaging.

Conclusion: Multi-shot DWI of the knee joint is feasible in routine imaging and reliably diagnoses, or rules out, active arthritis of the knee joint in paediatric patients without the need of gadolinium-based i.v. contrast injection. Possibly due to "T2w shine-through" artifacts, DWI does not reliably differentiate non-inflamed joints from knee joints with mild synovial irritation.

Keywords: Diffusion-weighted MRI, Juvenile idiopathic arthritis, Synovitis

Background

Juvenile idiopathic arthritis (JIA) is the most common entity of chronic arthritidis in children and adolescents with an incidence of about 4 to 10 patients per 100,000 children [1]. In most instances, MR imaging is more sensitive than physical examination for detecting active joint inflammation [2]. MRI is also useful for excluding non-rheumatological disease, for assessing inflammatory disease activity and for monitoring response to anti-inflammatory therapy [3]. Routine MR imaging of synovitis presently depends on T1-weighted scans with intravenous application of gadolinium-based contrast material [4]. In addition to known issues of allergic reactions and of gadolinium contrast injection in patients with impaired renal function, recent reports on cerebral gadolinium deposition after contrast-enhanced MRI [5, 6] have raised new concerns about the long-term safety of

* Correspondence: inu75@web.de
[1]Department of Diagnostic and Interventional Radiology, University Hospital Wuerzburg, 97080 Wuerzburg, Germany
[4]Department of Diagnostic and Interventional Radiology, University Hospital Ulm, Albert-Einstein-Allee 23, Ulm 89081, Germany

gadolinium-containing contrast agents. So there is a need for new gadolinium-free MRI techniques, also in young patients with arthritis. The first report on diffusion-weighted imaging (DWI) of synovitis in children was published in 2012 [7]. Since then, several studies have confirmed the feasibility and the potential diagnostic value of this technique [8–10]. However, standard DWI with single-shot diffusion-weighted imaging and echo-planar readout (single-shot DWI), as used in stroke imaging since the early 1990s, suffers from several technical limitations resulting in frequent imaging artifacts and low spatial resolution. In effect, discrimination of inflamed synovium is impossible or lacks diagnostic confidence in a significant proportion of patients [10, 11]. Recently, a refined DWI technique, that is readout-segmented multi-shot echo-planar DWI (multi-shot DWI), has become available on clinical scanners and promises higher spatial resolution, better delineation of small anatomical structures and less artifacts from magnetic field inhomogeneities [12, 13] and from the presence of joint effusion.

We undertook our study to investigate image quality and diagnostic performance of multi-shot DWI for synovial imaging in JIA patients with arthritis of the knee joint.

Methods

Patient population

Our study group includes 32 consecutive patients, that is 21 girls and 11 boys, who had both multi-shot DWI and contrast-enhanced MR imaging of the knee for routine diagnostic work-up between January 2014 and July 2016. Median patient age was 13 years, ranging from 2 to 14 years. Another eight patients, who had multi-shot DWI within this period of time, but no contrast-enhanced sequences, were excluded from the analysis for a lack of reference standard. Eventually, we analysed 24 JIA patients, diagnosed according to the International League of Associations for Rheumatology (ILAR) criteria [14], and another eight patients with subacute or chronic arthralgia, in whom JIA was eventually ruled out and who served as negative controls in our study. Of the 24 JIA patients, 15 patients had previously been diagnosed with JIA and were referred to follow-up MRI, 11 of these patients with on-going anti-inflammatory treatment (oral non-steroidal n = 6, methotrexate n = 4, adalimumab n = 1) and four patients without on-going treatment. Nine patients were newly diagnosed with JIA, with three patients being on oral non-steroidal anti-inflammatory treatment at the time of the MRI examination.

All study work was conducted in accordance with the Helsinki Declaration. Informed written consent was obtained from the legal guardians of all patients for all diagnostic procedures. A waiver was granted by the Institutional Review Board for the retrospective analysis of imaging data.

MRI examination

All patients underwent clinical routine MRI of the knee joint on the same 1.5 Tesla scanner (Magnetom Aera, Siemens Healthcare, Erlangen) in supine position with a cubital intravenous line in place. Standard sequences were first scanned as needed for clinical imaging (e.g. coronal T2w TIRM, sagittal PDw with fat saturation, T1w TSE). Diffusion-weighted scans were acquired prior to injection of contrast agent using the following typical parameters: transverse multi-shot DWI (RESOLVE, Siemens Healthcare, Erlangen, TR = 6600 ms, TE = 57 ms, 5 read-out segments, low b-value = 0 s/mm^2 (n = 11) or 50 s/mm^2 (n = 21) and high b-value = 800 s/mm^2, 3-scan trace-weighted, parallel imaging GRAPPA iPAT = 2, monopolar gradient scheme, one average for low b-value, two averages for b = 800 s/mm^2, epi factor 63, echo spacing 0.38 ms, 34 slices, voxel size 1.5 × 1.5 × 3 mm^3, field of view 200 mm, acquisition time 6 min 18 s). Scanning parameters were adapted as clinically needed for optimal fit in some patients. After intravenous injection of one weight-adapted standard dose of gadoterate meglumine (Dotarem, Guerbet, Paris, France), we acquired contrast-enhanced MRI (transverse T1w TSE with Dixon fat saturation), followed by additional coronal or sagittal scans, if clinically necessary. All but two patients were examined feet-first and with a dedicated multi-channel knee coil. Two young patients, 2 and 3 years of age, had MRI of the lower extremities including both knee joints scanned in supine position head-first with phased-array body coils in place and with sedation administered by a paediatric anesthesiologist.

Image processing and analysis

All image analysis was performed on a dedicated radiological workstation (Merlin Version 5.1., Phoenix PACS GmbH, Freiburg, Germany). A board-certified paediatric radiologist with 8 years of experience in paediatric extracranial DWI (1st reader), a senior resident radiologist trained in paediatric imaging (2nd reader) and a radiation oncologist with basic training in musculoskeletal MRI, reflecting three different levels of experience, independently completed all qualitative image analyses. Each reader, blinded to all clinical patient data and to the results of the other readers, assessed contrast-enhanced images and then diffusion-weighted images in separate reading sessions (Fig. 1). Each reader recorded the presence and the degree of synovitis on a modified 5-item Likert scale: 0 = non-diagnostic image quality; 1 = no signs of synovitis; 2 = minimal circumscript or linear

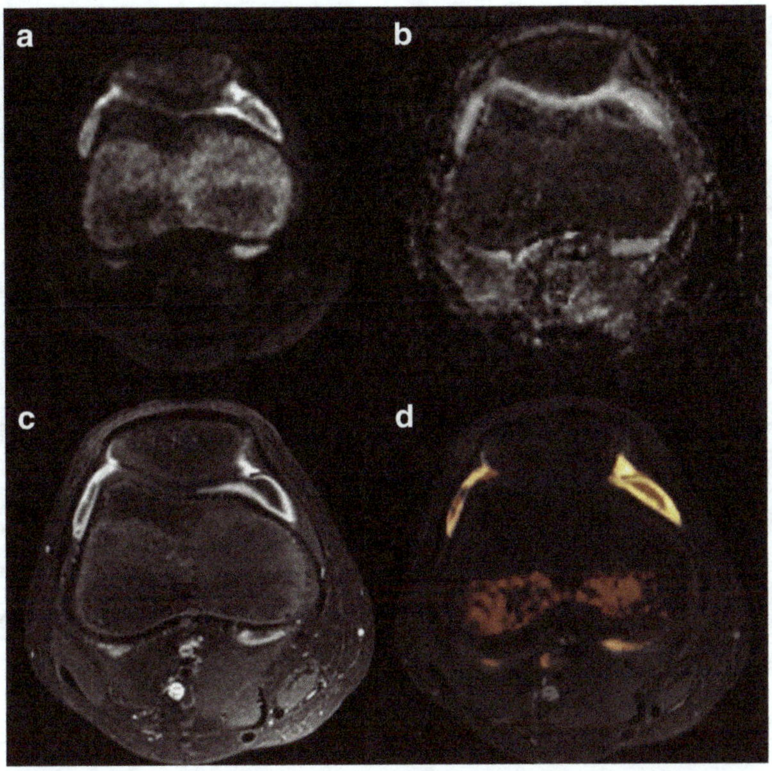

Fig. 1 Twelve-year-old male JIA patient, persisting clinical symptoms with methotrexate treatment. DWI b = 800 s/mm^2 (**a**), ADC map (**b**), contrast-enhanced MRI (**c**) and image fusion (**d**) of colorised overlay of DWI signal onto image (**c**) with 3D Fusion software (Siemens Medical) all show active synovitis and small amounts of joint effusion in the anterior and posterior joint space. Image acquisition with multi-shot read-out segmented DWI (RESOLVE, Siemens) is virtually free of artifacts

signal increase, not qualifying for active synovitis; 3 = active synovitis present, defined as marked linear signal increase of the synovial layer with 1–2 mm in thickness; 4 = active synovitis plus circumscript or diffuse synovial thickening in excess of 2 mm. Categories 3 and 4 were considered to represent active synovitis/arthritis, while category 1 was thought to exclude the presence of active synovitis, based on MR imaging criteria. Category 2 indicated mild synovial irritation not qualifying for active synovitis. Along with each rating on synovitis, the respective subjective level of diagnostic confidence (LoC) was documented on a modified 3-item Likert scale: 1 = undecided, questionable, low confidence; 2 = intermediate, diagnosis established with some confidence; 3 = certain diagnosis, high confidence. The contrast-enhanced MRI scan was considered the diagnostic standard of comparison.

The same experienced paediatric radiologist blinded to patient data and to the results of preceding qualitative image analysis also performed quantitative analysis using polygonal Regions of interest (ROIs) manually drawn on one representative cross-section of contrast-enhanced images, diffusion-weighted images (Fig. 2) and the corresponding ADC map. Signal intensities were measured for synovium, joint effusion, upper calf muscle, femoral epiphyseal bone marrow and popliteal lymph nodes on contrast-enhanced MRI, DWI at high b-values and on the ADC map. The apparent diffusion coefficient (ADC) was recorded as a quantitative measure of tissue diffusivity. We calculated signal intensity ratios for synovium vs. effusion, synovium vs. muscle etc., so as to quantify image contrast between different anatomical structures. Quantitative analysis was repeated by the same reader after one week for assessment of intra-observer variability.

Statistical analysis

Normally distributed data is presented as mean ± standard deviation and range, data deviating from normal distribution as median with inter-quartile range. The Wilcoxon paired-sample test was employed to compare means of two related data sets deviating from normal distribution. Kappa statistics were calculated to assess intra-observer and inter-observer agreement. The coefficient of variation was computed to quantify intra-observer variation in quantitative data. All data analyses were performed with SPSS Version 21 for Windows (IBM SPSS Statistics for Windows, Armonk, NY, USA).

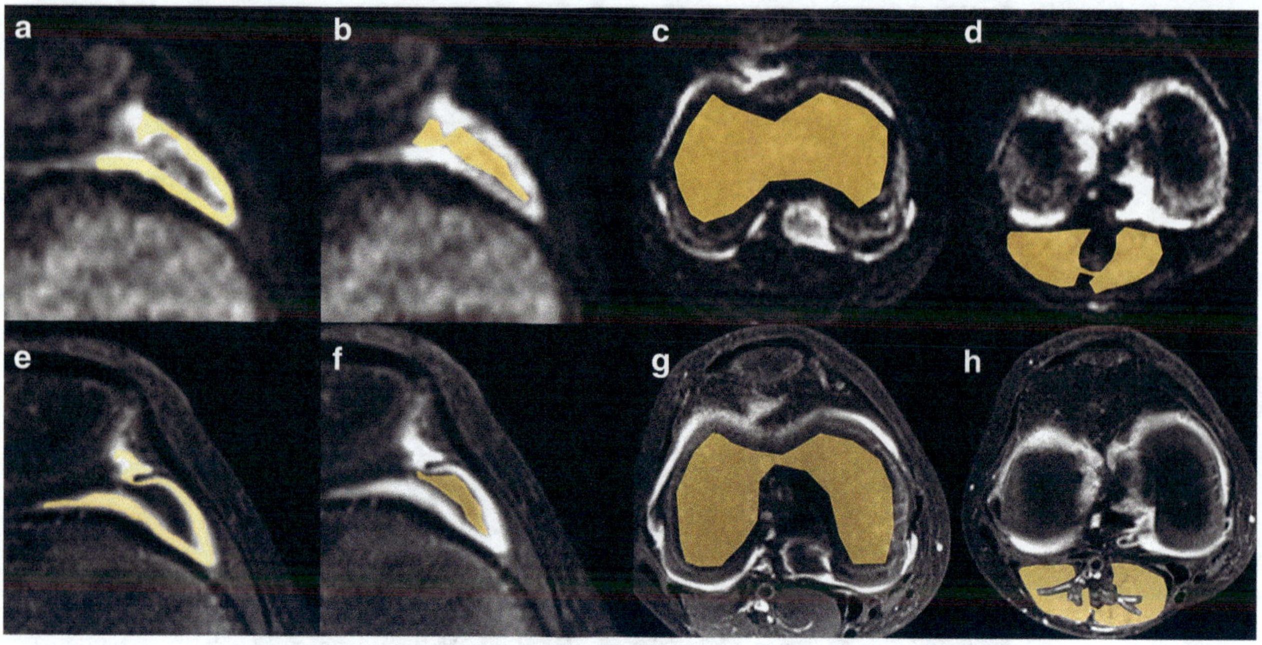

Fig. 2 Same patient as in Fig. 1. Region of interest (ROI) placement using half-translucent polygonal ROIs on DWI b = 800 s/mm^2 (**a**-**d**) and contrast-enhanced MRI (**e**-**h**) for manual segmentation of synovium (**a**, **e**), joint effusion (**b**, **f**), femoral epiphyseal bone marrow (**c**, **g**) and upper calf muscle (**d**, **h**)

Results

All MRI examinations were completed safely. All scans were consistently rated as diagnostic by all three readers.

Contrast-enhanced MRI as diagnostic standard

The reading completed by the 1st reader was considered the diagnostic standard of comparison. The 1st reader assigned patients to the categories of synovial signal as follows (Fig. 3): category 0 - no patients, as all scans were of sufficient diagnostic quality; category 1 - nine patients (28%) without any significant synovial contrast enhancement; category 2 - nine patients (28%) with minimal circumscript or linear synovial contrast uptake, not qualifying for active synovitis; category 3 - nine patients (28%) with marked synovial contrast uptake and mild synovial thickening not exceeding 2 mm; category 4 - five patients (16%) with strong synovial contrast uptake, marked synovial thickening and large joint effusion. Level of confidence (LoC) of the ratings by the 1st reader was high (LoC = 3) in 27 of 32 (84%) patients and medium (LoC = 2) in 5 (16%) patients. All patients in category 3 and 4 showed varying degrees of joint effusion. In contrast, none of the patients in category 1 and 2 had significant effusion. With regard to underlying pathology, none of the eight control patients without JIA had active synovitis (category 1 n = 6; category 2 n = 2). The 24 JIA patients were assigned to the categories of synovial signal as follows: categorry 1 - three patients with previously diagnosed JIA, all of them under ongoing anti-inflammatory treatment; category 2 - six patients, among these three newly diagnosed JIA patients and three of six patients under anti-inflammatory treatment; category 3 - nine patients, four of these newly diagnosed with JIA, and seven patients undergoing inflammatory treatment including four patients with persisting arthritis under methotrexate; category 4 - five patients, including one newly diagnosed two-year-old without previous anti-inflammatory treatment. Based on these findings, the categories 1&2 and 3&4 were combined into a dichotomous variable, presenting 0 = no arthritis and 1 = active arthritis, for further analysis.

Diagnosis of synovitis on DWI

Compared to the diagnostic standard of contrast-enhanced MRI, the reading of DWI completed by the 1st reader showed consistent ratings in the four categories of synovial signal in 26 of 32 cases (81%) with a $\kappa = 0.74$ ($p < 0.001$), indicating substantial agreement across all categories based on the criteria by Landis and Koch [15]. All disconcordances occured from "down-grading" on DWI, that is two cases of category 4 on contrast-enhanced MRI were rated as category 3 on DWI, and another 4 cases of category 2 on contrast-enhanced MRI were assessed as category 1 on DWI. Interestingly, the downgrades from category 4 to 3 all were high confidence (LoC = 3) ratings on DWI, while the downgrades from category 2 to 1 all occured with low confidence (LoC = 1) on DWI. There was full agreement between the ratings on contrast-

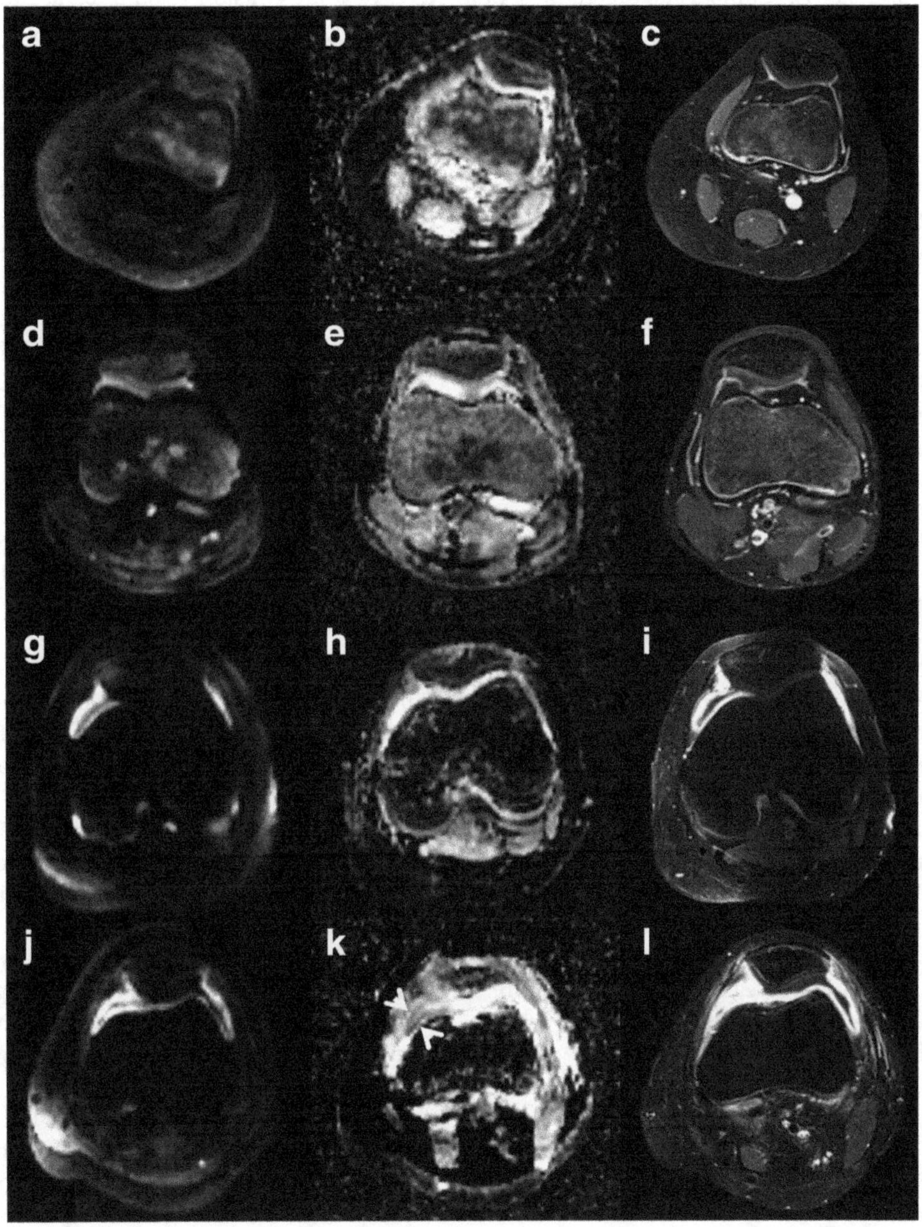

Fig. 3 Corresponding transverse cross-section of DWI b = 800 s/mm^2 (**a**, **d**, **g**, **j**), ADC map (**b**, **e**, **h**, **k**), contrast-enhanced T1w imaging (**c**, **f**, **i**, **l**) in four different patients, rated as not having synovitis (category 1, **a-c**), showing mild synovial irritation (category 2, **d-f**), active synovitis with joint effusion (category 3, **g-i**) and synovitis aggravated by synovial thickening (category 4, **j-l**) on contrast enhanced MRI as the diagnostic standard. The fourth patient (**j-l**) was rated as category 3 on DWI, since the synovial layer appears less prominent and since the ADC map nicely delineates synovium from joint effusion (arrow heads) and periarticular oedematous signal increase. Contrast-enhanced MRI may overestimate the extent of synovial proliferation in the presence of perisynovial inflammation and oedema in this patient

enhanced MRI and on DWI with regard to the presence or absence of active arthritis. The overall diagnostic level of confidence was lower on DWI, compared to contrast-enhanced MRI, including 14 ratings with high, 8 ratings with intermediate and 11 ratings with low diagnostic confidence. All low-confidence ratings pertained to choosing between categories 1 and 2.

Inter-observer agreement on contrast-enhanced imaging

Compared to the reference reading performed by the first observeron on contrast-enhanced MRI images, the ratings of the other observers showed moderate agreement. Kappa values across all categories were 0.50 ($p < 0.001$) for the 2nd reader and 0.48 ($p < 0.001$) for the 3rd observer. Agreement between 2nd and 3rd reader was 0.54 ($p < 0.001$). Comparing the ratings of the 2nd reader to the reference reading, there were one upgrade from category 1 to 2, six downgrades from category 2 to 1, three upgrades from category 3 to 4 and one downgrade from category 4 to 3. The 3rd reader passed higher ratings in seven patients (all upgrades from category 1 to 2) and lower ratings in five patients ($n = 1$ category 2 to 1; n = 1 category 3 to 2; $n = 3$ category 4 to 3). As compared to reference, one patient with active synovitis (category 3) was therefore misdiagnosed as not having synovitis. Deciding on the presence or absence of active arthritis, there was full agreement between the first and second reader ($\kappa = 1$) and disagreement in one case between the first and the third reader ($\kappa = 0.94$, $p < 0.001$) on contrast-enhanced MRI.

Inter-observer agreement on DWI

Compared to the reference reading on contrast-enhanced MRI performed by the first reader, the DWI ratings of the other readers showed fair to moderate agreement. Kappa values across all categories were 0.50 ($p < 0.001$) for the 2nd reader and 0.39 ($p < 0.001$) for the 3rd reader. Agreement of DWI ratings for the 2nd reader vs. 3rd reader was still fair with $\kappa = 0.25$ ($p < 0.002$). Comparing the DWI ratings of the 2nd reader to reference, there were one upgrade from category 1 to 2, six downgrades from category 2 to 1, four upgrades from category 3 to 4 and one downgrade from category 4 to 3. The 3rd reader passed higher ratings in eight patients ($n = 5$ category 1 to 2; $n = 1$ category 2 to 3; $n = 2$ category 3 to 4) and lower ratings in six patients (n = 1 category 2 to 1; $n = 4$ category 4 to 3). Therefore, the 3rd reader considered one patient without active synovitis as having synovitis.

With regard to the presence or absence of active arthritis on DWI, we thus found full agreement for the second reader ($\kappa = 1$) and discrepancy in one case for the third reader ($\kappa = 0.94$, $p < 0.001$) on diffusion-weighted imaging, as compared to the diagnostic standard.

Observer-dependent level of confidence

Diagnostic level of confidence (LoC) showed the following median values for confidence ratings: median LoC =3 on contrast-enhanced MRI and on DWI for the 1st reader, median LoC = 3 on contrast-enhanced MRI and median LoC = 2 on DWI for the 2nd reader and the 3rd reader. The proportion of high-confidence ratings (LoC = 3) was 84%, 81% and 72% on contrast-enhanced MRI and 44%, 32% and 0% on DWI for the 1st, 2nd and 3rd reader, respectively.

Quantitative analysis

Mean ADC (unit: 10^{-3} mm^2/s) of inflamed synovium (2.08 ± 0.24, range 1.64 to 2.42) was lower than mean ADC of joint effusion (2.85 ± 0.55, range 2.33 to 3.31), but higher than mean ADC of muscle (1.61 ± 0.29, range 1.36 to 1.88) and lymph nodes (1.11 ± 0.16, range 0.74 to 1.34). ADC of muscle tissue showed the smallest standard deviation and the smallest between-measurements coefficient of variation (3.0%) and was therefore chosen as standard internal reference for signal comparison. DWI showed high intrinsic signal for inflamed synovium and popliteal lymph nodes, compared to muscle signal. Median intensity ratios of synovium signal vs. muscle (2.7, interquartile range [IQR] 1.5) and of lymph nodes vs. muscle (2.8, IQR 1.8) were higher on DWI than on contrast-enhanced MRI (2.9, IQR 0.9, and 1.9, IQR 0.4, respectively) (both $p < 0.001$). In contrast, signal intensity ratio of synovium vs. joint effusion was significantly lower on DWI (1.5, IQR 0.5), compared to contrast-enhanced MRI (2.7, IQR 0.7) ($p < 0.001$). The coefficient of variation for two repeated measurements by the same reader ranged less than 10% for all measured tissues.

Discussion

In paediatric non-oncological MRI, imaging of synovitis is probably the most common of only few good indications for i.v. gadolinium-containing contrast injection. Although there has been research on gadolinium-free synovial scanning, such as arterial spin-labelling MRI [16] or DWI [7–10], the clinical impact of these techniques remains limited to date for various reasons, including lengthy image acquisition and post-processing, limited spatial resolution and proneness to imaging artifacts, among others. Single-shot echoplanar diffusion-weighted imaging has been state-of-the art in stroke imaging since the early 1990s and also visualises synovitis in knee joints [7, 10]. In extra-cranial anatomical regions, however, such DWI scans are frequently degraded by the presence of artifacts, such as ghosting, distortion or the so-called "T2w shine-through" arising from joint effusion which spoil diagnostic visibility of the synovial layer in about one-third of patients [11].

Based on our study results, the recently developed multi-shot DWI sequence (e.g. RESOLVE, Siemens), as used in our study, reliably visualises inflamed synovium in patients with active arthritis of the knee joint and is superior to the standard single-shot DWI. Multi-shot DWI is scanned in several steps, or "segments", and composes a qualitatively enhanced MR image with higher spatial resolution and less artifacts. In our study, voxel size was $1.5 \times 1.5 \times 3$ mm^3, as compared to 1.8 × 1.8 x (4 to 6) mm^3 with single-shot DWI in earlier studies [7, 11]. We observed less "T2w shine-through" artifacts, although these artifacts still occur in some patients. Limited diagnostic accuracy was observed in knee joints with little synovial inflammation in the presence of slightly increased amounts of synovial fluid (Fig. 4), as commonly seen with mild synovial irritation in patients with trauma, over-exertion or residual arthritis under anti-inflammatory treatment. This limitation would be even more serious when imaging small joints, such as wrist, finger or temporomandibular joints, where T2w shine-through artifacts could more easily mimick synovial signal increase and cause false-positive ratings [8, 9].

Using multi-shot DWI, mean ADC of synovium and of joint effusion fell within the range previously reported from single-shot DWI scans [7] and from an 1 Tesla open-bore scanner [10], while ADC of upper calf muscle tissue was substantially higher than the $1.17 \pm 0.12 \times 10^{-3}$ mm^2/s previously measured in skeletal muscle [17]. Generally, muscle tissue presents a good internal reference standard for ADC, as large and rather homogeneous tissue volumes can be measured with little partial volume effects and low between-measurement variation on the same scanner.

Qualitative evaluation of synovial signal was performed by three independent readers with different levels of expertise in musculoskeletal MRI. Diffusion-weighted imaging, as used in our study, counts among the technically advanced MRI acquisition methods. Spatial resolution is low, by comparison. And while DWI images contain a treasure of diagnostic information, the aesthetic effect of these images is not particularly striking. In our study, we were thus interested in knowing whether DWI of the knee joint is only for experts, or whether "normal" radiologists and radiologically trained non-radiologists can also work with such images. We thus chose three independent readers at respective levels of experience. Our results demonstrate that diagnostic accuracy indeed is a function of experience and also that the interpretation of diffusion-weighted images is generally more demanding, compared to contrast-enhanced MRI. Nevertheless, the crucial diagnostic decision of seeing or not seeing active arthritis was made with rather high accuracy and with low inter-observer variation. We are therefore convinced that, after some training, the new DWI technique presented in our study can readily be employed by radiologists in clinical routine imaging. The lower diagnostic confidence recorded for ratings on DWI is, in our view, directly related to the lower image contrast of inflamed synovium vs. effusion in combination with the still lower spatial resolution of DWI, as compared to contrast-enhanced MRI. In the absence of synovitis, there is no discernible DWI signal from the synovial membrane, which measures only a couple of cell layers in width. With increasing activity of synovitis, the synovial signal becomes visible and gradually more prominent. Eventually, synovial proliferation, as in chronic synovitis or pannus, produces strongly altered local diffusivity and shows most clearly. However,

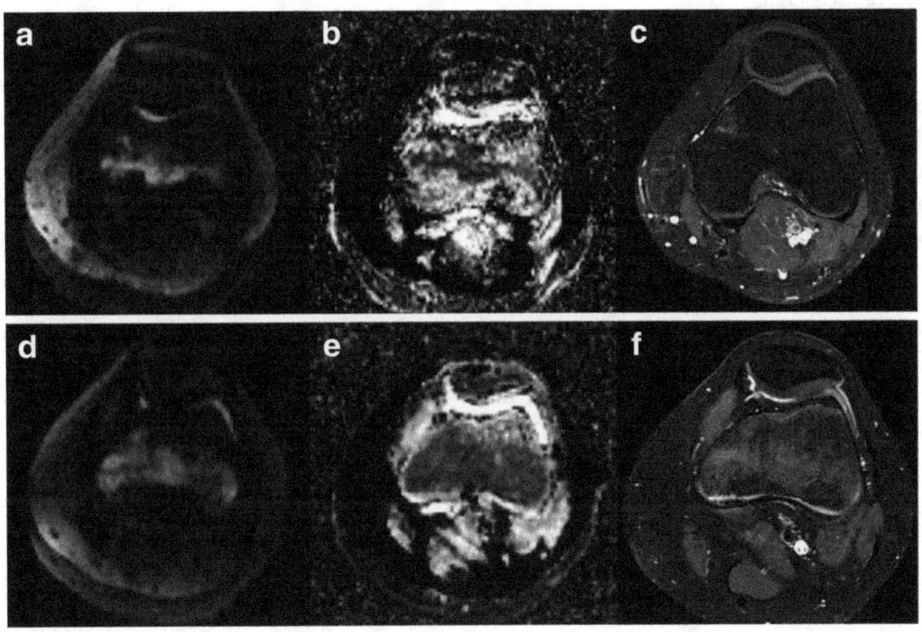

Fig. 4 Diagnostic dilemma in a 14-year-old female control patient without synovitis (**a-c**) and in a 13-year-old female patient (**d-f**) newly diagnosed with JIA based on International League of Associations for Rheumatology (ILAR) criteria [14]. While the first patient does not show any synovial contrast enhancement (category 1, **c**), there is mild synovial enhancement and some synovial fluid discernable in the JIA patient (category 2, **f**). Both patients, however, display retropatellar and parapatellar high signal on DWI b = 800 s/mm^2. Some signal increase as in (**a**) is frequently encountered in normal knee joints, possibly due to "T2w shine-through" of small amounts of physiological joint fluid, making diagnostic differentiation of synovial signal category 1 and 2 difficult, or impossible

the presence of joint effusion, which usually coincides with synovitis at varying degrees, makes things more complicated. By the so-called "T2w shine-through" artifact, effusion can produce some signal very close to synovitis on DWI. If there is little or no synovitis in the presence of small amounts of joint effusion, be it arthritic or non-arthritic in origin, it is difficult or impossible to decide whether the observed signal originates from synovitis or from T2 signal effects of the joint effusion. This presently limits the usefulness of DWI in joints with little inflammatory activity. In patients with severe synovitis and large effusion, the synovium is usually prominent enough to be easily distinguished from effusion. Advanced DWI techniques, such as intravoxel incoherent motion (IVIM) imaging [18, 19] visualize both synovial diffusivity and synovial perfusion. These techniques are probably superior to multi-shot DWI under difficult scanning conditions and promise to overcome the technical difficulties arising from joint effusion [20].

The main methodological limitation of our study is the retrospective data analysis. Diagnostic accuracy of DWI in patients with arthritis should be evaluated in a prospective setting with contrast-enhanced imaging as the diagnostic standard.

In summary, imaging of synovitis with multi-shot DWI is feasible in a clinical routine setting and holds considerable clinical potential to increase patient safety and comfort, to streamline MRI scan protocols for arthritis patients and to reduce cost.

Conclusion

Based on our study results, multi-shot DWI recommends itself as a non-invasive gadolinium-free MR scanning technique for imaging of synovitis. Using multi-shot echo-planar imaging with segmented-readout, DWI consistently produces images of good diagnostic quality and reliably visualises active synovitis in JIA patients with arthritis of the knee joint. "T2w shine-through" originating from joint effusion still limits diagnostic accuracy in patients with mild synovial irritation. The diagnostic utility of multi-shot DWI for imaging small joints should be investigated in future prospective studies.

Abbreviations

ADC: Apparent diffusion coefficient; DWI: Diffusion-weighted imaging; IQR: Inter-quartile range; JIA: Juvenile idiopathic arthritis; LoC: Level of confidence; ROI: Region of interest

Acknowledgements

The authors would like to thank the technicians of the MR imaging team for performing high-quality scans and for taking care of the patients during the examination.

Funding

The study work was supported by the German Research Foundation (DFG) grant NE1953/1-1.

Departments and institutions to which work is attributed

University Hospital of Wuerzburg, Department of Radiology and Department of Paediatrics; University Hospital of Ulm, Department of Diagnostic and Interventional Radiology.

Sources of support

Supported by the National German Research Foundation (DFG).

Authors' contributions

HN conceived and planned the study and requested IRB approval. AS, ML, AHW and HN collected imaging data and clinical data and performed the data analysis. TP was responsible for setting up MRI scanner hardware and software so as to accomodate both clinical needs and the study protocol and discussed the imaging findings from the physicist's perspective. All authors participated in drafting and revising the manuscript and approved the submitted version.

Consent for publication

All the authors have reviewed the final manuscript and given their consent for publication.

Competing interests

The authors declare that they have no competing interests.

Author details

[1]Department of Diagnostic and Interventional Radiology, University Hospital Wuerzburg, 97080 Wuerzburg, Germany. [2]Department of Radiation Oncology, University Hospital Wuerzburg, 97080 Wuerzburg, Germany. [3]Department of Paediatrics, University Hospital Wuerzburg, 97080 Wuerzburg, Germany. [4]Department of Diagnostic and Interventional Radiology, University Hospital Ulm, Albert-Einstein-Allee 23, Ulm 89081, Germany. [5]SRH Clinic of Radiology, 98527 Suhl, Germany.

References

1. Helmick CG, Felson DT, Lawrence RC, et al. Estimates of the prevalence of arthritis and other rheumatic conditions in the United States. Part I. Arthritis Rheum. 2008;58:15–25.
2. Hemke R, Maas M, van Veenendaal M, et al. Contrast-enhanced MRI compared with the physical examination in the evaluation of disease activity in juvenile idiopathic arthritis. Eur Radiol. 2014;24:327–34.
3. Damasio MB, Malattia C, Martini A, et al. Synovial and inflammatory disease in childhood: role of new imaging modalities in the assessment of patients with juvenile idiopathic arthritis. Pediatr Radiol. 2010;40:985–98.
4. Hemke R, Kuijpers TW, van den Berg JM, et al. The diagnostic accuracy of unenhanced MRI in the assessment of joint abnormalities in juvenile idiopathic arthritis. Eur Radiol. 2013;23:1998–2004.
5. Stojanov D, Aracki-Trenkic A, Benedeto-Stojanov D. Gadolinium deposition within the dentate nucleus and globus pallidus after repeated administrations of gadolinium-based contrast agents - current status. Neuroradiology. 2016;58:433–41.
6. Roberts D, Holden K. Progressive increase of T1 signal intensity in the dentate nucleus and globus pallidus on unenhanced T1-weighted MR images in the pediatric brain exposed to multiple doses of gadolinium contrast. Brain and Development. 2016;38:331–6.
7. Neubauer H, Evangelista L, Morbach H, et al. Diffusion-weighted MRI of bone marrow oedema, soft tissue oedema and synovitis in paediatric patients: feasibility and initial experience. Pediatr Rheumatol Online J. 2012;10:20.
8. Jeromel M, Jevtic V, Sersa I, et al. Quantification of synovitis in the cranio-cervical region: dynamic contrast enhanced and diffusion-weighted magnetic resonance imaging in early rheumatoid arthritis - a feasibility follow-up study. Eur J Radiol. 2012;81:3412–9.
9. Li X, Liu X, Du X, et al. Diffusion-weighted MR imaging for assessing synovitis of wrist and hand in patients with rheumatoid arthritis: a feasibility study. Magn Reson Imaging. 2014;32:350–3.

10. Barendregt AM, Nusman CM, Hemke R, et al. Feasibility of diffusion-weighted magnetic resonance imaging in patients with juvenile idiopathic arthritis on 1.0-T open-bore MRI. Skelet Radiol. 2015;44:1805–11.
11. Neubauer H, Holl-Wieden A, Hassold N et al. Diffusion-weighted MRI in Paediatric patients with Gonarthritis: a novel approach to imaging of Synovitis. Radiological Society of North America 2014 scientific assembly and annual meeting VSPD21-06, Chicago IL., 2014; http://archive.rsna.org/2014/14010339.html. Accessed 7 Oct 2017.
12. Naganawa S, Yamazaki M, Kawai H, et al. Anatomical details of the brainstem and cranial nerves visualized by high resolution readout-segmented multi-shot echo-planar diffusion-weighted images using unidirectional MPG at 3T. Magn Reson Med Sci. 2011;10:269–75.
13. Hayes LL, Jones RA, Palasis S, et al. Drop metastases to the pediatric spine revealed with diffusion-weighted MR imaging. Ped Radiol. 2012;42:1009–13.
14. Petty RE, Southwood TR, Manners P, et al. International league of associations for rheumatology classification of juvenile idiopathic arthritis: second revision. Edmonton 2001. J Rheumatol. 2004;31:390–2.
15. Landis JR, Koch GG. The measurement of observer agreement for categorical data. Biometrics. 1977;33:159–74.
16. Boss A, Martirosian P, Fritz J, et al. Magnetic resonance spin-labeling perfusion imaging of synovitis in inflammatory arthritis at 3.0T. Magn Reson Mater Phy. 2009;22:175–80.
17. Neubauer H, Evangelista L, Hassold N, et al. Musculoskeletal tumorous and tumour-like lesions: diagnostic utility of diffusion-weighted MRI for detection and differentiation in pediatric patients. World J Pediatr. 2012;8: 342–9.
18. Le Bihan D, Breton E, Lallemand D, et al. Separation of diffusion and perfusion in intravoxel incoherent motion MR imaging. Radiology. 1988;168: 497–505.
19. Zhao YH, Li SL, Liu ZY, et al. Detection of active Sacroiliitis with Ankylosing Spondylitis through Intravoxel incoherent motion diffusion-weighted MR imaging. Eur Radiol. 2015;25:2754–63.
20. Hilbert F, Holl-Wieden A, Sauer A, et al. Intravoxel incoherent motion MRI of the knee joint in children with juvenile idiopathic arthritis. Ped Radiol. 2017; 47:681–90.

10

Patient characteristics associated with response to NSAID monotherapy in children with systemic juvenile idiopathic arthritis

Anjali Sura[1*], Christopher Failing[1], Julie Sturza[1], Jasmine Stannard[2] and Meredith Riebschleger[1]

Abstract

Background: Systemic juvenile idiopathic arthritis (sJIA) is an auto-inflammatory disease characterized by fever, arthritis, and ≥1 of rash, generalized lymphadenopathy, hepato/splenomegaly, and serositis. Non-steroidal anti-inflammatory drugs (NSAIDs) are among the initial treatments of sJIA, but there is currently no evidence indicating which children should undergo a trial of NSAID monotherapy and which should not. Our objective is to identify presentation characteristics which are associated with response and lack of response to a trial of NSAID monotherapy.

Methods: This is a retrospective single-center cohort study of children diagnosed with sJIA from 2000 to 2014. Patient demographics and disease characteristics were investigated to identify predictors of response to NSAID monotherapy.

Results: Eighty-seven children were newly diagnosed with sJIA 2000-2014. Thirteen of the 51 children who received NSAID monotherapy achieved clinically inactive disease (CID) without other medications. Age at presentation (≤8 years old), initial joint count (≤5), and C-reactive protein (CRP) (≤13 mg/dL) at diagnosis were associated with achievement of CID on NSAIDs alone. Physicians were less likely to trial NSAID monotherapy if the patient had either serositis or macrophage activation syndrome (MAS) at diagnosis. Ultimate achievement of CID and time to CID were not significantly affected by whether the patient received a trial of NSAID monotherapy.

Conclusions: While a subset of children with sJIA can achieve CID with NSAID monotherapy, we recommend *against* a trial in patients who are >8 years old, with >5 joints involved, or with CRP > 13 mg/dL. Patients who undergo a trial of NSAID monotherapy should follow up within 2-4 weeks to evaluate for possible need for drug escalation. Clinical trials are necessary to confirm these findings.

Keywords: Systemic juvenile idiopathic arthritis (sJIA), Non-steroidal anti-inflammatory drugs (NSAIDs), NSAID monotherapy, Therapeutics, Risk stratification

* Correspondence: sethia@med.umich.edu
[1]University of Michigan, 1500 E Medical Center Dr, Ann Arbor, MI 48109, USA
Full list of author information is available at the end of the article

Background

Over the last 20 years, the outcomes of juvenile idiopathic arthritis (JIA) have markedly improved. Decreases in morbidity and mortality have occurred alongside increases in knowledge regarding the pathophysiology of JIA and the development of new medications that prevent long-term joint damage [1]. In the case of systemic JIA (sJIA), new agents have transformed treatment of the disease. In the past, many pediatric rheumatologists treated sJIA using a pyramid approach, starting with non-steroidal anti-inflammatory drugs (NSAIDs) and/or corticosteroids prior to initiating disease-modifying anti-rheumatic drugs (DMARDs) or biologic agents.

However, the Childhood Arthritis and Rheumatology Research Alliance (CARRA) Consensus Treatment Protocols (CTPs), published in 2012, does not include any arms with NSAID monotherapy [2]. This is contrary to the 2011 *ACR Recommendations for the Treatment of Juvenile Idiopathic Arthritis* and the 2013 update, which includes 4 options for the initial treatment of sJIA: NSAIDs, corticosteroids, DMARDs, and biologic agents [3]. Each of these drug classes has unique characteristics, such as potential adverse effects, mechanism of drug delivery (oral, subcutaneous, or infusion), and expected time to improvement. Drug class characteristics, child/caregiver preferences, and physician preferences contribute to the choice of a specific agent for a specific child. Unfortunately, the absence of comparative trials limits the ability to make evidence-based suggestions about the treatment of specific children, so recommendations to date have primarily relied on expert consensus. Based upon this expert consensus, the 2013 recommendations suggest that NSAID monotherapy be considered as a treatment option for children whose physician global rating of disease activity is less than 5 on a 10-point scale with any number of active joints. Given the emerging data indicating a window of opportunity in the early treatment of sJIA [4], transitioning to glucocorticoids, IL-1 blockade, or IL-6 blockade is recommended for any children who continue to have active disease after 1 month.

Identifying patient characteristics which are associated with a response to a trial of NSAID monotherapy can aid pediatric rheumatologists in choosing medications for the initial treatment of sJIA. This will help balance the risks and benefits of therapy for specific children. The objective of this cohort study is to review and analyze the treatment and outcomes of all children diagnosed with sJIA at a tertiary care center over a 15-year period with regard to treatment with NSAID monotherapy.

Methods

Subjects

After IRB exempt status was approved, an administrative data query was conducted and identified all children 0-18 years of age with a visit to the authors' health system associated with the ICD-9 code for sJIA (714.30) between 1/1/2000 and 12/31/2014. As this ICD-9 code (714.30) also includes children with polyarticular JIA and unspecified JIA, charts were initially screened for specific diagnosis of sJIA. Children were included in the cohort if they were diagnosed with sJIA during the study period, meeting the International League of Associations for Rheumatology (ILAR) criteria [5].

Data abstraction

Clinical data were obtained via review of the electronic medical record (EMR) using a standardized tool. Variables included patient demographics; characteristics of initial presentation, including history, physical exam findings, and the results of laboratory studies at diagnosis; medication regimens; responses to therapy; and escalation of therapy. We adapted the Wallace criteria [6] to define clinically inactive disease (CID) as absence of arthritis, systemic features, and laboratory abnormalities, if labs were performed. Physician global assessment of disease activity was not consistently recorded in the EMR so this criterion was not included in our definition. MAS was defined by the PRINTO criteria (fever, ferritin >684 ng/dl, and any 2 of the following: platelet count $<181 \times 10^9$/L, aspartate aminotransferase (AST) > 48 U/L, triglycerides >156 mg/dl, fibrinogen <360 mg/dl [7].

Statistical analyses: Children were divided into 3 comparison groups for analyses:

(1) Children who achieved CID with NSAID monotherapy,
(2) Children who received a trial of NSAID monotherapy at diagnosis but required additional medications, therefore failing NSAID monotherapy, and
(3) Children who did not receive NSAID monotherapy at diagnosis

By definition, patients who received NSAID monotherapy did not receive any corticosteroids through their NSAID trial. If corticosteroids, DMARDs, or biologic medications were added to a patient's regimen, it was considered a failure of NSAID monotherapy.

All analyses were conducted with SAS 9.4 (SAS Institute Inc., Cary, NC, USA). CRP at diagnosis was unknown for 6 of the 51 children in the cohort, and was imputed via multiple imputation using SAS Proc MI using the white blood cell count (WBC), hemoglobin (Hg), and platelet level.

In order to determine which patient demographic and disease presentation variables (initial joint count, presence of specific diagnostic criteria, lab values at diagnosis) were predictive of assignment of NSAID monotherapy as well as NSAID monotherapy success, we began by examining the bivariate relations between these variables and either the assignment to or response to NSAID monotherapy. Logistic regression was used for continuous variables and chi-square or Fisher's exact test for categorical variables. Use of a single multivariate regression model was not practical given the high ratio of possible predictors to number of study participants. Continuous predictor variables were transformed into dichotomous variables to create clinically meaningful categories.

To create a multivariate model predictive of NSAID monotherapy response, we began with the patient demographic or disease presentation variable with the strongest bivariate association with NSAID monotherapy response and continued to add patient demographic or disease presentation variables in order of strength of bivariate association with NSAID monotherapy response. Any p-values <0.25 were included in the multivariate model, based on the Wald test from logistic regression [8].

Results

We identified 1717 potential subjects using the administrative query. Of those, 87 children were diagnosed with sJIA during the study period and met ILAR criteria for sJIA. All children included in the cohort had both systemic and articular features present. Fifty-one children received a trial of NSAID monotherapy and 13 of those (25.5%) achieved CID with NSAID monotherapy. Of the children who were given a trial of NSAID monotherapy, 35 (69%) were prescribed naproxen at a mean dose of 18 mg/kg/day, 12 (24%) were prescribed indomethacin at a mean dose of 2.5 mg/kg/day, 3 (6%) were prescribed sulindac at a mean dose of 10 mg/kg/day, and 1 (2%) was prescribed ibuprofen at an unknown dose.

Results from the tests of bivariate associations with both the assignment of NSAID monotherapy as well as the response to NSAID monotherapy are shown in Table 1. Patients with serositis at diagnosis were significantly less likely to receive a trial of NSAID monotherapy ($p = 0.003$). Other patient demographic or disease characteristics (such as initial joint count and rash) were not associated with whether a child received a trial of NSAID monotherapy.

When evaluating disease characteristics of patients who achieved CID with NSAID monotherapy, initial joint count was the only statistically significant predictor ($p = 0.01$). Age at presentation, ferritin, and CRP were trending towards significance ($p = 0.10$, $p = 0.08$, $p = 0.14$ respectively).

A multivariate model combined the three most significant/suggestive factors: age at presentation, initial joint count, and CRP at diagnosis. Ferritin was not included since it was unavailable in 45% of patients. In combination within the same patient, these three variables yield a very strong association with response to NSAID monotherapy ($p = 0.002$).

In the group of patients who failed NSAID monotherapy, 30 out of 37 patients (81%) achieved CID, while in the group of patients who did not receive NSAID monotherapy, 28 out of 34 (82%) patients achieved CID ($p = 0.89$). For those who failed NSAID monotherapy trial, median time to CID was 764 days, while for those who were not tried on NSAID monotherapy, the median time to CID was 267 days ($p = 0.60$). There was a significant difference within the group that received NSAID monotherapy, with the successful NSAID monotherapy group having a shorter time to CID than those who failed NSAID monotherapy ($p = 0.0001$). Within the group that failed NSAID monotherapy, the median time to drug escalation was 32 days. Regarding time to first follow-up, there was a significant difference, with patients successful on NSAID monotherapy taking longer to follow-up than those who failed NSAID monotherapy ($p = 0.004$). There was no difference in time to first follow-up visit between the group that received a trial of NSAID monotherapy versus not. There was also no difference between the groups with regard to disease duration prior to diagnosis or total follow-up time. Regarding the patient with 0 days to remission, that patient had a delay in presentation to a pediatric rheumatologist, and so was diagnosed retrospectively after symptoms had already resolved.

Two of the 51 patients who received NSAID monotherapy met criteria for MAS at diagnosis. One was 11 years old and had a CRP of 20.2 mg/dL at diagnosis. The second patient was 15 years old, with arthritis in 10 joints, and with a CRP of 7.4 mg/dL at diagnosis. Both patients' regimens were escalated to include steroids and methotrexate within 2 weeks, and anakinra was added 1 month later with excellent response in both. The remaining children who developed MAS after diagnosis had already been escalated to corticosteroids, DMARDs, and/or biologics at the time their MAS developed.

Anakinra became widely used as a treatment for sJIA in 2007. Prior to 2007, 30 of 39 patients (77%) received NSAID monotherapy trial. After 2007, 21 of 41 patients (51%) received NSAID monotherapy trial. This difference is statistically significant ($p = 0.02$).

Discussion

NSAID monotherapy is able to achieve CID in a small subset of children with sJIA. This study helps pediatric rheumatologists risk-stratify their patients at diagnosis when choosing whether to pursue a trial of NSAID monotherapy. Factors associated with achievement of CID with NSAID monotherapy include age ≤ 8 years at presentation, joint count ≤ 5, and CRP ≤ 13 mg/dL. When combined in a multivariate model, having all of these characteristics in the same patient have a very strong association with response to NSAID monotherapy ($p = 0.002$). Ferritin was also trending towards significance,

Table 1 Correlation of demographic features and disease characteristics with response to NSAID monotherapy

	Responded to NSAID monotherapy	Failed NSAID monotherapy	Did not receive a trial of NSAID monotherapy	p-value comparing trial (columns 1 and 2) vs no trial (column 3)	p-value comparing responded to trial (column 1) vs. failed trial (column 2)
Patients	13	38	36		
Demographic features					
Male, *n* (%)	7 (54%)	15 (39%)	17 (47%)	0.71	0.52
Age at presentation, mean (SD)	4.8 (3.6)	7.1 (4.7)	6.1 (4.6)	0.68	**0.10***
Age ≤ 8 years at presentation, *n* (%)	11 (85%)	21 (55%)	27 (75%)	0.23	**0.10***
Disease characteristics					
Initial joint count, mean (SD)	1.8 (1.6)	5.7 (9.0)	4.7 (6.3)	0.98	**0.01****
Joint count ≤5, *n* (%)	13 (100%)	29 (76%)	29 (81%)	0.83	**0.09***
Characteristic rash, *n* (%)	13 (100%)	34 (89%)	33 (92%)	0.93	0.56
Generalized lymphadenopathy, *n* (%)	2 (15%)	6 (16%)	9 (25%)	0.28	1.00
Hepatosplenomegaly, *n* (%)	2 (15%)	7 (18%)	5 (14%)	0.64	1.00
Serositis, *n* (%)	0 (0%)	1 (3%)	8 (22%)	**0.003****	1.00
CRP ≤13 mg/dL*, *n* (%)	12 (92%)	26 (68%)	17 (59%)	**0.14***	**0.14***
MAS at diagnosis, *n* (%)	0 (0%)	2 (5%)	7 (19%)	**0.03****	1.00
MAS ever, *n* (%)	0 (0%)	6 (16%)	11 (31%)	**0.03****	0.32
WBC (K/μL), mean (SD)	16.7 (±7.0)	16.4 (±7.0)	19.6 (±10.1)	0.15	0.89
Hg (g/dL), mean (SD)	10.4 (±0.9)	10.1 (±1.5)	9.9 (±1.6)	0.45	0.47
Platelets (K/μL), mean (SD)	492 (±193)	486 (±222)	519 (±248)	0.57	0.93
ESR (mm), mean (SD)	80 (±26)	77 (±26)	75 (±31)	0.69	0.81
Ferritin (ng/mL), mean (SD)	410 (±722)	3042 (±4813)	3060 (±3777)	0.55	**0.07***
Outcomes					
Days to clinically inactive disease, median (range)	49 (28-356)	764 (13-3806)	267 (0-2716)	0.60	**0.0001****
Days to medication escalation, median (range)	n/a	32 (2-146)	n/a	n/a	n/a
Days to first follow-up, median (range)	48 (28-252)	21 (6-327)	27 (9-188)	0.33	**0.004****
Days of disease duration prior to diagnosis, median (range)	55 (26-492)	46 (14-484)	81 (11-848)	0.25	0.60
Days of total follow-up, median (range)	1000 (154-3164)	1693 (0-4229)	956 (188-4678)	0.45	0.37

P-values below 0.25 have one asterisk (*) and were considered trending (based on Wald test from logistic regression). *P*-values below 0.05 have two asterisks (**) and were considered statistically significant. All *p*-values below 0.25 are bolded

but was unknown for 45% of patients who received NSAID monotherapy trial, so was not included in the multivariate model.

Conversely, children in our cohort who were older at diagnosis (> 8 years old), with more joints involved (>5), or with a higher CRP at diagnosis (>13), were less likely to respond favorably to NSAID monotherapy. When these variables are taken individually, joint count was independently statistically significant while age and CRP were trending towards significance. We recommend against NSAID monotherapy in a patient with sJIA with any of these unfavorable characteristics. In addition, we found that providers are less likely to trial NSAID monotherapy in the presence of serositis or MAS, and we agree with avoiding NSAID monotherapy in these groups, as these are indicators of more severe disease.

Of note, our study cohort spans the years 2000-2014, and anakinra became widely used as a first-line agent to treat sJIA in 2007. The introduction of anakinra did alter prescribing patterns at our institution. Prior to the anakinra era, 77% of patients received a trial of NSAID monotherapy. After 2007, this dropped to 51% of patients receiving a trial of NSAID monotherapy. This is consistent with our institutional practice becoming more aggressive with the initial treatment of sJIA.

There was no statistically significant difference in whether a patient achieved CID based on whether they received a trial of NSAID monotherapy or not. There was also no statistically significant difference in the time to CID between the group that received a trial of NSAID monotherapy and the group that did not. Despite this lack of statistical significance, the difference between 9 months versus 2 years of active disease is clinically significant for patients, their families, and their treating physicians. This leads us to the conclusion that if indicated, NSAID monotherapy trial should be very short, and if desired results are not achieved quickly, escalation should be aggressive. The group that is predisposed to achieve CID with NSAID monotherapy does so quickly (median time to CID was 49 days), and so if a significant response is not achieved within 2-4 weeks, medications should be transitioned to alternative first- and second-line agents, including corticosteroids. This adheres to the current ACR guidelines (2). In our cohort, there was no difference in time to first follow-up between patients who received versus did not receive a trial of NSAID monotherapy. However, there was a difference in time to follow-up between patients who achieved CID on NSAID monotherapy versus those who did not achieve CID, with those failing NSAID monotherapy having sooner follow-up. Therefore, all patients should receive a standard 2-4 week follow-up after initial diagnosis to determine whether medication regimen requires escalation; this recommendation is also consistent with the current ACR guidelines [2].

The two patients with MAS at diagnosis who received NSAID monotherapy had presenting characteristics (older age, high joint count, and elevated CRP) which were associated with poor response to this treatment (in addition to their presence of MAS). In retrospect, they should have initially been treated more aggressively. Fortunately, their medication regimens were quickly escalated and their disease came under good control within 6 weeks. The remainder of the patients in the NSAID monotherapy group who developed MAS did so after their medications had already been escalated to corticosteroids, DMARDs, and/or biologics. As previously stated, children with MAS either at presentation or at any point during their disease are not candidates for NSAID monotherapy.

This study has several limitations. The cohort was of modest size, so the number of characteristics that could be considered for analysis was limited. Selection bias was present in that providers chose to pursue NSAID monotherapy in only 51 out of 87 children diagnosed with sJIA during the study period. Disease activity scores could not be generated due to lack of patient global assessment in the majority of electronic medical records. Since this is an observational study, it is subject to the risk of unidentified confounders as well. CRP was not obtained for all patients at diagnosis, so the value was imputed for some subjects. ESR and ferritin were available for an even smaller number of patients at diagnosis, so these values could not be included in the multivariate model. Despite these limitations, this study represents an important first step in beginning to stratify initial therapy for sJIA based on clinical presentation. It will be critical to validate our findings in a larger cohort of patients, ideally in the setting of a clinical trial.

Conclusions

- We retrospectively evaluated NSAID monotherapy in children with systemic juvenile idiopathic arthritis (sJIA), and examined patient characteristics to determine which aspects at diagnosis were associated with achievement of clinically inactive disease (CID).
- We found that NSAID monotherapy *should not* be considered in children with sJIA who are >8 years old at diagnosis, with >5 joints involved, or with an initial C-reactive protein (CRP) > 13 mg/dL based on our data. We also do not recommend NSAID monotherapy trial in children with serositis or MAS at diagnosis.
- If NSAID monotherapy trial is pursued, patients should follow up within 2-4 weeks to evaluate whether escalation of therapy is warranted.

Abbreviations

AST: Aspartate aminotransferase; CARRA: Childhood arthritis and rheumatology research alliance; CID: Clinically inactive disease; CRP: C-reactive protein; CTPs: Consensus treatment protocols; DMARDs: Disease-modifying anti-rheumatic drugs; EMR: Electronic medical record; ESR: Erythrocyte sedimentation rate; Hg: Hemoglobin; ICD-9: International statistical classification of diseases and related health problems – 9; IL-1: Interleukin-1; IL-6: Interleukin-6; ILAR: International league of associations for rheumatology; JIA: Juvenile idiopathic arthritis; MAS: Macrophage activation syndrome; NSAIDs: Non-steroidal anti-inflammatory drugs; PRINTO: Pediatric rheumatology international trials organization; sJIA: Systemic juvenile idiopathic arthritis; WBC: White blood count

Acknowledgements
Not applicable

Funding
Not applicable.

Authors' contributions

AS collected data from EMR, interpreted data, and was a major contributor in writing the manuscript. CF collected data from EMR. JS (Julie Sturza) performed statistical analysis of data. JS (Jasmine Stannard) collected data from EMR. MR collected data from EMR, interpreted data, and was a major contributor in writing the manuscript. All authors read and approved the final manuscript.

Authors' information
Not applicable.

Consent for publication
Not applicable.

Competing interests
The authors declare that they have no competing interests.

Author details
[1]University of Michigan, 1500 E Medical Center Dr, Ann Arbor, MI 48109, USA. [2]IHA Rheumatology Consultants, 4990 W Clark Rd, Suite 300, Ypsilanti, MI 48197, USA.

References

1. Prince F, Otten M, Suijlekom-Smit L. Diagnosis and management of juvenile idiopathic arthritis. BMJ. 2011;342:95–102.
2. Dewitt EM, Kimura Y, et al. Consensus treatment plans for new-onset systemic juvenile idiopathic arthritis. Arthritis Care Res (Hoboken). 2012;64(7): 1001–10.
3. Ringold S, et al. 2013 update of the 2011 American College of Rheumatology Recommendations for the treatment of juvenile idiopathic arthritis. Arthritis Rheum. 2013;65(10):2499–512.
4. Vastert SJ, de Jager W, et al. Effectiveness of first-line treatment with recombinant interleukin-1 receptor antagonist in steroid-naive patients with new-onset systemic juvenile idiopathic arthritis: results of a prospective cohort study. Arthritis Rheumatol. 2014;66(4):1034–43.
5. Petty RE, Southwood TR, Manners P, Baum J, Glass DN, Goldenberg J, et al. International league of associations for rheumatology classification of juvenile idiopathic arthritis: second revision, Edmonton, 2001. J Rheumatol. 2004;31:390–2.
6. Wallace CA, et al. Clinically inactive disease in a cohort of children with new-onset polyarticular juvenile idiopathic arthritis treated with early aggressive therapy: time to achievement, total duration, and predictors. J Rheumatol. 2014;41:1163–70.
7. Boom V, Anton J, Lahdenne P, Quartier P, Ravelli A, Wulffraat NM, Vastert SJ. Evidence-based diagnosis and treatment of macrophage activation syndrome in systemic juvenile idiopathic arthritis. Pediatr Rheumatol Online J. 2015;13(1):55.
8. Bursac Z, Gauss CH, Williams DK, Hosmer D. Purposeful selection of variables in logistic regression. Source Code Biol Med. 2008;3:17.

11

Successful treatment of methotrexate intolerance in juvenile idiopathic arthritis using eye movement desensitization and reprocessing – treatment protocol and preliminary results

Lea Höfel[1,2], Bruno Eppler[1,2], Magdalena Storf[1,2], Elizabeth Schnöbel-Müller[2], Johannes-Peter Haas[1,2] and Boris Hügle[1*]

Abstract

Background: Methotrexate (MTX), commonly used in juvenile idiopathic arthritis (JIA), frequently has to be discontinued due to intolerance with anticipatory and associative gastrointestinal adverse effects. Eye Movement Desensitization and Reprocessing (EMDR) is a psychological method where dysfunctional experiences and memories are reprocessed by recall combined with bilateral eye movements. The objective of this study was to assess efficacy of EMDR for treatment of MTX intolerance in JIA patients.

Methods: We performed an open prospective study on consecutive JIA patients with MTX intolerance. Intolerance was determined using the Methotrexate Intolerance Severity Score (MISS) questionnaire prior to treatment, directly after treatment and after four months. Health-related quality of life was determined using the PedsQL prior to and four months after treatment. Patients were treated according to an institutional EMDR protocol with 8 sessions over two weeks. Changes in MISS and PedsQL were analyzed using non-parametric statistics.

Results: Eighteen patients with MTX intolerance (median MISS at inclusion 16.5, IQR = 11.75–20.25) were included. Directly after treatment, MTX intolerance symptoms were significantly improved (median MISS 1 (IQR = 0–2). After four months, median MISS score was at 6.5 (IQR = 2.75–12.25, $p = 0.001$), with 9/18 patients showing MISS scores ≥6. Median PedsQL after 4 months improved significantly from 77.6% to 85.3% ($p = 0.008$).

Conclusion: MTX intolerance in children with JIA was effectively treated using an EMDR protocol, with lasting effect over a period of 4 months. EMDR treatment can potentially increase quality of life of affected patients and enable continued MTX treatment.

Keywords: Juvenile idiopathic arthritis, Methotrexate, Intolerance, Adverse effects, EMDR

* Correspondence: huegle.boris@rheuma-kinderklinik.de
[1]German Center for Pediatric and Adolescent Rheumatology (DZKJR), Gehfeldstrasse 24, 82467 Garmisch-Partenkirchen, Germany
Full list of author information is available at the end of the article

Background

Methotrexate (MTX) is the most commonly used medication in the treatment of children with inflammatory joint diseases, especially for polyarticular juvenile idiopathic arthritis (JIA) [1, 2]. Treatment with low-dose MTX therapy exhibits few serious adverse effects; treatment is usually discontinued due to intolerance symptoms such as anticipatory nausea and refusal to take the medication [3, 4]. The origin of MTX intolerance is still unclear, and common countermeasures have been shown to be ineffective in suppressing MTX intolerance [5, 6]. Current studies demonstrate high rates of intolerance for JIA patients on treatment with low-dose MTX, while high-dose regimens e.g. in the treatment of childhood cancer, are usually much more responsive to medication with antiemetics [6–9].

EMDR (Eye Movement Desensitization and Reprocessing) is a psychological method that has historically been applied to the treatment of posttraumatic stress disorder, but has since then been developed into an overall approach for other adverse life experiences. The eight-phase treatment approach is composed of standardized protocols and procedures, using intensive recall of unprocessed memories while applying bilateral eye movements, taps, or tones [10]. As a result, affective distress is relieved, negative beliefs are reformulated, and physiological arousal is reduced.

The efficacy of EMDR for trauma-related disorders has been shown in controlled trials for the treatment of trauma in children and adolescents, but also in other fields of stress related psychological disorders, such as post-operative pain or seizure-related post-traumatic stress [11–13].

While EMDR has not been used for the treatment of MTX intolerance so far, a treatment approach would be based on the hypothesis that MTX treatment in JIA patients is a repetitive stressful or even traumatic event leading to anticipatory and associative adverse effects that prevent healthy information processing. The objective of this study was to describe the EMDR protocol for the treatment of MTX intolerance, as well as to determine efficacy of EMDR when used to treat MTX intolerance in children with JIA on continued MTX treatment.

Methods

Patients

Consecutive patients admitted to the German Center for Pediatric and Adolescent Rheumatology from October 2016 until May 2017 for planned EMDR treatment were included in this study. Inclusion criteria were 1) diagnosis of JIA according to ILAR criteria [14], 2) age between 8 and 17 years, 3) symptoms of MTX intolerance, as determined by questionnaire (see below), and 4) necessity of MTX treatment for at least 6 more months as determined by the treating physician. Intolerance to MTX was determined using the Methotrexate Intolerance Severity Score (MISS) questionnaire, previously developed and validated in JIA [7]. The MISS consists of four domains: abdominal pain, nausea, vomiting and behavioral symptoms, assessing symptoms after MTX administration, anticipatory and associative symptoms. The behavioral symptoms domain includes restlessness, irritability and refusal of MTX, which develop in response to MTX-induced gastrointestinal symptoms and anticipation thereof. A patient could score 0 (no symptoms), 1 (mild symptoms), 2 (moderate symptoms) or 3 (severe symptoms) points on each item. MTX intolerance was defined as ≥6 points, including at least one anticipatory, associative or behavioral symptom [3]. Exclusion criteria were 1) other diseases leading to nausea and/or abdominal complaints, 2) concomitant medications possibly inducing nausea (excepting biologics and non-steroidal anti-inflammatory drugs) and 3) pre-existing contraindications that would prevent EMDR treatment such as dissociative disorders, personality disorders or severe somatic disorders (e.g. cardiac arrhythmias).

Written consent was obtained from the parents prior to inclusion in the study. The study was approved by the ethics committee of the Medical Faculty of the Ludwig-Maximilian University, Munich, Germany.

Intervention

Treatment was performed by two pediatric psychologists (BE and MS) trained in EMDR technique following an institutional EMDR protocol. The standard EMDR protocol, which includes the 8 phases "history taking", "preparation", "assessment", "desensitization", "installation", "body scan", "closure" and "reevaluation" was adapted for the treatment of MTX intolerance [15]. The protocol is described in detail in Additional file 1: Table S1.

Treatment started with an initial session consisting of a structured psychosocial and medical history, including preexisting traumatic experiences and the development of the MTX intolerance reaction as well as education about the method. At the end of the first session, a 'calm place' exercise was conducted in order to address potential paradoxical anxiety responses, using a slow bilateral stimulation while the patients envisioned a place where they felt calm and peaceful (phases 1 and 2 of the protocol).

Subsequently, five sessions lasting 60 min each were held over a time period of 10–12 days according to the standard EMDR protocol (phases 3–8 of the protocol), concluding with the forthcoming and thus anticipated MTX application.

The final two sessions consisted of the application of Methotrexate, without supervision of the therapist, and a final session following the MTX application, where the positive experiences were installed and a possible "worst case" scenario in the future was reprocessed to lessen residual anticipatory anxiety or avoidance (future template). Parents were present at the first session, during the application of MTX and for the closing meeting.

Data acquisition and analysis

Primary outcome was improvement of MTX intolerance measured by MISS 4 months after therapy. MISS was measured prior to the first therapy session, directly after the last therapy session and 4 months later [7]. Health-related quality of life was also measured prior to therapy and 4 months after therapy, using the PedsQL 4.0 Generic Core Scales [16]. The following data was extracted from patient files: age, gender, body weight and height (to calculate methotrexate dose per body surface area), age at diagnosis, duration of disease, methotrexate dose, route of administration and folic acid supplementation and were analyzed using descriptive statistics. MISS score changes over time and changes of PedsQL over time were compared using non-parametric Wilcoxon Signed Rank tests. Statistical analysis was performed using SPSS version 21.0 (SPSS Inc., Chicago, IL, USA).

Results

Eighteen patients were included in the study. Demographic and clinical data of the patients are shown in Table 1. Patients did not change route or dose of MTX administration during the study.

Methotrexate intolerance and change of MISS score over time

All patients showed MTX intolerance prior to treatment (defined as MISS score ≥ 6), with a median MISS score of 16.5 (IQR = 11.75–20.25, mean: 15.6). Directly after EMDR treatment, median MISS score decreased significantly to 1 (IQR = 0–2, mean: 1.0, $p < 0.001$). No patient had MISS scores ≥6 at this time, and all reported subjective improvement compared to prior to EMDR treatment when MTX medication was applied. 4 months after treatment, median MISS score was at 6.5 (IQR = 2.75–12.25, mean: 8.3, $p = 0.001$) (Fig. 1). 9/18 patients (50%) showed MISS scores ≥6 at this time.

Quality of life and change of PedsQL score over time

Median health related quality of life as measured by the PedsQL questionnaire was 77.6% (range 46.7% – 100%) prior to treatment. 4 months after treatment, PedsQL was significantly improved with a median PedsQL score of 85.3% (range 64.1% – 100%, $p = 0.008$) (Fig. 2). The median Physical Health Summary Score of the PedsQL improved from 76.3% (range 40.6% – 100%) to 82.7% (range 59.4% – 100%, $p = 0.026$), while the median Psychosocial Health Summary Score of the PedsQL improved from 77.3% (range 37.5% – 100%) to 86.4% (range 59.4% – 100%, $p = 0.007$).

Table 1 Baseline demographic data of patient cohort

Characteristics	*N* = 18
Gender, female	16 (89%)
Age, mean ± SD	13,9 ± 2.9 years
JIA subtype	
Oligoarticular, persistent	5 (28%)
Oligoarticular, extended	6 (33%)
Polyarticular, rheumatoid-factor negative	4 (22%)
Psoriatic arthritis	2 (11%)
Enthesitis-associated arthritis	1 (6%)
Disease characteristics	
ANA positive	14/18 (78%)
HLA-B27 positive	4/18 (22%)
Age at diagnosis, mean ± SD	6.8 ± 4.4 years
Disease duration, mean ± SD	7.1 ± 4.1 years
Medications	
MTX route of administration, subcutaneous	11/18 (61%)
MTX duration use, mean ± SD	59 ± 40 months
MTX dose, mean ± SD	12.3 ± 1.6 mg/sqm/week
Additional medication	
TNFα inhibitors	7/18 (39%)
NSAIDs, regularly	2/18 (11%)
Folic acid	16/18 (89%)

Discussion

Methotrexate is a commonly used and highly effective drug in the treatment of children with rheumatic diseases, with very limited adverse effects. Discontinuation

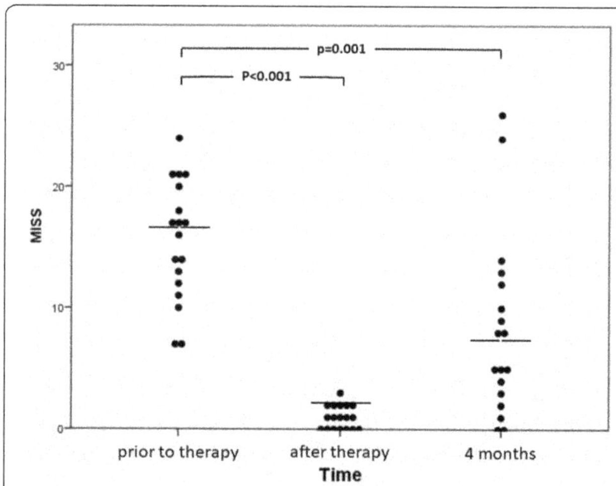

Fig. 1 MISS scores of the cohort prior to, directly after and four months after EMDR treatment

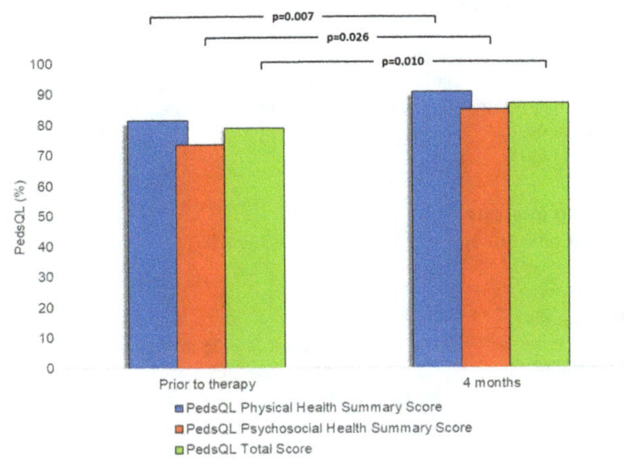

Fig. 2 PedsQL scores of the cohort prior to, and four months after EMDR treatment

of an obviously effective and, besides the intolerance, well-tolerated medication can be extremely frustrating for patients, parents and care providers alike. In this study we demonstrate that treatment with EMDR has the potential to significantly alleviate MTX intolerance symptoms, with a sustained effect over 4 months. We were also able to show that quality of life in treated patients had improved after 4 months, with the largest improvement found in the physical health subscore of the PedsQL. This either results from MTX intolerance being experienced primarily as a physical phenomenon by the affected patients or, EMDR treatment having a more pronounced effect on the physical sensations of MTX intolerance.

These preliminary results indicate that EMDR treatment has had a beneficial effect on patients with MTX intolerance; besides improving the quality of life, this treatment also has the potential to prevent medication changes which do not only carry increased risk for the patients, but frequently lead to the incurrence of substantial costs to the families and the coverage provider alike.

The concept of EMDR is based on the Adaptive Information Processing Method, stating that, when experiences are processed in a healthy way, multiple elements of the experience such as thoughts, images, emotions and sensations are stored in our memory and helpful associations are forged with stored experiences and reactions in memory. If a disturbing or traumatic event occurs, this information processing may not be complete. Strong feelings or dysfunctional coping mechanisms may interfere with information processing. This interference then prevents the access to more adaptive and healthy information that is stored in our memory networks. One might be stuck in the experience loop of a visual flashback or an emotion without being able to adapt and learn from it. The experience is then unprocessed and the physiological system is not able to return to a healthy, stable baseline – the emotions are not in balance.

EMDR enables the processing of dysfunctional and traumatic memories, using an intensive recall combined with bilateral stimulation usually evoked by eye movement to dissolve the memories by reprocessing them. As a result, affective distress is relieved, negative beliefs are reformulated, and physiological arousal is reduced. Unprocessed memory content and dysfunctional experiences and memories are reprocessed several times in order to enable healthy information processing [15]. The traumatic memory is desensitized by short imaginal exposure to this memory and subsequent bilateral stimulation, which is repeated until the accompanying subjective sense of disturbance has disappeared. Bilateral stimulation by eye movement is supposed to counteract the ‚frozen information', enabling dissolution of traumatic memories, neutralization of the negative affect and reduction of physiological arousal [10].

EMDR has proven an effective treatment of traumatic stress disorder in adults and children [17–20]. Whilst EMDR is most frequently used in the treatment of trauma- and stress-related disorders, its usefulness has been demonstrated in the treatment of other kinds of dysfunctional memories and inefficient information processing of further adverse life experiences [11, 12].

For this study, we assumed that MTX intolerance is based on dysfunctional or incomplete information processing evoked by e.g. strong negative feelings or adverse anticipation of side effects that can be considered similar to a trauma- or stressor-related disorder. This is in keeping with the adaptive information processing model of EMDR, which states that dysfunctionally stored and not fully processed memories are the cause of various mental disorders, or more broadly "that after a certain event, a certain psychopathology appears, which can be effectively addressed by EMDR therapy" [21]. Being diagnosed with a rheumatic disorder and being treated with MTX might not necessarily qualify as severe mental or emotional stress or physical injury alone [22]. However, patients have experienced MTX-related adverse effects or might have been told of the possibility of these occurring, and thus anticipate them in the future, with regular weekly re-enforcements and virtually no chance for escape. The behavioral distress such as showing panic or resistance at the sight of the medication frequently reported in children with MTX intolerance fits well within the symptom clusters of trauma- and stress related disorders [4, 7].

While patients improved significantly directly after EMDR treatment, a significant number showed symptoms of MTX intolerance at follow-up 4 months later. Continuous treatment with MTX could arguably re-initiate the same process that led to the intolerance symptoms in the first place; however, in most cases the EMDR treatment, including techniques imparted on the affected patients, seem to provide a measure of protection. A possibly neglected factor is the education of the parents; personal communications in selected cases suggested an influence of parental expectations on recurrence of MTX intolerance symptoms. Possible improvements to the EMDR protocol in the future include one or several regularly scheduled follow-up treatment sessions as well as an in-depth education of the parents included in the primary protocol.

MTX intolerance as a unified construct of the anticipatory and associative side effects associated with prolonged use of MTX has only recently been described, and the MISS questionnaire tries to capture this construct [7]. So far, genetic studies have been unsuccessful in finding a causal link to MTX intolerance [5, 23, 24]. Interaction between the patient and his parents, physicians and other caregivers as well as psychological and social background factors can all influence frequency and severity of MTX intolerance symptoms, and therefore the efficacy of any intervention. A limitation of this study was patient selection, including only patients with sufficiently severe symptoms of MTX intolerance to be willing to undergo two weeks of (partially in-patient) treatment. This was not a randomized trial but a mere 'proof of concept', and there was no control group with 'treatment as usual'; however, it has previously been shown that untreated or conventionally treated MTX intolerance tends to get worse over time rather than improve on its own [6]. The significant benefits the patient received from the treatment in this study argues for the efficacy of the EMDR approach in the treatment of MTX intolerance. Further studies are necessary to elucidate not only the cause of MTX intolerance, but also the exact benefits of EMDR treatment for MTX intolerance.

Conclusion

Patients with JIA showing MTX intolerance profited significantly from EMDR treatment directly after the treatment and over a period of 4 months, allowing continuation of MTX treatment with improved quality of life. To our knowledge, this is the first report of an efficacious measure against MTX intolerance, which is developing into one of the largest problems in the day-to-day treatment of JIA patients in the clinic. Further studies should investigate long-term efficacy of this treatment approach, if re-treatment is necessary, and if yes, in what format.

Acknowledgements
The authors would like to thank the participating patients and their parents.

Funding
This work was supported in part by an unrestricted grant from the Verein 'Hilfe für das rheumakranke Kind e.V.'.

Authors' contributions
LH, BE and BH designed the study, recruited the patients and performed the statistical analysis, LH, MS and BE performed the EMDR treatment on the patients. ESM and JPH participated in the design and coordination of the study and helped draft the manuscript. All authors read and approved the final manuscript.

Competing interests
The authors are not aware of any conflict of interest.

Author details
[1]German Center for Pediatric and Adolescent Rheumatology (DZKJR), Gehfeldstrasse 24, 82467 Garmisch-Partenkirchen, Germany. [2]Center for Pain Treatment in Young People, Garmisch-Partenkirchen, Germany.

References

1. Beukelman T, Patkar NM, Saag KG, Tolleson-Rinehart S, Cron RQ, DeWitt EM, Ilowite NT, Kimura Y, Laxer RM, Lovell DJ, et al. 2011 American College of Rheumatology recommendations for the treatment of juvenile idiopathic arthritis: initiation and safety monitoring of therapeutic agents for the treatment of arthritis and systemic features. Arthritis Care Res (Hoboken). 2011;63:465–82.
2. Ravelli A, Davi S, Bracciolini G, Pistorio A, Consolaro A, van Dijkhuizen EHP, Lattanzi B, Filocamo G, Verazza S, Gerloni V, et al. Intra-articular corticosteroids versus intra-articular corticosteroids plus methotrexate in oligoarticular juvenile idiopathic arthritis: a multicentre, prospective, randomised, open-label trial. Lancet. 2017;389:909–16.
3. Ortiz-Alvarez O, Morishita K, Avery G, Green J, Petty RE, Tucker LB, Malleson PN, Cabral DA. Guidelines for blood test monitoring of methotrexate toxicity in juvenile idiopathic arthritis. J Rheumatol. 2004;31:2501–6.
4. van der Meer A, Wulffraat NM, Prakken BJ, Gijsbers B, Rademaker CM, Sinnema G. Psychological side effects of MTX treatment in juvenile idiopathic arthritis: a pilot study. Clin Exp Rheumatol. 2007;25:480–5.
5. Scheuern A, Fischer N, McDonald J, Brunner HI, Haas JP, Hugle B. Mutations in the MTHFR gene are not associated with methotrexate intolerance in patients with juvenile idiopathic arthritis. Pediatr Rheumatol Online J. 2016;14:11.
6. Scheuern A, Tyrrell PN, Haas JP, Hugle B. Countermeasures against methotrexate intolerance in juvenile idiopathic arthritis instituted by parents show no effect. Rheumatology (Oxford). 2017;
7. Bulatovic M, Heijstek MW, Verkaaik M, van Dijkhuizen EH, Armbrust W, Hoppenreijs EP, Kamphuis S, Kuis W, Egberts TC, Sinnema G, et al. High prevalence of methotrexate intolerance in juvenile idiopathic arthritis: development and validation of a methotrexate intolerance severity score. Arthritis Rheum. 2011;63:2007–13.
8. van Dijkhuizen EH, Pouw JN, Scheuern A, Hugle B, Hardt S, Ganser G, Kummerle-Deschner JB, Horneff G, Holzinger D, Bulatovic Calasan M, Wulffraat NM. Methotrexate intolerance in oral and subcutaneous administration in patients with juvenile idiopathic arthritis: a cross-sectional, observational study. Clin Exp Rheumatol. 2016;34:148–54.
9. Holmboe L, Andersen AM, Morkrid L, Slordal L, Hall KS. High dose methotrexate chemotherapy: pharmacokinetics, folate and toxicity in osteosarcoma patients. Br J Clin Pharmacol. 2012;73:106–14.
10. Shapiro F. The role of eye movement desensitization and reprocessing (EMDR) therapy in medicine: addressing the psychological and physical symptoms stemming from adverse life experiences. Perm J. 2014;18:71–7.
11. Dautovic E, de Roos C, van Rood Y, Dommerholt A, Rodenburg R. Pediatric seizure-related posttraumatic stress and anxiety symptoms treated with EMDR: a case series. Eur J Psychotraumatol. 2016;7:30123.
12. Maroufi M, Zamani S, Izadikhah Z, Marofi M, O'Connor P. Investigating the effect of eye movement desensitization and reprocessing (EMDR) on postoperative pain intensity in adolescents undergoing surgery: a randomized controlled trial. J Adv Nurs. 2016;72:2207–17.
13. Dorsey S, McLaughlin KA, Kerns SEU, Harrison JP, Lambert HK, Briggs EC, Revillion Cox J, Amaya-Jackson L. Evidence base update for psychosocial treatments for children and adolescents exposed to traumatic events. J Clin Child Adolesc Psychol. 2017;46:303–30.

14. Petty RE, Southwood TR, Manners P, Baum J, Glass DN, Goldenberg J, He X, Maldonado-Cocco J, Orozco-Alcala J, Prieur AM, et al. International league of associations for rheumatology classification of juvenile idiopathic arthritis: second revision, Edmonton, 2001. J Rheumatol. 2004;31:390–2.
15. Leeds AM. A guide to standard EMDR Therapy Protocols for Clinicians, Supervisors, and Consultants. 2nd edition edn. New York: Springer Publishing Company; 2016.
16. Varni JW, Seid M, Rode CA. The PedsQL: measurement model for the pediatric quality of life inventory. Med Care. 1999;37:126–39.
17. Gillies D, Maiocchi L, Bhandari AP, Taylor F, Gray C, O'Brien L. Psychological therapies for children and adolescents exposed to trauma. Cochrane Database Syst Rev. 2016;10:CD012371.
18. Rodenburg R, Benjamin A, de Roos C, Meijer AM, Stams GJ. Efficacy of EMDR in children: a meta-analysis. Clin Psychol Rev. 2009;29:599–606.
19. Bradley R, Greene J, Russ E, Dutra L, Westen D. A multidimensional meta-analysis of psychotherapy for PTSD. Am J Psychiatry. 2005;162:214–27.
20. Shapiro F. EMDR 12 years after its introduction: past and future research. J Clin Psychol. 2002;58:1–22.
21. Hase M, Balmaceda UM, Ostacoli L, Liebermann P, Hofmann A. The AIP model of EMDR therapy and pathogenic memories. Front Psychol. 2017;8: 1578.
22. Association AP. Diagnostic and statistical manual of mental disorders. 5th ed. DC: Washington; 2013.
23. Hugle B, Scheuern A, Dollinger S, Fischer N, Haas JP. Cathechol-O-methyltransferase Val158Met polymorphism is associated with nocebo effects, but not with methotrexate intolerance in patients with juvenile idiopathic arthritis. Scand J Rheumatol. 2017:1–2.
24. van Dijkhuizen EH, Bulatovic Calasan M, Pluijm SM, de Rotte MC, Vastert SJ, Kamphuis S, de Jonge R, Wulffraat NM. Prediction of methotrexate intolerance in juvenile idiopathic arthritis: a prospective, observational cohort study. Pediatr Rheumatol Online J. 2015;13:5.

Vitamin D and juvenile idiopathic arthritis

Sarah L. Finch[1], Alan M. Rosenberg[2] and Hassan Vatanparast[3*]

Abstract

Background: Vitamin D has been implicated in the pathogenesis of autoimmune diseases. While the roles of vitamin D in other autoimmune diseases have been investigated, less is known about the role of vitamin D in chronic childhood arthritis.

Main body: This review summarizes and evaluates evidence relating to 25-hydroxyvitamin D (25(OH)D) and chronic childhood arthritis. A scoping literature review was conducted using Ovid Medline, Ovid Embase, Cumulative Index to Nursing and Allied Health Literature, Web of Science and Scopus. Further, we geo-mapped the results of the studies to identify the patterns of the association between vitamin D and chronic childhood arthritis across the globe. Of 38 studies reporting 25(OH)D concentrations in childhood chronic arthritis, 32 (84.2%) reported that a significant number of children had suboptimal (< 75 nmol/L) status.

Conclusion: The data indicate suboptimal vitamin D status in children with chronic arthritis. Further, the association between low vitamin D and increased arthritis activity follow a north-south geographical gradient.

Keywords: Vitamin D, Childhood arthritis, Juvenile idiopathic arthritis

Background

Arthritis is among the most common chronic diseases in children. Juvenile Idiopathic Arthritis (JIA) is the current nomenclature applied to denote a group of clinically distinguishable subsets that share chronic, childhood-onset arthritis of unknown cause as a unifying feature. The etiologies of JIA are unknown and the pathogeneses unclear but are likely multifactorial. Among epidemiologic studies there is substantial variability in the frequencies with which JIA and its respective subtypes are reported to occur; chronic arthritis prevalence rates range from 0.07 to 4.01/1000 children and annual incidences from 0.008 to 0.226/1000 children [1]. Putative explanations for the disparities in reported juvenile arthritis prevalence rates include, as examples, differences in diagnostic criteria applied (specifically, JIA or the earlier Juvenile Rheumatoid Arthritis (JRA) [2] or Juvenile Chronic Arthritis (JCA) [3] classification systems) and in case ascertainment methods.

While methodologic inconsistencies among JIA epidemiologic studies might account for perceived prevalence differences, actual differences might occur as a consequence of genetic, ethnic, environmental, and lifestyle influences. Vitamin D status is potentially governed by these same factors; vitamin D receptor genotype, ethnically related skin tone and clothing, environmental variations in exposure to ultraviolet B radiation relating to the latitude of residence and season, and vitamin D nutritional intake are factors that modulate vitamin D concentrations.

As an immune and inflammatory mediator, vitamin D is implicated in the pathogenesis of autoimmune diseases including, as examples, multiple sclerosis, type 1 diabetes, rheumatoid arthritis, Crohn's disease, and chronic childhood arthritis [4–6]. Cells involved in innate and adaptive immune responses such as macrophages, dendritic cells, T cells, and B cells express enzymes required to activate and respond to vitamin D [7–9]. Cytochrome p450 27B1 (CYP27B1) is the enzyme required to synthesize 1,25-dihydroxyvitamin D (1,25(OH)2D), the active form of vitamin D, from circulating 25-hydroxyvitamin D (25(OH)D). The actions of 1,25(OH)2D are mediated by its binding to the vitamin D receptor (VDR), a nuclear transcription factor. VDR then binds to the Vitamin D Response Element (VDRE), a genetic sequence located in the promotor region of genes regulated by vitamin D [7–9]. Vitamin D tends to suppress the immune response [6]. Consequently, low vitamin D concentrations are associated with an increase in pro-inflammatory mediators and more active disease [6, 10] consistent, for example, with the observation that low serum 25(OH)D is associated with increased disease activity in rheumatoid arthritis [11].

* Correspondence: vatan.h@usask.ca
[3]College of Pharmacy & Nutrition and School of Public Health, University of Saskatchewan, 104 Clinic Place, Saskatoon, SK S7N 2Z4, Canada

Reports of relationships between vitamin D and chronic childhood arthritis are derived from studies having different methodologic approaches, originating from multiple geographic regions, and comprising demographically disparate populations. Since the last analysis of these reports in 2013 [12] the number of studies reporting 25(OH)D concentrations in children with chronic arthritis have increased from 14 to 38. An updated, systematic analysis of pertinent literature should help to further refine understanding of the relationships between vitamin D and juvenile arthritis, contribute to optimizing management of vitamin D status in children with arthritis, and clarify vitamin D's potential role in mediating disease pathogenesis.

Scoping reviews are methodologic approaches for thoroughly distilling and synthesizing information derived from different studies having varied designs. The purposes of scoping reviews are to not only capture key concepts that can guide care but also to recognize knowledge gaps that can inspire future research priorities [13].

Although nomenclature applied to chronic childhood arthritis classification systems has changed over the years, JIA is the current terminology. For clarity, this review will hereafter use the term JIA to encompass the forms of chronic childhood arthritis also included in the JCA and JRA classification systems. However, in this review, when quoting the literature, we use the terminology for chronic childhood arthritis (JCA, JRA, or JIA) that was applicable at the time the cited reference was published [14].

Here we report the results of a vitamin D- JIA scoping review that summarizes, synthesizes, evaluates, and interprets pertinent evidence from the literature to address the following research questions: 1) What is the relationship between vitamin D status and the occurrence of JIA? 2) What is the relationship between vitamin D status and childhood arthritis activity? 3) What is the relationship between vitamin D status in JIA and medication use? 4) What is the relationship between vitamin D status and geographic and demographic characteristics in children with JIA?

Methodology

To ensure a comprehensive literature scan, this scoping review applied the iterative methodological framework escribed by Arksey and O'Malley, with refinements by Levac et al. and Colquhoun et al. [14–16]. Five biomedical literature search engines were accessed, in the following sequence: Medline (using Ovid), Embase (using Ovid), Cumulative Index to Nursing and Allied Health Literature (CINHAL), Web of Science, and Scopus. Reference lists within each of the publications retrieved from the web-based searches were scanned to ensure that no relevant citations were missed. Medical Subject Heading (MeSH) terms used for retrieval were "vitamin D" and "juvenile arthritis". The search term "juvenile arthritis" was general enough to capture citations that referred to JCA, JRA and JIA classification terms (Table 1). Search results, which included published articles, letters, and abstracts

Table 1 Comparison of classification systems of chronic childhood arthritis[a]

	American College of Rheumatology 1977 [2]	European League Against Rheumatism 1978 [3]	International League Against Rheumatism 1994 and 2001 [17]
Classification Title	Juvenile Rheumatoid Arthritis	Juvenile Chronic Arthritis	Juvenile Idiopathic Arthritis
Symptom duration	Minimum 6 weeks	Minimum 3 month	Minimum 6 weeks
Subtypes	Systemic	Systemic	Systemic
	Polyarticular	Polyarticular	Polyarthritis RF negative
		JRA (RF positive Polyarticular)	Polyarthritis RF positive
	Pauciarticular	Pauciarticular	Oligoarthritis
			Persistent
			Extended
		Juvenile psoriatic	Psoriatic arthritis
		Juvenile ankylosing spondylitis	Enthesitis-related arthritis
		Arthritis associated with inflammatory bowel disease	
			Undifferentiated arthritis

[a]Prior to 1997, two chronic childhood arthritis classification systems were used. The American College of Rheumatology (ACR) [2] classification criteria referred to chronic childhood arthritis as Juvenile Rheumatoid Arthritis (JRA) and the European League Against Rheumatism (EULAR) applied the term Juvenile Chronic Arthritis (JCA) [3]. Differences between the two classification systems hindered exchange and comparison of data between the two systems [61]. To reconcile differences between ACR and EULAR criteria, the International League Against Rheumatism (ILAR) JIA criteria were introduced. This table provides a comparison of diagnostic criteria [17]. The ILAR classification system defines JIA as all forms of inflammation of one or more joints beginning in children younger than age16 years [17]. JIA is further classified into seven categories based on inclusion and exclusion criteria according to features present within the first six months of disease. The seventh category includes those who do not fit into one category, meet criteria for more than one category, or have exclusion criteria that preclude assigning a category

from conference proceedings, were collated and duplicates of articles removed. Publication titles and abstracts were then screened for relevance to the subject of vitamin D in children with idiopathic chronic arthritis as defined by JIA, JCA, or JRA classification criteria [2, 3, 17]. The full texts of relevant articles were then reviewed.

Inclusion criteria for the review were 1) study conducted in humans, 2) 25(OH)D concentrations reported, 3) participants having a diagnosis of JCA, JRA, or JIA, and 4) JCA, JRA, JIA diagnosis without an associated coexistent autoimmune disease. Exclusion criteria were 1) study conducted in animals, 2) the presence of an associated autoimmune disease 3) pregnant or lactating subjects, 4) 25(OH)D concentrations not reported), and 5) review articles. The process applied to identify eligible articles for the review is shown in Fig. 1 [18]. Articles in any language were eligible; however, no non-English language articles without at least an English abstract were found. From all relevant articles retrieved the following information was extracted: juvenile arthritis classification system (JCA, JRA, or JIA); sample size; sex ratio; patient age (at baseline or time of study if the study was cross-sectional); geographic location (country, city, and latitude and longitude), year of study; 25(OH)D concentration; study conclusion; and, if applicable, control group sample size, characteristics, and 25(OH)D concentration. The latitudes and longitudes reported were that of the city where the study was conducted; if unavailable, the province, state or region's center latitude was used and, as a last resort, the country's central latitude was used. 25(OH)D status by season of measurement was not reported in any of the articles found and therefore could not be considered.

Geographic Information Systems (GIS) mapping was performed using ArcGIS version 10.4 to visualize studies by juvenile arthritis classification, 25(OH)D status, location, and latitude. For all reported studies, an additional map comparing the difference in 25(OH)D concentration between those reporting active versus inactive disease was made.

Defining vitamin D status

Vitamin D deficiency is defined as a serum 25(OH)D concentration less than 30 nmol/L, a 25(OH)D concentration between 30 and 50 nmol/L is considered insufficient, greater than 50 nmol/L is considered sufficient and a 25(OH)D status greater than 125 nmol/L is considered at risk of adverse effects [19]. These values are based on the Institute of Medicine (IOM) review of published research focused on determining the optimal vitamin D concentration for maximal calcium absorption, prevention of rickets, reduction of fracture risk and prevention of osteomalacia in healthy populations [19]. In the most recent review of vitamin D requirements, the IOM concluded that there was inadequate information to make intake recommendations in relation to other biologic roles of vitamin D [19]. The current recommended dietary allowances (RAD) of vitamin D are 400 IU from 0 to 12 months of age and 600 IU per day from 1 to 18 years of age [19].

The Endocrine Society has published clinical practice guidelines for patients at risk of vitamin D deficiency [20]. The Society recommends that at-risk populations, including "obese children and adults and children and adults on anticonvulsant medications, glucocorticoids, antifungals such as ketoconazole, and medications for acquired immune deficiency syndrome be given at least two to three times more vitamin D for their age group to satisfy their body's vitamin D requirement" [20]. The optimal 25(OH)D concentration suggested by the Endocrine Society is 75 nmol/L. To meet this concentration it is recommended that 400–1000 IU be given between 0 to 12 months of age, 600–1000 IU per day from 1 to 8 years of age, and 1500–2000 IU for children between ages 9–18 years [20]. These recommendations, however, are not specific for children with chronic arthritis.

Results of scoping review and discussion

Considerations when evaluating the role of vitamin D in JIA include vitamin D requirements for this population and the role that vitamin D plays in disease activity. Using the specified MeSH search terms (vitamin D and childhood arthritis), 386 reports (full-text articles, conference abstracts, and letters to the editor) were identified. Thirty-eight studies met the inclusion criteria and are the subject of this review (Table 2). One meta-analysis reported cumulative 25(OH)D concentrations from fourteen studies comprising children with JIA, JCA, and JRA and other rheumatic conditions; this meta-analysis was not included in our scoping review but is referenced in the discussion [12]. This present review summarizes accumulated evidence on vitamin D and chronic childhood arthritis by disease activity and latitude. Additionally, this study provides new information about differences in 25(OH)D status between healthy controls and children with JIA.

Vitamin D status in relation to chronic childhood arthritis classification

Twenty-one of the 38 studies (55.3%) reported 25(OH)D status for patients with JIA [21–40], eight (21.1%) for patients with JRA [41–48] and five (13.2%) for JCA patients [49–53]. Additionally, there were four studies that included patients with juvenile arthritis and other rheumatic diseases [54–57]. As the JRA classification system tended to be applied in North America and the JCA classification in Europe, there was a corresponding hemispheric-specific division in the geographic region from which JRA and JCA articles originated. Studies originated from 17 countries at latitudes ranging from 3°S to 61°N (Table 2). There were no eligible studies found that reported data below a latitude of 39°N prior to the

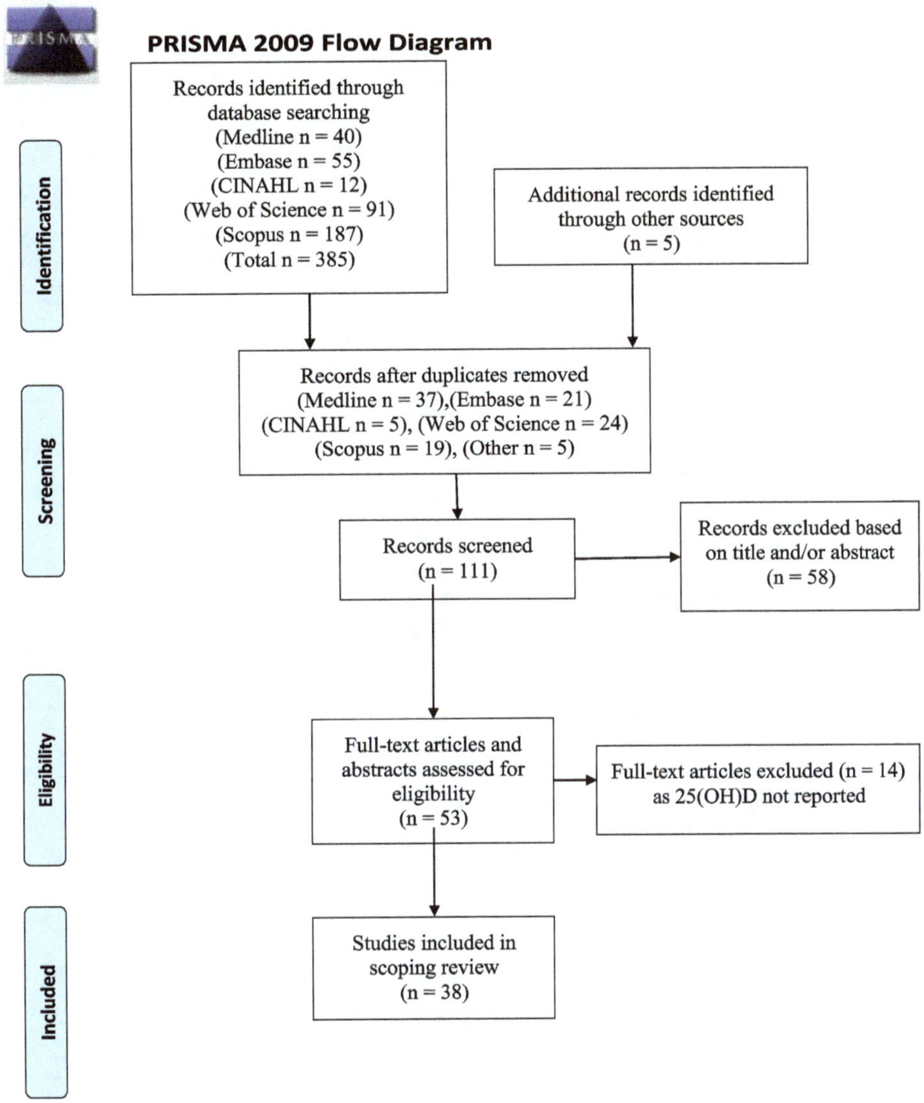

Fig. 1 Articles identified from the retrieved publications reference lists are identified as "other" in the flow diagram

introduction of the ILAR JIA disease classification systemic and no eligible JRA studies above 42°N.

The 2013, systematic literature review of 19 childhood arthritis studies reported vitamin D status (14 reporting 25(OH)D and 11 reporting 1,25(OH)D) suggested that at that time there was no clear link between vitamin D status and children with chronic arthritis [12]. The review also contained a meta-analysis comprising three studies that reported the prevalence of vitamin D insufficiency to be 82% in JIA [12]. Only three studies reported in the meta-analysis were conducted using ILAR JIA criteria [12].

Comparison of study design

Seventeen studies used a cross-sectional design ($n = 17$; 44.7%) [27–30, 32–35, 37, 42, 44, 51, 53, 57–59], 16 (42.1%) a case-control design [21–26, 31, 39, 41, 43, 47–50, 60] and the remainder (5; 13.2%) were randomized controlled trials [40, 45, 46, 54, 55]. The primary objective of the majority of studies was to investigate the relationship between juvenile arthritis and bone health ($n = 20$; 52.6%). In all studies where sex distribution was reported, there were significantly more female participants than males, an observation consistent with the overall preponderance of females in JIA [61]. With the exception of one study [35], the age range of the participants was 0–21 years.

25(OH)D status

Of the 38 studies reviewed, six (15.8%) had mean 25(OH)D concentrations above 75 nmol/L [28, 42, 44, 45, 53, 54]. Seventeen studies (44.7%) had mean 25(OH)D concentrations between 50 and 75 nmol/L [22, 23, 25, 27,

Table 2 Summary of current literature of 25(OH)D status and chronic childhood arthritis

Study Location and Reference	Disease	Sample size (number female)	Age (years) Mean ± SD or range	25(OH)D (nmol/L) Mean ± SD or range	Results relating to vitamin D	Control Group Results	Vitamin D Intake
Study Design: Meta-Analysis							
Meta-Analysis Nisar et al. 2013 [12]	JRA JCA & JIA	$n = 529$	0–18	61.4	Mean of 14 studies 61.4 nmol/L (Range 28.7–139.8) prevalence reported from 3 studies 82% insufficient.		
Study Design: Randomized Controlled Trial							
Cincinnati, Ohio USA Stark et al. 2006 40°N [45]	JRA	$n = 49$	4–10 y	79.9 ± 25.0 (39.9–142.3)	Behaviour intervention to increase calcium intake successful.		
Ioannina, Greece Siampoulou et al. 2001 39°N [40]	JIA	n = 10 (6F)	13.1 ± 2.5	53.9 ± 8.5	All patients were vitamin D replete 25(OH)D > 17.5 nmol/L, most were measured between February to May.		
Missouri, USA Hillman et al. 2008 37°N [54]	Children with arthritis	$n = 18$	3–15	82.1 ± 38.7	Supplemental vitamin D improved status, but supplemental vitamin D or calcium did not improve bone mass.		
Kansas, USA Warady et al. 1994 39°N [55]	Rheumatic disease (6 with JRA)	$n = 10$ (7F) 6 JRA	13.(10.9–18.0)	70.1 ± 21.2	Children with rheumatic disease would benefit from receiving calcium and vitamin D supplements.		
Illinois, USA Reed et al. 1991 40°N [46]	JRA	$n = 13$ (12F)	5–18	70.0 ± 40	Vitamin D may help prevent bone loss in children with active disease.		
Study Design: Case-Control							
Istanbul, Turkey Dagdeviren-Cakir et al. 2016 41°N [21]	JIA	Active disease: $n = 64$ (41) Remission: 53(35)	Active disease: 9.7 ± 4.3 Remission: 9.8 ± 4.3	Active disease: 46.5 ± 23.0 Remission: 47.3 ± 27.5	Vitamin D concentrations in children with JIA were significantly lower than healthy children. Of those who were measured while in remission there was no difference in 25(OH)D concentrations.	Healthy control $n = 100$ 66.8 ± 26.6 nmol/L.	
Mexico city, Mexico Hernandez Rosiles et al. 2015 19°N [39]	JIA	$n = 37$ (27)	12.5 ± 3.1	55.0 ± 13.9	No difference between children with JIA and controls.	Healthy controls $n = 79$ 59.0 ± 7.7 nmol/L.	
Fortaleza, Brazil De Sousa-Studart et al. 2015 3°S [22]	JIA	$n = 51$ (31 F)	13.4 ± 4	55.4 ± 25.0	25(OH)D similar for disease activity status, JIA category, and arthritis severity measure.	Age sex-matched controls 25(OH)D, 75.9 ± 14.0 nmol/L.	
	JIA	$n = 53$	Not reported	Median 42.6	A significant difference between JIA and control 25(OH)D $p < 0.01$.	Control $n = 106$ 25(OH)D 49.9 nmol/L.	

Table 2 Summary of current literature of 25(OH)D status and chronic childhood arthritis *(Continued)*

Study Location and Reference	Disease	Sample size (number female)	Age (years) Mean ± SD or range	25(OH)D (nmol/L) Mean ± SD or range	Results relating to vitamin D	Control Group Results	Vitamin D Intake
Hangzhou, China (article in Chinese, English Abstract) Wang et al. 2015 30°N [60]					No correlation between 25(OH)D and JIA subtypes, ACR pediatric 30, CRP or ESR.		
Florence, Italy Stagi et al. (2014) 43°N [23]	JIA	n = 152 (115F)	16. ± 7.4	54.4 ± 20.5	JIA had reduced 25(OH)D and higher PTH compared to controls. Active disease or frequent flare-ups resulted in lower vitamin D than non-active and no frequent flare-ups.	Control group 25(OH)D 74.4 ± 28.0 nmol/L $p < 0.005$.	Intake JIA 164 ± 84 IU/day control 160 ± 72 IU/day.
New Delhi, India Dey et al. 2014 28°N [31]	JIA	n = 35	3–16	22.0 ± 18.0	Decreased dietary intake of vitamin D and calcium, decreased weight bearing physical activity and sunlight exposure were the major factors for low BMD. Duration of disease 2.30 ± 1.91 yrs.	Age sex-matched controls 25(OH)D 37.9 ± 10.0 nmol/L sig nificant difference.	Intake JIA 123 ± 53.6 (50–207) control 309 ± 62.38 (213–387) IU/day.
Lodz, Poland Szyamanska-Kaluza et al. 2013 51°N [24]	JIA	$n = 50$ (40)	9.4 ± 5.52	43.4 ± 21.1	Vitamin D deficiency is common in this population. No correlation between disease activity, type of JIA or metabolites of vitamin D.	Control $n = 28$ Age, gender matched, hospitalized children 43.4 ± 40.7 nmol/L.	
Sao Paulo, Brazil Munekata et al. 2013 23°S [25]	JIA-polyarticular	$n = 30$ (23F)	14 (4–20)	64.1 ± 21.6	High frequency of 25(OH)D deficiency in both control and JIA groups; no difference between the two. No association of 25(OH)D with disease activity.	Control group age-sex matched (n = 30). 16 non-Caucasian; mean disease duration 5y (1–12) control 2 5(OH)D 67.2 ± 19.0 nmol/L.	
Oslo, Norway Lien et al. 2005 59°N [26]	JIA	$n = 108$	6 to 18	49.7 ± 16.5	No difference in 25(OH)D between control and JIA groups.	Control n = 108 25(OH)D 50.4 ± 8.1 nmol/L D	Intake JIA 164 ± 84 IU control 160 ± 72 IU
London, UK Rooney et al. 2000 51°N [49]	JCA	$n = 34$ (23F)	9.2 (4.6–13.6)	Estimated from graph 45 (14.5–62.5)	Vitamin D status was significantly lower in JCA patients than age-matched controls before treatment, Steroid-treated children have low vitamin D. All but three children re ceived corticosteroids.	Control group 25(OH)D estimate 75 nmol/L.	
Florence, Italy Falcini et al. 1998 43°N [48]	JCA	n = 47 (34)	15 months-12 years(7.13 ± 4.1)	61.4 ± 20.5	The lower serum concentrations of osteocalcin in active disease support the hypothesis that both bone formation and resorption are reduced in JRA	Controls $n = 47$ 25(OH)D 56.7 ± 21.5 nmol/L.	
Missouri, USA Pepmueller et al. 1996 37°N [43]	JRA	$n = 41$	4–18.5	45.7 ± 23.5	Suggest an association between decreased bone mineralization in	Control $n = 62$ 65.5 ± 23.5 nmol/L significant difference.	Vitamin D intake in

Table 2 Summary of current literature of 25(OH)D status and chronic childhood arthritis *(Continued)*

Study Location and Reference	Disease	Sample size (number female)	Age (years) Mean ± SD or range	25(OH)D (nmol/L) Mean ± SD or range	Results relating to vitamin D	Control Group Results	Vitamin D Intake
					JRA and low bone formation that is related to disease severity.		JRA 464 ± 262 IU Intake of controls not reported.
Ioannina, Greece Tzoufi et al. 1994 39°N [50]	JCA	n = 35 (14)	8.8 ± 4.1	39.8 ± 20.5	Disease activity of JCA appears to be associated with lower vitamin D.	Mean disease duration 3.4 years Control *n* = 15 25(OH)D 68.1 ± 15.5 nmol/L control group taking corticosteroids n = 4 25(OH)D 51.4 ± 24.5 nmol/L.	
Missouri, USA Hillman et al. (1994) 37°N [47]	JRA	*n* = 44 (28)	11.8 ± 3.8	66.6 ± 26.7	Lower bone mineral content and bone biomarkers in JRA patients that controls but higher vitamin D in JRA.	N = 37 controls 25(OH)D 53.2 ± 18.7 nmol/L.	
Milano, Italy Bianchi et al. 1990 45°N [41]	JIA	*n* = 36 (64%)	9.96 (5–17)	45.9 nmol/L Reported from Nissar et al. Review	Suggests severe JRA has an influence on bone mass possibly mediated by a decrease in active vitamin D metabolites.	Study duration one year, controls only measured at baseline 25(OH)D 92 ± 17.5 nmol/L *N* = 20	
Huddinge, Sweden Johansson et al. 1986 59°N [52]	JCA	26 (all female)	11–16	63.2 ± 36.4	Statistically lower than controls, however no evidence of deficiency.	Healthy controls n = 28 76.2 ± 28.0 nmol/L	
Study Design: Cross Sectional							
Chongqing, China Tang & Mingyue Conference Abstract 2016 29°N [27]	JIA	*n* = 76 (36)	8.49 ± 3.09	52.8 ± 15.3 nmol/L	JIA patients have reduced serum 25(OH)D3, particularly those with active disease or/and using glucocorticoid.		
Riyahad, Saudi Arabia Alhomaidah et al. 2016 24°N [28]	JIA	*n* = 22 (13)	12.4	14 > 75 nmol/L 8 < 75 nmol/L	Vitamin D insufficiency is frequent in children with JIA.		
Bialystok, Poland (abstract only) Goralczyk et al. 2015 53°N [29]	JIA	*n* = 189 (113)	3–17.7	40.6 ± 23.5	67% 25(OH)D < 50 nmol/L. Obese children had significantly reduced 25(OH)D compared to normal weight peers. Negative relationship between MTX use and 25(OH)D.		
Oporto, Portugal Peixoto et al. 2013 Conference Abstract 41°N [30]	JIA	*n* = 40 (31)	22.3 (4–63)	10 > 75 nmol/L, 19 between 50 and 75 nmol/L, 11 < 20 nmol/L	Prevalence of vitamin D deficiency/ insufficiency among JIA patients is very high.		
Antalya, Turkey Comak et al. 2014 36°N [32]	JIA	n = 47 (29)	9.3 ± 3.9	44.2 ± 29.0	Only 27.7% patients had 25(OH)D > 50 nmol/L. There was a significant negative correlation between vitamin D concentration and disease activity ($p = 0.01$, $r = -0{,}37$).		

Table 2 Summary of current literature of 25(OH)D status and chronic childhood arthritis *(Continued)*

Study Location and Reference	Disease	Sample size (number female)	Age (years) Mean ± SD or range	25(OH)D (nmol/L) Mean ± SD or range	Results relating to vitamin D	Control Group Results	Vitamin D Intake
Salé, Morocco Bouaddi et al. (2014) 34°N [33]	JIA	n = 40 (18)	11 ± 4.23	55.4 ± 27.2	25(OH)D < 75 nmol/L in 75% of sample. Poly arthritis and oligoarthritis 25(OH)D status negatively associated with disease activity in univariate but not multivariate analysis.	Median disease duration two years.	
Helinski, Finland Miettinen et al. 2013 Letter to the Editor 60°N [34]	JIA	n = 136	1–18	M: 63.9 ± 18.0 F: 62.9 ± 20.0	Suggest that JIA subtype may be associated with 25(OH)D concentration in female patients. Seasonal difference with female patients.		
CambridgeUK Nisar et al. 2013 Conference Abstract 52°N [35]	JIA	n = 37 (31)	0–10 (n = 13), 11–20 (n = 12) and > 21 years (n = 12)	49.6 nmol/L (range 13.2–112.0 nmol/L).	Half of patients with JIA have low Vitamin D levels which are inversely related to disease activity and disease duration.		
Boston, USA Pelajo et al. 2012 42°N [36]	JIA	n = 154 (61%)	10.6	72.9 ± 23.0	13% deficient, 42% insufficient. Age, ethnicity, season, BMI associated with 25(OH)D but not vitamin D deficiency.No association with whole sample; small negative association for new onset JIA; mean time since onset 28 months.		
Helinski, Finland Markula-Patjas et al. 2012 60°N [37]	JIA	n = 50 (41)	14.8 (7.0–18.7)	53 nmol/L (20–95 nmol/L)	62% sufficient, 24% insufficient and 14% deficient.		52% taking vitamin D supplement % of DRI median and IQR 187 (57,331).
Saskatchewan, Canada McNally et al. 2009 52°N [59]	Pediatric arthralgia	n = 730 25(OH)D n = 73	< 18	59.9	Significantly more reported fall and winter as season of onset – more referrals from northern SK 40% < 50 nmol/L 42% 50–75 nmol/L Association between psychological stress, school absenteeism vitamin D insufficiency and arthralgia.		
Helinski, Finland Valta et al. 2007 60°N	JIA Glucocorticoid treated	n = 62 (43)	Median 11.8 (4.6–17.9	Median 49 nmol/L 16 (23%) ≤ 37.5 nmol/L	Osteoporosis is a concern in glucocorticoid treated children with JIA.		32% prescribed 400–800 IU vitamin D daily Mean intake 316 IU

Table 2 Summary of current literature of 25(OH)D status and chronic childhood arthritis *(Continued)*

Study Location and Reference	Disease	Sample size (number female)	Age (years) Mean ± SD or range	25(OH)D (nmol/L) Mean ± SD or range	Results relating to vitamin D	Control Group Results	Vitamin D Intake
							(range 44–1204 IU).
Ohio, USA Henderson et al. 1997 40°N [44]	JRA	$n = 48$ (37)	8.1 ± 1.9	89.4 ± 28.7	Serum 1,25-dihydroxyvitamin D concentrations were able to accurately segregate 79.6% of the JRA subjects into either the low or normal BMD groups.		%RDA 87.6 ± 52.7.
Illinois, USA Reed et al. 1993 40°N [42]	JRA	$n = 27$ (23)	2.9–16	84.9 ± 11.0	No difference in vitamin D status between active and inactive groups. Children with JRA who have improvement in their disease activity have an improvement in BMD heralded by an increase in serum osteocalcin values 4–87 months from disease onset.		
Harrow, UK Reeve et al. 1993 51°N [53]	JCA- treated with glucocorticoids	Prednisone n = 17 Deflazacort $n = 17$	Prednisone 10.6 ± 3.7 Deflazacort 10.3 ± 3.9	Prednisone 140.8Deflazacort 115.6	25(OH)D was surprisingly high, there was no difference between the two groups $p = 0.8$.		
Chicago, Illinois Reed et al. 1990 40°N [57]	Chronic Rheumatic Disease	$n = 113$ (82) JRA $n = 83$	1.5 to 21	Range of groups 44.9 ± 15.0 to 54.9 ± 22.5	No difference between those with active and inactive disease.		
London, UK Elsasser et al. 1982 51°N [51]	JCA	$n = 63$ serum 25(OH)D $n = 29$	Not reported	24.5 nmol/L (9 > 25 nmol/L, 20 < 25 nmol/L)	There was a marginally significant correlation between TBD and 25(OH)D concentrations ($r = 0.37$. $P < 0.05$). Only nine children had acceptable vitamin D status.		

30, 33, 34, 36, 37, 39, 40, 46–48, 55, 59] and 15 (39.5%) had values below 50 nmol/L [21, 24, 26, 29, 31, 32, 35, 38, 41, 43, 49–51, 57, 60]. Of those 15 studies, 10 reported the mean 25(OH)D value, the median value reported for one study and a range or cutoff was provided for four studies). Of the 14 studies (36.8%) that published mean 25(OH)D status of healthy control groups, nine (64.3%) had mean control values significantly greater than the population with childhood arthritis [21–23, 31, 41, 43, 49, 50], three (21.4%) had concentrations that were statistically similar [25, 39, 60], and two studies (14.3%) had mean 25(OH)D values significantly below the juvenile arthritis comparison groups [47, 48]. One study compared 25(OH)D concentrations in children with JIA to hospitalized children and found no statistically significant difference between the two groups [24]. Mean 25(OH)D status of most studies (32 of the 38; 84.2%) was below the optimal concentration of 75 nmol/L in children with arthritis [20].

Geography in relation to 25(OH)D status in chronic childhood arthritis

Vitamin D status in children with JIA appears to follow a north-south gradient (Fig. 2). While this could be due to the diagnostic resources of the countries reporting values, the gradient does appear to be present in Europe where access to care and diagnostic resources are similar. Interestingly, the relationship between reduced vitamin D status and increased disease activity also appears to be present and follow a north-south gradient (Fig. 3). More studies are required to confirm this relationship worldwide, especially in locations around the equator as well as in the southern hemisphere where thus far only two studies have taken place [22, 25].

The major source of vitamin D for most people is endogenous vitamin D synthesis induced by sunlight exposure [62]. Above 33° latitude UVB radiation is not intense enough for the cutaneous synthesis of vitamin D all year long [63, 64]. At latitudes 42° and 53° North, between October to April, UVB radiation is not intense enough to elicit endogenous vitamin D synthesis [65] thus potentiating the risk of vitamin D deficiency, [63].

The prevalence of JIA, as well as the dominating subtype, varies with latitude [1]. As illustrated in Fig. 2, seven reviewed studies (18.4%) were conducted in populations residing at latitudes at or below 33° [22, 25, 27, 28, 31, 39, 60], 19 studies (50.0%) were conducted between 33 and 50° [21, 23, 30, 32, 36, 40–48, 50, 54, 55, 57, 66], and 12 at a latitude above 50° [24, 26, 29, 34, 35, 37, 38, 49, 51, 53, 59]. For those below 33°, 1 study (14.3%) reported a mean 25(OH)D concentration > 75 nmol/L, 4 (57%) reported a concentration between 50 and 75 nmol/L, and two (29%) reported values less than 50 nmol/L. For the studies that took place between 33 and 45° latitude, four studies (21.1%) reported a 25(OH)D concentration > 75 nmol/L (21%), nine (47.4%) reported a concentration between 50 and 75 nmol/L(47%) and six (31.6%) reported values less than 50 nmol/L. From the studies that took place above 45° latitude, one study (8.3%) reported a 25(OH)D concentration > 75 nmol/L, four (21.1%) reported a concentration between 50 and 75 nmol/L (33%) and seven (36.8%) reported values less than 50 nmol/L (39%).

Current chronic childhood arthritis diagnostic criteria

Of the 21 studies that applied the current chronic childhood arthritis criteria used by ILAR to diagnose children with JIA, only one study reported mean 25(OH)D concentrations above 75 nmol/L (15%) [28]. The majority of the studies ($n = 11$; 52.4%) reported mean concentrations between 50 and 75 (52%) nmol/L [22, 23, 25, 27, 30, 33, 34, 36, 37, 40, 67], and the remaining studies ($n = 9$; 42.9%) reported a mean concentration below 50 nmol/L (43%) [21, 24, 26, 29, 31, 32, 35, 38, 60]. As latitude increased, the percentage of studies that reported mean 25(OH)D in the 50–75 nmol/L range decreased.

Vitamin D and disease activity

No single measure has been established as an accurate indicator of childhood arthritis disease activity. While C-reactive protein and Erythrocyte Sedimentation Rate are indicators of inflammation, they alone do not fully reflect overall disease activity. In the studies reviewed, a variety of validated composite scores were used to measure function or disease activity, including the Childhood Health Assessment Questionnaire (CHAQ), the Juvenile Arthritis Disease Activity Score - 27 (JADAS-27) and American College of Rheumatology Pediatric 30 Criteria (ARC Peds 30) [68–70].

Fifteen of the 38 studies comprising this present review (39.5%) evaluated the relationship between vitamin D and disease activity (Fig. 3). Seven studies (18.4%) reported that patients with active disease or those with elevated inflammatory biomarkers had lower 25(OH)D concentrations than those patients who were in remission or who had less disease activity [23, 27, 30, 32, 35, 41, 50]. One study (26.3%) showed the opposite relationship; those with active disease had higher vitamin D concentrations than those with inactive disease [34]. Of the seven studies (18.5%) that reported no relationship between 25(OH)D and disease activity [21, 22, 25, 33, 36, 42, 57] one found a relationship between 25(OH)D concentrations and disease activity in the univariate but not the multivariate analysis [33]. Except for one study conducted in Turkey [21], all other studies conducted in Europe that explored disease activity reported an inverse association between vitamin D and disease activity.

Long-term cohort studies can further clarify the relationship between vitamin D concentration and disease

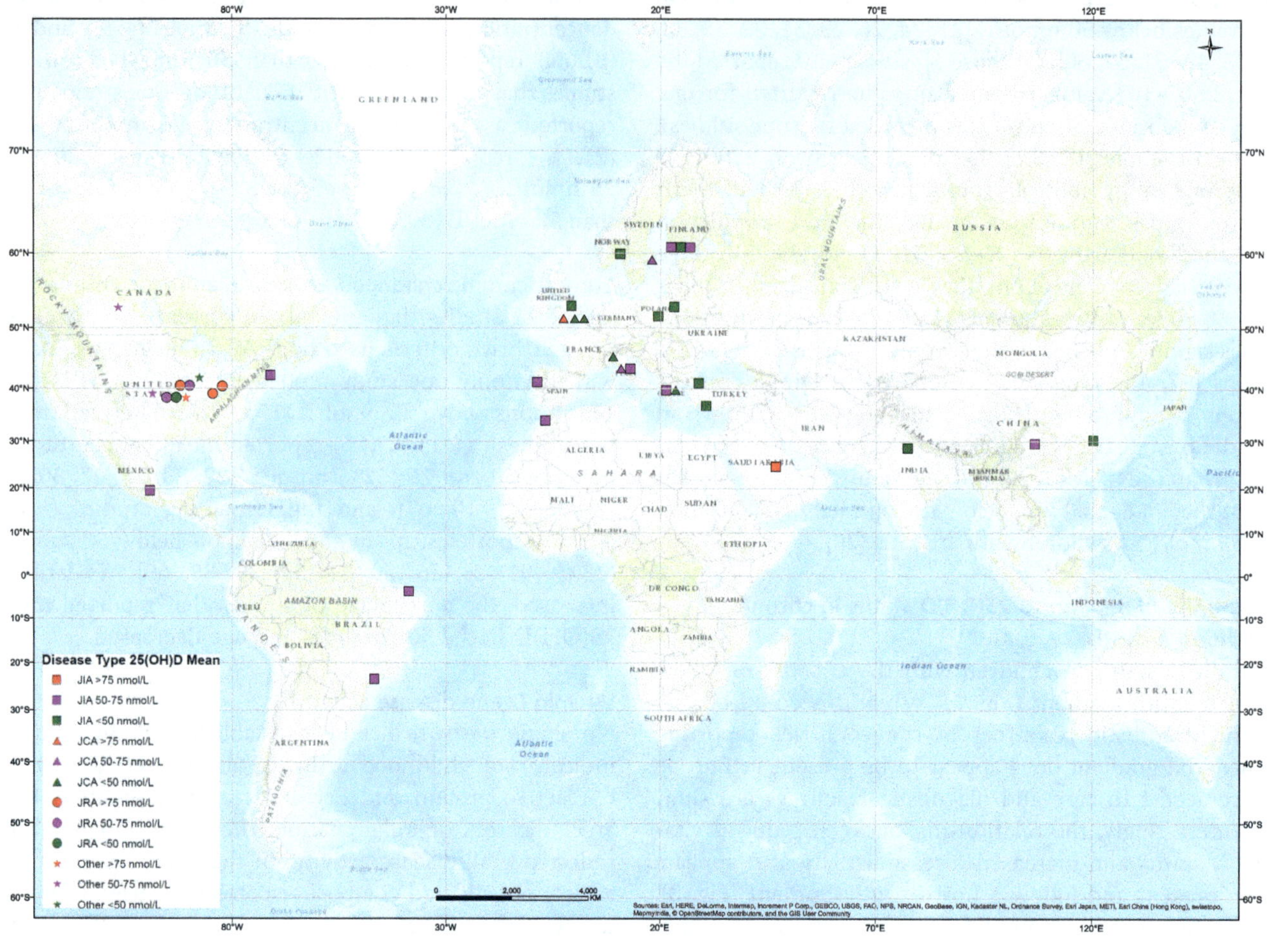

Fig. 2 Disease type by 25(OH)D group. Note: Overlapping points are spread out. Map Produced by The Spatial Initiative, University of Saskatchewan, 2018

duration or frequency of relapse. Such an association was explored in a cross-sectional study which found significantly reduced 25(OH)D status in JIA patients ($n = 152$) compared with 188 age-and-sex-matched controls [23]. Active disease or frequent relapse was associated with reduced vitamin D status compared to patients with no active disease or frequent flare-ups. The authors questioned whether JIA patients with more severe disease require higher supplementation of vitamin D to maintain normal 25(OH) D concentrations. As latitude increases more studies report a difference in vitamin D status between patients with active versus inactive disease in comparison to lower latitudes as illustrated in Fig. 3.

To date, the evidence to support a relationship between vitamin D and disease activity with autoimmune diseases in humans is correlative and not causative [71]. Long-term, adequately powered randomized studies which control for confounding variables (sun exposure, season, and vitamin D intake) are required to confirm a causative relationship between vitamin D and disease activity.

Potential requirements of vitamin D intake

Vitamin D intake was only measured in seven studies [23, 26, 31, 37, 38, 43, 44]. All of these studies reported a mean or median vitamin D intake that was less than the Estimated Average Requirement (EAR) of 400 IU per day set by the IOM [19]. This is the amount of vitamin D that is expected to be sufficient for 50% of the population [19]. This indicator is used to evaluate the prevalence of inadequacy at the population level. The recommendation at the individual level is the Recommended Dietary Allowance (RDA) which ranges from 400 to 600 IU based on age groups. Two studies reported intake of vitamin D supplements by study participants but neither had a mean 25(OH)D that reached the optimal concentration [38, 44]. Three studies reported intake of both children with JIA and healthy controls [23, 26, 31]. Vitamin D intake and status was similar for two JIA patient groups [23, 26], and lower intake resulted in lower vitamin D status in the third group [31]. In comparison to the control groups, Lien et al. found similar intake and 25(OH)D status between those with

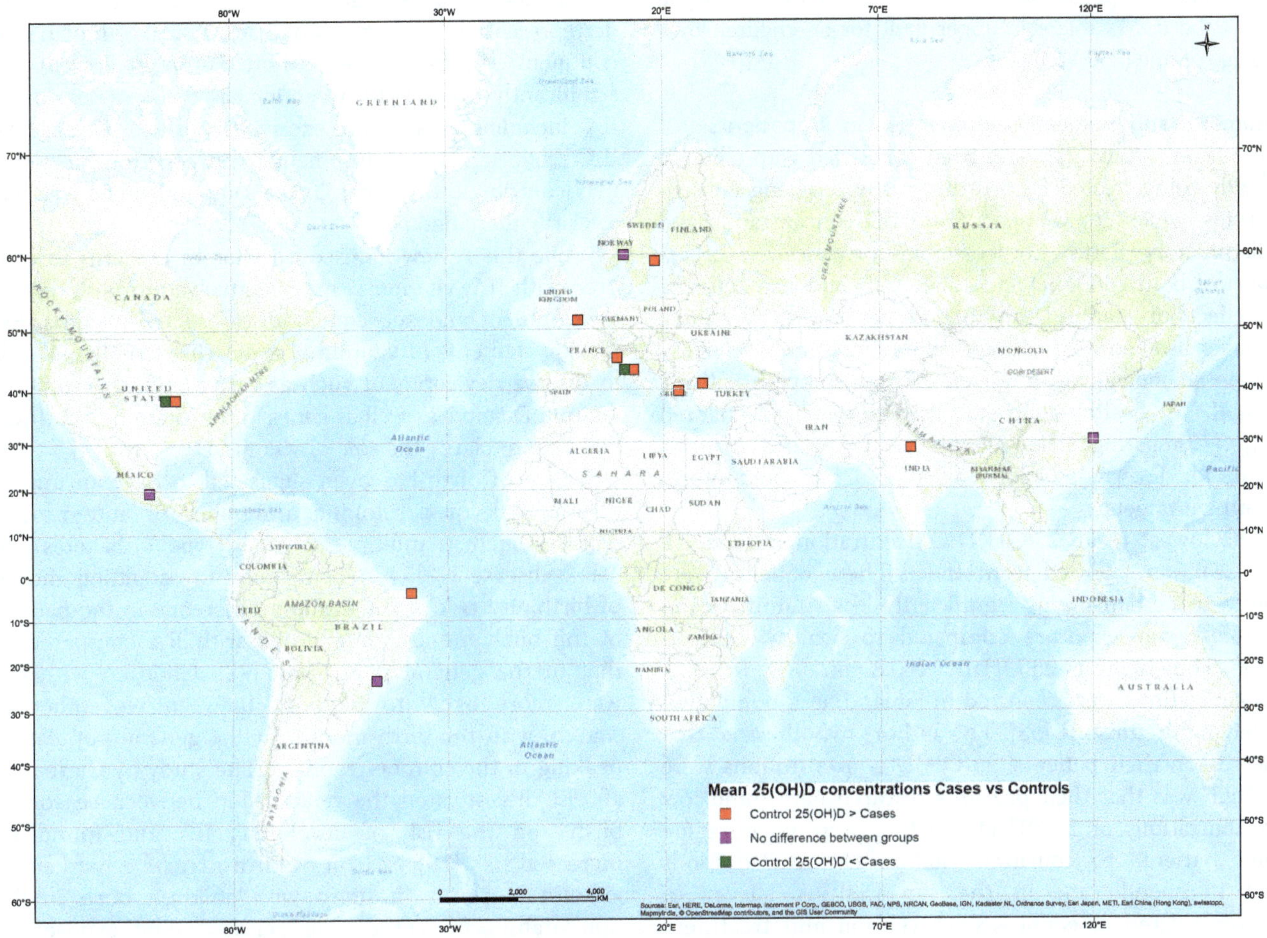

Fig. 3 Difference in 25(OH)D concentration in active vs inactive chronic childhood arthritis patients. Note: Overlapping points are spread out. Map Produced by The Spatial Initiative, University of Saskatchewan, 2018

JIA and controls [26]. Stagi et al. reported similar intake of vitamin D and higher 25(OH)D in controls, and in the study reported by Dey et al. the intake of control participants was two times higher than the participants with JIA and the control group had higher 25(OH)D concentrations [23, 31].

It has been theorized that there may be an increased utilization of vitamin D during active inflammation, possibly caused by \the presence of vitamin D receptor polymorphisms in patients with autoimmune diseases [6, 72]. Additional studies investigating vitamin D intake from all sources (both food and supplements) are required to determine if children with chronic arthritis require additional vitamin D to maintain serum concentrations in comparison to healthy children. Understanding this relationship will be important in the use of vitamin D as a potential adjunct therapy. Additionally, improved understanding of vitamin D needs in children with chronic arthritis will help to clarify the role of vitamin D in the underlying disease processes so that therapies that target specific vitamin D responsive immune pathways can be developed. By exploring the factors that influence vitamin D status (genetics, environment, and nutrition), we will be better able to discern an association between vitamin D and JIA.

Two articles have discussed vitamin D requirements for children with rheumatic conditions not in the context of corticosteroids. In 2011, von Scheven and Burnham suggested that in the absence of specific guidelines for children with rheumatic conditions that the American Academy of Pediatrics guidelines of 400 IU per day be used as a suggested minimum dosing regimen [4]. The authors cautioned that providing large doses of vitamin D can result in providing "too much of a good thing" and that studies comparing children with rheumatic diseases to healthy children are required. The second article was published by Vojinovic and Cimaz in 2015 and recommends that the guidelines set out by the Endocrinology Society for patients receiving corticosteroids be followed for all children with rheumatic diseases [73]. This would result in a dose of 2–3 times the current recommendation and would be approximately 2000 IU/day. This dose is still below the IOM's tolerable upper limit for all children over the age of one (2500 IU) [19].

Vitamin D and medication interactions in JIA patients

All but one study [24], have been conducted with children already being treated for arthritis, many receiving corticosteroids, which could impact 25(OH)D concentration and inflammatory status. Corticosteroids promote the breakdown of both 25(OH)D and 1,25(OH)D and also counteract effects of vitamin D on bone formation [74, 75]. These patients also had varying disease duration. A study of newly diagnosed individuals, however, did not compare patients with JIA to healthy controls but to hospitalized children [24] . Comparing children with JIA to healthy controls allows for discerning biologic differences that could inform treatment targets.

The lowest mean 25(OH)D concentration, 22 nmol/L ($n = 35$) was reported from India. These patients were found to be consuming significantly less vitamin D and had less sun exposure compared to healthy controls [31]. The highest 25(OH)D, 140.8 nmol/L ($n = 17$), concentrations were reported in Finland, in a population receiving Prednisone [53]. The authors hypothesized that the reason their patients' 25(OH)D concentrations were so high was that their previous research had found low concentrations of 25(OH)D and they were encouraging their patients to consume vitamin D fortified foods and to spend time in the sun [53]. A survey of steroid-related osteoporosis, prevention and treatment practices of pediatric rheumatologists in North America was conducted by Soybilgic et al. in 2014 [76]. They found that the majority of pediatric rheumatologists are recommending vitamin D for patients who were on long-term corticosteroids [76]. The role of vitamin D in mediating bone health, especially in relation to corticosteroids, has been established [75]. Both short and long-term corticosteroid intake even at small doses impact bone health in patients with autoimmune diseases [74]. The role and an appropriate amount of vitamin D intake or 25(OH)D target for inflammation or disease activity have yet to be established.

Additional research directions

Considering ethnicity when comparing incidence and prevalence amongst populations would be useful in understanding if the regional differences observed are due to environmental or genetic factors or a combination of the two. Evidence from a multiethnic cohort study of 1082 children at The Hospital for Sick Children, Toronto, Canada investigated the influence of ethnicity on the risk of developing JIA [77]. When the diversity of the study population was compared to that of the general Toronto region population, there was an overrepresentation of patients of European and Indigenous descent and an underrepresentation of patients of Black, Asian, or Indian subcontinent ethnicity in their cohort. European descent was significantly associated with an increased risk of developing JIA, including all subtypes except RF-positive polyarticular JIA. Exploring the environmental and genetic factors that may contribute to JIA risk in the same individual will help to clarify these findings.

While this review focused on vitamin D status in children with JIA, vitamin D may be involved in both disease development and subsequent disease activity status. Exploring elements of vitamin D status that may have a role in disease development such as early life and gestational vitamin D status as well as genes in the vitamin D pathway will help to clarify the role of vitamin D.

Season of birth has been suggested to have an impact on the risk of developing a number of autoimmune diseases such as multiple sclerosis, type 1 diabetes and celiac disease [78]. A recent study investigating month of birth and risk of JIA found a difference in the pattern of the birth month for children with JIA compared to that of the general population [78]. Children with JIA were more likely to be born between November to March, with the birth month for the general population peaking in the summer months. The study by Carlens et al. also investigated the relationship between season of birth and the risk of developing JIA and found no increased risk [79]. Season of birth may be a marker for vitamin D status in utero with children born in the non-vitamin D synthesizing periods being exposed to less vitamin D during their time in utero than those who are born during the vitamin D synthesizing seasons.

The Childhood Arthritis Risk factor Identification sTudY (CLARITY) explored the use of nutritional supplements during pregnancy and the risk of developing JIA [80]. The use of vitamin D and fish oil during pregnancy in case mothers was not significantly different from controls following covariate adjustments [80]. A case-cohort investigation from Denmark, comparing 25(OH)D status in children diagnosed with either oligoarticular or polyarticular JIA using dried blood spot samples that were collected at birth did not find any association between 25(OH)D status at birth and risk of developing JIA [81]. Concentrations of 25(OH)D fluctuated significantly by season of birth and year of birth (calendar year). There was no follow up to determine if 25(OH)D status or season during the first few months of life impacted risk of JIA or whether other subtypes of JIA were impacted by season of birth of 25(OH)D status at birth.

Certain VDR gene polymorphisms may be associated with different biologic response to vitamin D. The Cdx2 polymorphism of the VDR gene specifically the GG genotype, have been suggested to be more represented in patients with JIA compared to healthy controls who more often have the GA genotype [82]. Recently the idea of investigating epistasis (gene-gene interactions) amongst genes in the inflammatory and vitamin D pathway and how their interactions contribute to JIA risk was explored by Ellis et al. [86]. This is the first study to explore this interaction, and the authors suspect that through exploring these interactions there is the opportunity to account for the missing heritability that has been observed with complex diseases with genetic components [86]. Their work found evidence of epistasis amongst tyrosine-protein phosphatase non-receptor type 2 (PTPN2) gene and the vitamin D binding protein gene in contributing to the risk of JIA [86]. The role of genes in the vitamin D pathway on both disease development and disease activity are still in the early stages of investigation. Also how they impact the biological response involving vitamin D and inflammation remains unclear. Investigating genetic, nutritional and environmental factors that influence vitamin D in JIA could help inform ways in which vitamin D status influences the occurrence and activity of JIA. Understanding if genetic variants increase the risk of disease development will help tailor vitamin D management in individual patients and contribute to improving control of disease activity and improve outcomes.

A north-south gradient of incidence and a mechanism for the suppression of inflammation in relation to 25(OH)D status has been suggested. However, no study has summarized the current evidence of chronic childhood arthritis diagnosis by 25(OH)D status in relation to latitude and disease activity. This first step is important for the development of future studies leading to the exploration of potential optimal target concentrations of vitamin D for the reduction of inflammation in children with chronic arthritis.

Limitations

This scoping review has limitations due to the limited amount of comparative data. Season of measurement and JIA subtype could not be considered due to a lack of reporting in most reviewed articles. With the exception of one study, all studies reviewed used various unreported types of medication in patients who had had JIA for varying durations. These variables can make it difficult to interpret the relationship between vitamin D and disease activity in relation to both inflammation status and risk of relapse. Of the studies that investigated the relationship between vitamin D and function or disease activity, various measures were used. The most common included the CHAQ, JADAS-27 and ARC Peds 30. The JADAS-27 and ACRS Peds 30 both include active joint counts in their scoring which confounds comparisons of disease activity between patients with different JIA that are defined by numbers of joints involved. Subtypes [17, 83, 84]. Many studies included multiple subtypes of JIA measured by the same disease activity score that included an active joint count. This review was unable to explore the relationship between vitamin D status and ethnicity, vitamin D receptor genes or other genes that influence vitamin D metabolism.

Conclusion

This is the first scoping review to summarize research relating to vitamin D and JIA in the context of vitamin D status, latitude, disease activity. It is also the first to map the results according to geography. Thirty-two studies (84.2%) reported a mean 25(OH)D concentration below 75 nmol/L or the optimal value. This suggests that whether due to inadequate intake or increased utilization the majority of children with juvenile arthritis do not have optimal 25(OH)D status as defined by the Endocrine Society [20]. The optimal concentration of 25(OH)D and the corresponding dietary requirements for patients with chronic childhood arthritis has yet to be determined. Further, the relationship between vitamin D status and disease activity in children with JIA is still unclear. Studying newly diagnosed patients who are treatment naive for longer periods of time would help characterize this relationship as there would be fewer confounders associated with patients who have had the disease for varying durations (medication, lifestyle modifications, and disease duration). Thus far, we know that there is a role for vitamin D in the inflammatory pathways, a high prevalence of 25(OH)D insufficiency among children with JIA, and an established link of vitamin D with other autoimmune diseases. We do not, however, know the optimal vitamin D status for children with JIA, whether reduced vitamin D is caused by increased utilization or reduced vitamin D status in children with JIA, the impact of vitamin D in disease activity or the role of VDR polymorphisms with JIA. Larger, long-term studies of new-onset JIA are required to explore the association. The relationship between vitamin D status and JIA over time in newly diagnosed individuals has yet to be investigated. Investigating the genetic and environmental role that vitamin D plays in the prevention and control of JIA in the same children will help to tease out the multifaceted role played by vitamin D in this disease. Being able to suggest specific targets for vitamin D status as a potential adjunct therapy in the treatment of JIA and understanding how genetic variants increase the risk of disease development will enhance the quality of life of patients and their families.

Abbreviations

1,25(OH)2D): 1,25-dihydroxyvitamin D; 25(OH)D: 25-dihydroxyvitamin D; CINHAL: Cumulative Index to Nursing and Allied Health Literature; CLARITY: Childhood Arthritis Risk factor Identification sTudY; CYP27B1: Cytochrome p450 27B1; GIS: Geographic Information Systems;

IOM: Institute of Medicine; JCA: Juvenile Chronic Arthritis; JIA: Juvenile Idiopathic Arthritis; JRA: Juvenile Rheumatoid Arthritis; MeSH: Medical Subject Heading; VDR: Vitamin D receptor

Acknowledgments
We acknowledge the help of Vicky Duncan, Librarian, University of Saskatchewan, in designing the outline of the search procedure, and Dr. Weiping Zeng of the Spatial Analysis Initiative/Social Science Research Laboratory at the University of Saskatchewan for creating maps. This research was supported, in part, by the Jim Pattison Children's Hospital Foundation of Saskatchewan.

Funding
The University of Saskatchewan Scholarship for Sarah Finch.
The Jim Pattison Children's Hospital Foundation.

Authors' contributions
The co-authors designed the review. SF drafted the manuscript under the direct supervision of HV and AR. HV and AR provided critical review and feedback throughout different stages of the manuscript preparation. All authors read and approved the final manuscript.

Competing interests
The authors declare that they have no competing interests.

Author details
[1]College of Pharmacy and Nutrition, University of Saskatchewan, Saskatoon, Canada. [2]Department of Pediatrics, University of Saskatchewan, Saskatoon, Canada. [3]College of Pharmacy & Nutrition and School of Public Health, University of Saskatchewan, 104 Clinic Place, Saskatoon, SK S7N 2Z4, Canada.

References

1. Manners PJ, Bower C. Worldwide prevalence of juvenile arthritis - why does it vary so much? J Rheumatol. 2002;29:1520–30.
2. Brewer EJ Jr, Bass J, Baum J, Cassidy JT, Fink C, Jacobs J, Hanson V, Levinson JE, Schaller JSJ. Current proposed revision of JRA criteria. JRA criteria Subcommittee of the Diagnostic and Therapeutic Criteria Committee of the American rheumatism section of the Arthritis Foundation. Arthritis Rheum. 1977;20:195–9.
3. Woods P. Special meeting on nomenclature and classification of arthritis in children. Basel: EULAR Publishers; 1978. p. 47–50.
4. Von Scheven E, Burnham JM. Vitamin D supplementation in the pediatric rheumatology clinic. Curr Rheumatol Rep. 2011;13:110–6.
5. Agmon-Levin N, Theodor E, Segal RM, Shoenfeld Y. Vitamin D in systemic and organ-specific autoimmune diseases. Clin Rev Allergy Immunol. 2013; 45:256–66.
6. Cutolo M, Pizzorni C, Sulli A. Vitamin D endocrine system involvement in autoimmune rheumatic diseases. Autoimmun Rev. 2011;11:84–7.
7. Hewison M. Vitamin D and the immune system: new perspectives on an old theme. Rheum Dis Clin N Am. 2012;38:125–39.
8. Adorini L, Penna G. Control of autoimmune diseases by the vitamin D endocrine system. Nat Clin Pract Rheumatol. 2008;4:404–12.
9. Holick MF. Vitamin D: Extraskeletal Health. Rheum Dis Clin N Am. 2012; 38:141–60.
10. Baeke F, Takiishi T, Korf H, Gysemans C, Mathieu C. Vitamin D: modulator of the immune system. Curr Opin Pharmacol. 2010;10:482–96.
11. Sabbagh Z, Markland J, Vatanparast H. Vitamin D status is associated with disease activity among rheumatology outpatients. Nutrients. 2013; 5:2268–75.
12. Nisar MK, Masood F, Cookson P, Sansome A, Ostör AJK. What do we know about juvenile idiopathic arthritis and vitamin D? A systematic literature review and meta-analysis of current evidence. Clin Rheumatol. 2013;32:729–34.
13. Daudt HM, van Mossel C, Scott SJ. Enhancing the scoping study methodology: a large, inter-professional team's experience with Arksey and O'Malley's framework. BMC Med Res Methodol. 2013;13:48.
14. Arksey H, Malley LO. Scoping studies: towards a methodological framework. Int J Soc Res Methodol. 2005;8:19–32.
15. Levac D, Colquhoun H, O'Brien KK. Scoping studies: advancing the methodology. Implement Sci. 2010;5:69.
16. Colquhoun HL, Levac D, O'Brien KK, Straus S, Tricco AC, Perrier L, et al. Scoping reviews: time for clarity in definition, methods, and reporting. J Clin Epidemiol. 2014;67:1291–4.
17. Petty R, Southwood T, Manners P. International league of associations for rheumatology. International league of associations for rheumatology classification of juvenile idiopathic arthritis. J Rheumatol. 2004;31:390–2.
18. Moher D, Liberati A, Tetzlaff J, Altman DG. Systematic reviews and meta-analyses: the PRISMA statement. Annu Intern Med. 2009;151:264–9.
19. Institute of Medicine. Food and nutrition board, dietary reference intakes for calcium and vitamin D. Washington: National Academy Press; 2010.
20. Holick MF, Binkley NC, Bischoff-Ferrari HA, Gordon CM, Hanley DA, Heaney RP, et al. Evaluation, treatment, and prevention of vitamin D deficiency: an Endocrine Society clinical practice guideline. J Clin Endocrinol Metab. 2011; 96:1911–30.
21. Dağdeviren-çakır A, Arvas A, Barut K, Gür E, Kasapçopur Ö. Serum vitamin D levels during activation and remission periods of patients with juvenile idiopathic arthritis and familial Mediterranean fever. Turk J Pediatr. 2016;58: 125–31.
22. de Sousa Studart SA, Leite AC, Marinho AL, Pinto AC, Rabelo Júnior CN, de Melo NR, et al. Vitamin D levels in juvenile idiopathic arthritis from an equatorial region. Rheumatol Int. 2015;35:17–23.
23. Stagi S, Bertini F, Cavalli L, Matucci-cerinic M, Brandi ML, Falcini F. Determinants of vitamin D levels in children, adolescents, and young adults with juvenile idiopathic arthritis determinants of vitamin D levels in children, adolescents, and young adults with juvenile idiopathic arthritis. J Rheumatol. 2014;41:1884–92.
24. Szymańska-Kałuża J, Biernacka-ZielińskaM, Stańczyk J, Smolewska E. Vitamin D level in children with juvenile idiopathic arthritis and its correlation with clinical picture of the disease. Reumatologia. 2013;51:271–6.
25. Munekata RV, Terreri MTRA, Peracchi OAB, Len C. Serum 25-hydroxyvitamin D and biochemical markers of bone metabolism in patients with juvenile idiopathic arthritis. Braz J Med Biol Res. 2013;46:98–102.
26. Lien G, Selvaag AM, Flatø B, Haugen M, Vinje O, Sørskaar D, et al. A two-year prospective controlled study of bone mass and bone turnover in children with early juvenile idiopathic arthritis. Arthritis Rheum. 2005;52:833–40.
27. Tang X. Mingyue L. Association between vitamin D concentrations with disease activity and bone mineral density of juvenile idiopathic arthritis patients. International Journal of Rheumatic Diseases. Conference: 18th Asia Pacific League of Associations for Rheumatology Congress, APLAR. China. 2016. Conference Start 20160926. Conference End: 20160929. 2016;19:158.
28. Alhomaidah D, Alsagheir A, Al-mayouf SM. ScienceDirect coexistence of endocrinopathies in children with rheumatic diseases. Int J Pediatr Adolesc Med. 2016;3:119–22.
29. Goralczyk A, Konstantynowicz J, Abramowicz P, Dobrenko E, Babinska-Malec E. Deficits of vitamin D are strongly associated with methotrexate treatment in patients with juvenile idiopathic arthritis. Bone Abstr. 2015;183
30. Peixoto D, Teixeira F, Lucas R, Costa J, Costa L, AD. Vitamin D status in patients with juvenile idiopathic arthritis. Ann. Rheum. Dis. Conf. Annu. Eur. Congr. Rheumatol. Eur. Leag. Against Rheum. EULAR. 2012;2013:71.
31. Dey S, Jahan A, Yadav TP, Bhagwani DK, Sachdev N. Measurement of bone mineral density by dual energy X-ray absorptiometry in juvenile idiopathic arthritis. Indian J Pediatr. 2014;81:126–32.
32. Çomak E, Doğan ÇS, Uslu-gökçeoğlu A, Akbaş H, Özdem S. Association between vitamin D deficiency and disease activity in juvenile idiopathic arthritis. Turk J Pediatr. 2014;56:626–31.
33. Bouaddi I, Rostom S, El Badri D, Hassani A, Chkirate B, Abouqal R, et al. Vitamin D concentrations and disease activity in Moroccan children with juvenile idiopathic arthritis. BMC Musculoskelet Disord. 2014;15:115.
34. Miettinen ME, Kinnunen L, Harjutsalo V, Reinert-Hartwall L, Lamberg-Allardt C, Toumilehto J, Saila H. Serum 25-hydroxyvitamin D in juvenile idiopathic arthritis patients in Finland-letters to the editors. Clin Exp Rheumatol. 2013;31:988.

35. Nisar M, Cookson P, Masood F, Sansome A, Ostor A. Is there a link between vitamin D and juvenile idiopathic arthritis? Ann Rheum Dis Conf Annu Eur Congr Rheumatol Eur Leag Against Rheum EULAR. Conference Start: 20130612. Conference End:20130615.2013:72.
36. Pelajo CF, Lopez-Benitez JM, Kent DM, Price LL, Miller LC, Dawson-Hughes B. 25-hydroxyvitamin D levels and juvenile idiopathic arthritis: is there an association with disease activity? Rheumatol Int. 2012;32:3923–9.
37. Markula-patjas KP, Valta HL, Kerttula LI, Soini IH, Honkanen VEA, Mäkitie OM, et al. Prevalence of vertebral compression fractures and associated factors in children and adolescents with severe juvenile idiopathic arthritis prevalence of vertebral compression fractures and associated factors in children and adolescents with severe Juvenil. J Rheumatol. 2012;39:365–73.
38. Valta H, Lahdenne P, Jalanko H, Aalto K. Bone health and growth in glucocorticoid-treated patients with juvenile idiopathic arthritis. J Rheumatol. 2007;34:831–6.
39. Rosiles VH, Salazar CD, Velazquez RM, Ruiz RR, CP. Determination of 25(OH)D serum levels in children with systemic lupus erythematosus and juvenile idiopathic arthritis. Bol Med del Hosp Infant Mex. 2015;72:99–105.
40. Siamopoulou A, Challa A, Kapoglou P, Cholevas V, Mavridis AK, Lapatsanis PD. Effects of intranasal salmon calcitonin in juvenile idiopathic arthritis: an observational study. Calcif Tissue Int. 2001;69:25–30.
41. Bianchi ML, Bardare M, Caraceni MP, Cohen E, Falvella S, Borzani M, et al. Bone metabolism in juvenile rheumatoid arthritis. Bone Miner. 1990;9:153–62.
42. Reed AM, Haugen M, Pachman LM, Langman CB. Repair of osteopenia in children with juvenile rheumatoid arthritis. J Pediatr. 1993;122:693–6.
43. Pepmueller PH, Cassidy JT, Allen SH, Hillman LS. Bone mineralization and bone mineral metabolism in children with juvenile rheumatoid arthritis. Arthritis Rheum. 1996;39:746–57.
44. Henderson CJ, Cawkwell GD, Specker BL, Sierra RI, Wilmott RW, Campaigne BN, et al. Non-corticosteroid-treated prepubertal children with juvenile rheumatoid arthritis. Arthritis Rheum. 1997;40:1967–75.
45. Stark LJ, Davis AM, Janicke DM, Mackner LM, Hommel KA, Bean JA, Lovell D, Heubi JE, KH. A randomized clinical trial of dietary calcium to improve bone accretion in children with juvenile rheumatiod arthritis. Pediatrics. 2006;148:501–7.
46. Reed A, Haugen M, Pachman LM, Langman CB. 25-Hydroxyvitamin D therapy in children with active juvenile rheumatoid arthritis: short-term effects on serum osteocalcin levels and bone mineral density. J Pediatr. 1991;119:657–60.
47. Hillman L, Cassidy JT, Johnson L, Lee D, Allen SH. Vitamin D metabolism and bone mineralization in children with juvenile rheumatoid arthritis. J Pediatr. 1994;124:910–6.
48. Falcini F, Ermini M, Bagnoli F. Bone turnover is reduced in children with juvenile rheumatoid arthritis. J Endocrinol Investig. 1998;21:31–6.
49. Rooney M, Davies UM, Reeve J, Preece M, Ansell BM, WP. Bone mineral content and bone mineral metabolism: changes after growth hormone treatment in juvenile chronic arthritis. J Rheumatol. 2000;27:1073–81.
50. Tzoufi M, Siamopoulou-Mavridou A, Challa A, Lapatsanis PD. Changes of mineral metabolism in juvenile chronic arthritis. Acta Paediatr Suppl. 1994; 394:52–7.
51. Elsasser U, Wilkins B, Hesp R, Thurnham DI, Reeve J, Ansell BM. Bone rarefaction and crush fractures in juvenile chronic arthritis. Arch Dis Child. 1982;57:377–80.
52. Johansson U, Portinsson S, Akesson A, Svantesson H, Ockerman PA, Akesson B. Nutritional status in girls with juvenile arthritis. Hum Nutr - Clin Nutr. 1986;41:57–67.
53. Reeve J, Loftus J, Hesp R, Ansell BM, Wright DJ, Woo PMM. Biochemical prediction of changes in spinal bone mass in juvenile chronic (or rheumatoid) arthritis treated with glucocorticoids. J Rheumatol. 1993;20:1189–95.
54. Hillman LS, Cassidy JT, Chanetsa F, Hewett JE, Higgins BJ, Robertson JD. Percent true calcium absorption, mineral metabolism, and bone mass in children with arthritis: effect of supplementation with vitamin D3 and calcium. Arthritis Rheum. 2008;58:3255–63.
55. Warady BD, Lindsley CB, Robinson FG, LB. Effects of nutritional supplementation on bone mineral status of children with rheumatic diseases receiving corticosteroid therapy. J Rheumatol. 1994;21:530–5.
56. McNally JD, Menon K, Chakraborty P, Fisher L, Williams KA, Al-Dirbashi OY, et al. The Association of Vitamin D Status with Pediatric Critical Illness. Pediatrics. 2012;130:429–36.
57. Reed A, Haugen M, Pachman LM, Langman CB. Abnormalities in serum osteocalcin values in children with chronic rheumatic diseases. J Pediatr. 1990;116:574–80.
58. Pelajo CF, Lopez-Benitez JM, Miller LC. Obesity and disease activity in juvenile idiopathic arthritis. Pediatr Rheumatol. 2012;10:3.
59. McNally JD, Matheson LA, Rosenberg AM. Epidemiologic considerations in unexplained pediatric arthralgia: the role of season, school, and stress. J Rheumatol. 2009;36:427–33.
60. Wang Y, Lu MP, Teng LP, Guo L, Xu YP, Zou LX, et al. Association of vitamin D concentrations with juvenile idiopathic arthritis. Zhongguo Dang Dai Er Ke Za Zhi. 2015;17:375–8.
61. Borchers AT, Selmi C, Cheema G, Keen CL, Shoenfeld Y, Gershwin ME. Juvenile idiopathic arthritis. Autoimmun Rev. 2006;5:279–98.
62. Holick MF. Biological effects of sunlight, ultraviolet radiation, visible light, infrared radiation and vitamin D for health. Anticancer Res. 2016;36:1345–56.
63. Tsiaras WG, Weinstock MA. Factors influencing vitamin d status. Acta Derm Venereol. 2011;91:115–24.
64. Wacker M, Holick MF. Sunlight and vitamin D: a global perspective for health. Dermatoendocrinol. 2013;5:51–108.
65. Webb AR, Kline L, Holick MF. Influence of season and latitude on the cutaneous synthesis of vitamin D3: exposure to winter sunlight in Boston and Edmonton will not promote vitamin D3 synthesis in human skin. J Clin Endocrinol Metab. 1988;67:373–8.
66. Rosiles VH, Salazar CD, Velazquez RM, Ruiz RR, Clark P. Determination of 25(OH)D serum levels in children with systemic lupus erythematosus and juvenile idiopathic arthritis. Bol Med Hosp Infant Mex. 2015;72:99–105.
67. Duffy CM. Measurement of health status, functional status, and quality of life in children with juvenile idiopathic arthritis: clinical science for the pediatrician. Rheum Dis Clin N Am. 2007;33:389–402.
68. Ringold S, Wallace CA. Measuring clinical response and remission in juvenile idiopathic arthritis. Curr Opin Rheumatol. 2007;19:471–6.
69. Ringold S, Weiss PF, Beukelman T, Dewitt EM, Ilowite NT, Kimura Y, et al. 2013 update of the 2011 American College of Rheumatology recommendations for the treatment of juvenile idiopathic arthritis: recommendations for the medical therapy of children with systemic juvenile idiopathic arthritis and tuberculosis screening among c. Arthritis Care Res. 2013;65:1551–63.
70. Dankers W, Colin EM, van Hamburg JP, Lubberts E. Vitamin D in autoimmunity: molecular mechanisms and therapeutic potential. Front Immunol. 2017;7:697.
71. Cutolo M, Otsa K, Uprus M, Paolino S, Seriolo B. Vitamin D in rheumatoid arthritis. Autoimmun Rev. 2007;7:59–64.
72. Vojinovic J, Cimaz R. Vitamin D—update for the pediatric rheumatologists. Pediatr Rheumatol Online J. 2015;13:18.
73. Gröber U, Spitz J, Reichrath J, Kisters K, Holick MF. Vitamin D: update 2013 - from rickets prophylaxis to general preventive healthcare. Dermatoendocrinol. 2013;5:331–47.
74. Gröber U, Kisters K. Influence of drugs on vitamin D and calcium metabolism. Dermatoendocrinol. 2012;4:158–66.
75. Soybilgic A, Tesher M, Wagner-Weiner L, Onel KB. A survey of steroid-related osteoporosis diagnosis, prevention and treatment practices of pediatric rheumatologists in North America. Pediatr. Rheumatol. Online J. 2014;12:24.
76. Saurenmann RK, Rose JB, Tyrrell P, Feldman BM, Laxer RM, Schneider R, et al. Epidemiology of juvenile idiopathic arthritis in a multiethnic cohort: ethnicity as a risk factor. Arthritis Rheum. 2007;56:1974–84.
77. Ellis JA, Ponsonby A-L, Pezic A, Chavez RA, Allen RC, Akikusa JD, et al. CLARITY - ChiLdhood arthritis risk factor identification sTudY. Pediatr Rheumatol Online J. 2012;10:–37.
78. Thorsen S, Pipper C, Alberdi-Saugstrup M, Nielsen S, Cohen A, Lundqvist M, et al. No association between vitamin D levels around time of birth and later risk of developing oligo- and polyarticular juvenile idiopathic arthritis: a Danish case–cohort study. Scand J Rheumatol. 2016;9742:1–8.
79. Falcini F, Marini F, Rigante D, Bertini F, Lepri G, Stagi S, et al. PReS-FINAL-2053: vitamin D receptor polymorphisms in a cohort of Italian patients with juvenile idiopathic arthritis. Pediatr Rheumatol. 2013;11:P66.
80. Ellis JA, Scurrah KJ, Li YR, Ponsonby A-L, Chavez RA, Pezic A, et al. Epistasis amongst PTPN2 and genes of the vitamin D pathway contributes to risk of juvenile idiopathic arthritis. J Steroid Biochem Mol Biol. 2015;145:113–20.
81. Consolaro A, Bracciolini G, Ruperto N, Pistorio A, Magni-Manzoni S, Malattia C, et al. Remission, minimal disease activity, and acceptable symptom state in juvenile idiopathic arthritis: defining criteria based on the juvenile arthritis disease activity score. Arthritis Rheum. 2012;64:2366–74.
82. Giannini EH, Ruperto N, Ravelli A, Lovell DJ, Felson DT, Martini A. Preliminary definition of improvement in juvenile arthritis. Arthritis Rheum. 1997;40:1202–9.

13

A wearable activity tracker intervention for promoting physical activity in adolescents with juvenile idiopathic arthritis

Liane D. Heale[1*], Saunya Dover[2], Y. Ingrid Goh[1,2], Victoria A. Maksymiuk[1], Greg D. Wells[1] and Brian M. Feldman[1,3]

Abstract

Background: Children and adolescents with juvenile idiopathic arthritis (JIA) are less physically active than their healthy peers and are at high risk of missing out on the general health benefits of physical activity. Wearable activity trackers are a promising option for intervening in this population with potential advantages over traditional exercise prescriptions. The objectives of this study were to: (1) determine the feasibility of a wearable activity tracker intervention in adolescents with JIA; and (2) estimate the variability in response to a wearable activity tracker intervention on the physical activity levels of adolescents with JIA.

Methods: Participants aged 12–18 years with JIA were recruited during their routine rheumatology clinic visits at a tertiary care hospital. Participants completed the 3-Day Physical Activity Recall self-reported questionnaire at baseline, 1 week and 5 week follow-up. At the 1 week follow up, participants were instructed to start wearing an activity tracker for 28 consecutive days. Participants completed a feasibility questionnaire at their end of study visit. Participant demographics, adherence rates and feasibility outcomes were summarized using descriptive statistics. The effect of wearing a tracker on moderate-to-vigorous physical activity (MVPA) and total metabolic equivalents (METs) per day were analyzed using a paired t-test.

Results: Twenty-eight participants (74% female; median age 15.1, range 12.8–18.6) were included in the analysis. All of the participants were able to synchronize the activity tracker to a supported device, use the activity tracker correctly and complete the study measurements. On average, participants had activity logged on their smartphone application for 72% of the intervention period. The standard deviation of the change in mean METs/day was 12.148 and for mean MVPA blocks/day was 3.143 over the study period.

Conclusion: Wrist worn activity tracking is a feasible intervention for adolescent patients with JIA. More research is needed to examine the effect of activity tracking on physical activity levels.

Keywords: Physical activity, Juvenile idiopathic arthritis, Exercise, Health behaviors, Activity tracker, Adolescent

* Correspondence: ldheale@gmail.com
[1]Division of Rheumatology, The Hospital for Sick Children, 555 University Ave, Toronto, ON M5G 1X8, Canada
Full list of author information is available at the end of the article

Background

Regular physical activity is associated with health benefits in all children. Higher levels of physical activity are associated with improved body composition [1], metabolic profile [2] and measures of bone health [3, 4]. Conversely, low levels of physical activity are associated with increased cardiovascular disease risk factors [4, 5]. In addition to physical health benefits, habitual physical activity is associated with improved measures of mental health including increased self-esteem, cognitive performance, academic achievement, and reduction in depression [4] and anxiety [6].

A 2011 report indicated that Canadian youth are not meeting Canadian Physical Activity Guideline recommendations for optimal health [7]. Similar results have also been reported in youth studies in the United States [8, 9] and globally [10]. For most measures of health, aerobic-based activities provide the greatest benefit [4]. For optimal bone health, high-impact weight bearing activities are required [4]. Currently, the Canadian Physician Activity Guidelines [11] and the WHO Global Recommendations on Physical Activity for Health [12] recommend that children and youth aged 5–17 accumulate at least 60 min of moderate-to-vigorous physical activity (MVPA) daily. They should also participate in vigorous-intensity activities and activities that strengthen muscle and bone at least 3 days per week. Unfortunately, less than 10% of Canadian youth are adhering to these recommendations [7].

Children and adolescents with juvenile idiopathic arthritis (JIA) are even less physically active than their healthy peers [13–15]. Using accelerometers to objectively measure physical activity, Bohr et al. reported lower levels of total activity, and MVPA when children and adolescents with JIA were compared with age and gender-matched controls [13]. Adolescents with JIA also have lower levels of sports participation [16]. These low levels of physical activity persist despite adequate disease control [13]. As a consequence, young people with JIA have reduced cardiorespiratory fitness [14, 15] and bone mineral density [17] when compared with age-matched controls.

The impact of physical activity on JIA disease course and symptomatology has not been established. Despite theoretical advantages of reducing loss of proteoglycans and cartilage damage, and optimizing bone mineral density, there is no established relationship between physical activity levels and disease activity or functional ability [14, 15, 18]. The relationship between physical activity and pain in JIA is also complex and results of studies have been conflicting [19].

While the effect of physical activity on disease activity is unknown, randomized controlled trials with exercise interventions in JIA were well tolerated and resulted in improvements in cardiovascular fitness [20, 21].

Considering the low levels of physical activity reported in the JIA population in childhood and the tendency for a precipitous decline in physical activity during adolescence [22], young people with JIA are at high risk of missing out on the general health benefits of physical activity. Because of this, physical activity interventions are critical for this vulnerable population.

Wearable activity trackers are a promising option for intervening in this population with potential advantages over traditional exercise prescriptions. Wearable technology is increasing in popularity and offers real-time feedback (in the form of progress towards an activity goal) that has the potential to motivate patients. The trackers also offer social platforms that could inspire healthy competition with peers. In addition, activity trackers can provide physicians with objective measurements of patients' progress and response to medical therapies.

While a recent systematic review suggested that activity trackers have the potential to increase physical activity levels of healthy youth, it concluded that there is a paucity of research on the feasibility and effectiveness of activity trackers in this age group [23]. Furthermore, although some research has examined the feasibility of activity trackers in youth with chronic disease [24, 25], to the best of our knowledge there are no studies to date that have described their use in the adolescent JIA population.

Thus, the primary objectives of this study are to: (1) determine the feasibility of a wearable activity tracker (the Misfit Flash™) intervention in adolescents with JIA; and (2) estimate the variability in the effect size of an activity tracker intervention on the physical activity levels of adolescents with JIA, for use in planning a definitive trial. Exploratory objectives include determining the effects of an activity tracker on patient-reported health outcomes, pain, active joint count and physician global rating of disease activity.

Methods

Design

In this feasibility pilot, a single-group pre- and post-intervention study design was used to determine the feasibility of studying the effect of a wearable activity tracker on physical activity levels, patient reported health outcomes, pain, active joint count and physician global rating of disease activity. Participants completed study measurements at three time points: with a clinic visit at study enrollment; over the telephone and with online questionnaires 1 week after study enrollment and with a clinic visit after at least 28 days of wearing the activity tracker (Table 1).

Table 1 Overview of data collection at study visits

	Baseline	1 week	≥ 5 weeks
Demographics	X		
3DPAR	X	X	X
PROMIS® scales	X	X	X
Pain Scale	X		X
CHAQ	X		X
Joint Count	X		X
Physician Global Rating	X		X
Activity tracker start and stop		START	STOP

Study subjects

Boys and girls aged 12–18 years who met ILAR classification criteria for JIA [26] were selected for inclusion in the study if (1) their disease status was considered stable by their rheumatologist; (2) they were unlikely to require modification to medication therapy for the duration of the study; and (3) they had access to a smart phone or tablet compatible with the activity tracker chosen for this study – the Misfit Flash™.

Patients were excluded from participation if they (1) had moderate or high disease activity based on 2011 American College of Rheumatology recommendations for the treatment of JIA [27]; (2) had changes to their JIA medications in the 3 months prior to study enrollment; (3) had significant cardiovascular, respiratory or metabolic comorbidity; and (4) were already using an activity tracker at the time of enrolment.

Recruitment

Participants were recruited during their routine clinic visits in the general rheumatology clinics and medical day care unit at The Hospital for Sick Children. This study was approved by the Research Ethics Board at The Hospital for Sick Children. All participants provided written informed consent.

A convenience sample was used with enrollment of consecutive patients fulfilling study criteria. The planned sample size was 30 participants, a sufficient number for our feasibility aims.

Measurements

Physical activity

The 3-Day Physical Activity Recall (3DPAR) was completed at all three study time points. The 3DPAR is a self-report instrument that was designed to capture habitual physical activity of adolescents and has been validated in subsequent studies in this age group [28, 29].

The 3DPAR instrument requires the recall of activity performed during each of the three previous days, beginning with the most recent day. Each day is segmented into 34 30-min time blocks (7:00 a.m. to midnight). The instrument provides a list of common activities grouped into the following categories: sleep/bathing, eating, work, after-school/spare time/hobbies, transportation, and physical activities/sports [30]. For each block of the day, participants were asked to report the main activity in which they participated during each 30-min time period. Participants also rated the relative intensity of each activity as light, moderate, hard, or very hard. A member of the research team facilitated completion of the questionnaire at all study time points.

Following completion of the questionnaire, each 30-min block was assigned a metabolic equivalent (MET) value based on the specific activity and level of intensity reported by the participant [30]. MET values were summed over each of the 3 days for a measure of total daily physical activity (METs/day). In addition, the number of 30-min blocks in which energy expenditure was estimated at three METs or greater (i.e., MVPA blocks) were summed for each individual day (MVPA blocks/day). Three-day averages for METs/day, MVPA blocks/day were then calculated.

Self-reported pain, fatigue and depressive symptoms

Participants completed the Patient Reported Outcomes Measurement Information System (PROMIS®) questionnaires at all study time points. The PROMIS® tool provides a measure of patient-reported health status for physical, mental and social well-being. Participants completed the short form tools in the following domains: (1) pain interference, (2) fatigue, and (3) depressive symptoms. Participants were asked to rank the frequency with which they experienced symptoms in the past 7 days. Scores for each symptom range from 0 – never experienced the symptom, to 4 – almost always experienced the symptom. A total score was calculated by taking the sum of the scores (0–4) for each item in that domain. There are 8 items in the pain interference and depressive symptoms domains; thus, scores ranged from 0 to 32. Total scores in the 10-item fatigue domain ranged from 0 to 40.

Clinical assessment

Participants had a clinical assessment at study enrollment and study completion. As part of routine follow up visits in the rheumatology clinic, physicians recorded the total number of active and swollen joints and provided a physician global rating of participant disease activity. Participants were asked to rate their pain in the past week on a 10-cm visual analog scale from 0 (no pain), to 10 (very severe pain). They completed the Child Health Assessment Questionnaire (CHAQ) [31] as a self-report measure of their functional impairment.

Dropout

We tracked participant dropout as part of our feasibility aims. At the conclusion of the study, we asked participants if they had any illness or injury that interfered with their ability to participate in physical activity during the study.

Intervention

The Misfit Flash™ is a wearable activity tracker that measures step counts, tracks activity and estimates calories burned. The device can be worn with a wrist band or a clasp for attaching to shoes or clothing, depending on the activity type. It is water resistant up to 30 m and has a battery life of up to 6 months. The Misfit Flash™ synchronizes with compatible smartphones to provide feedback on activity levels and progress towards daily activity goals.

Participants and their parents were educated on the general use of the Misfit Flash™ through verbal and written information at the first clinic visit. A member of the research team offered assistance as needed with synchronizing the Misfit Flash™ to the participant's smartphone. Demographic information including date of birth, gender, height and weight was entered in the program by each participant. A daily activity goal was set by each participant without input from the research team. For example, a daily goal of "active" corresponds to 1000 Misfit Flash™ points and can be achieved with a variety of activities such as 30 min of running or 45 min of swimming.

Participants were asked to wear the Misfit Flash™ for 24 h per day, 7 days a week for at least 28 consecutive days following the telephone interview 1 week after study enrollment. Participants were asked to return the device at the final study visit.

Statistical analysis

Using descriptive statistics, the feasibility was measured by our ability to reach our desired sample size of 30 participants, as well as the proportion of those participants completing the study measurements and returning the device at study completion. Adherence with the activity tracker was assessed as the proportion of days with missing or incomplete data for each participant. The rate of device malfunction was also calculated.

Standardized response means were determined as a measure of responsiveness of the outcome variables to clinical change. The standard deviation of the paired score change was determined as a measure of variability. The standardized response mean was calculated as the difference in the mean values of self-reported 30-min blocks of MVPA and total METs per day from week one to week five divided by the standard deviation of the paired score change. The standardized response mean of the difference in the mean values of participant PROMIS® scores, pain scale, CHAQ and active joint count from baseline to week five were also determined with standard deviations calculated. A Bayes factor favouring the alternative hypothesis over the null hypothesis of no change (BF_{10}) was used as a test of significance with a percent error calculated. To rule in favour of the alternative hypothesis, a $BF_{10} \geq 3$ is considered significant.

Results

Thirty-one patients met inclusion criteria and were willing to participate in the study. Of the 31 participants in the study, 28 were included in the estimation of effect size. One participant was diagnosed with inflammatory bowel disease during the study period and two participants withdrew due to school and extra-curricular commitments. Baseline characteristics for the participants included in the analysis are displayed in Table 2.

Values are the number of study participants (percent of sample size) unless otherwise specified.

Feasibility

All of the participants were able to synchronize the Misfit Flash™ to a supported device, use the Misfit Flash™ correctly and complete the study measurements. Twenty-six participants had usable wear time data. One participant lost the device and another lost smart phone privileges and was unable to access the application. On average, participants had activity logged on their Misfit Flash™ application for 72% of the days in the intervention period. Five participants (19%) wore their Misfit Flash™ every day of the study period. Fifteen participants (58%) wore the Misfit Flash™ for at least 80% of the days

Table 2 Baseline characteristics for study participants ($n = 31$)

	Study Participants ($n = 31$)
Age in years, median (range)	15.1 (12.8–18.6)
Female (%)	23 (74)
JIA Subtype, n (%)	
Oligoarticular	7 (22.6)
Polyarticular (RF[a] positive)	11 (35.5)
Polyarticular (RF[a] negative)	4 (12.9)
Enthesitis Related	2 (6.5)
Psoriatic	4 (12.9)
Systemic	3 (9.7)
Medications, n (%)	
NSAID[a]	9 (29)
Prednisone	1 (3.2)
Non-biologic DMARD[a]	17 (54.9)
Biologic DMARD[a]	16 (51.6)

[a] *RF* rheumatoid factor, *NSAID* non-steroidal anti-inflammatory drug, *DMARD* Disease-modifying antirheumatic drugs

of the study period. The majority of participants (55%) returned the Misfit Flash™ at the completion of the study.

The device malfunction rate for the Misfit Flash™ was 53%. Eight participants (29%) reported the battery died and their device stopped working during the study period. Four participant's devices stopped working after wearing them in the water and three participants reported that the activity tracker disc fell out of the wrist band. Despite the technical issues, all but one participant (96%) reported that they enjoyed using the Misfit Flash™ and 89% were interested in continuing to use an activity tracker after completing the study.

Nine participants reported that illness, injury or pain prevented them from being active at some point in the study period. One patient had arthritis-related knee and ankle pain in the last week of the study period.

Activity tracker and physical activity level

There was no significant difference in the mean METs/day and mean number of MVPA blocks/day from week 1 to week 5 (Table 3). The standard deviation of the change in METs/day was 12.148 and for MVPA blocks/day was 3.143 over the study period (Table 3). Bayesian repeated measures ANOVA, showed no effect of sex on the change in METs/day and number of MVPA blocks/day over time (Figs. 1 and 2).

The majority of participants (71%) reported that they felt like they were more physically active as a result of the Misfit Flash™ when asked at the completion of the study.

Activity tracker and self-reported symptoms and clinical parameters

There was no significant difference in the mean PROMIS® scores from the baseline visit to week five (Table 3). There was also no significant difference in the mean CHAQ disability index, pain scale or active joint count from the baseline visit to week five (Table 3).

Discussion

Overall, the Misfit Flash™ wearable activity tracker is a feasible intervention for adolescents with JIA. While we have estimated the variability of the change in physical activity parameters for use in planning a definitive trial, device malfunction issues should be addressed beforehand.

As a result of a short recruitment window and a convenience sample, the oligoarticular JIA subtype was under-represented in our sample. There was also a high proportion of patients receiving both non-biologic and biologic disease modifying anti-rheumatic drugs. Although we sampled from all of the JIA clinics including subspecialty (i.e. juvenile spondyloarthropathy and systemic JIA) clinics, young people with ERA were under-represented in our sample. With no established difference in physical activity levels based on JIA subtype or disease activity level [8], we believe that these factors do not materially affect our physical activity results or the generalizability of our feasibility aims.

Two participants withdrew from the study due to school and extra-curricular commitments. As busy schedules and time demands are common aspects of adolescents' lives, ensuring that participants have adequate time and energy to engage in the intervention will be a challenge for future studies that other researchers should note and anticipate. Involving adolescents in the study design process could help address this and other potential issues for this age group.

In our review of the literature, we found one similar feasibility study that used a 2-week FitBit® intervention in 17 pediatric patients with acute lymphoblastic leukemia during the maintenance phase of their therapy [24]. They also reported a high proportion (94%) of

Table 3 Changes from baseline in mean values of study variables and clinical parameters

Measure	$Mean_{baseline}$	$Mean_{week5}$	$SD_{baseline}$	SD_{week5}	SRM	SD_{change}	BF_{10}	%error
MET[a]	65.728	66.710	12.270	11.090	0.135	12.148	0.253	0.012
MVPA[a]	3.722	3.905	3.045	2.787	0.114	3.143	0.237	0.009
CHAQ	0.333	0.392	0.679	0.639	−0.090	0.299	0.250	0.022
Pain[b]	1.319	1.890	2.171	2.550	0.281	2.523	0.463	0.012
Swollen Joint Count	0.310	0.500	0.541	1.051	0.287	0. 693	0.476	0.012
Physician Global Assessment	0.429	0.711	1.016	1.217	0.355	0.604	1.025	0.003
Fatigue[c]	46.400	43.805	12.791	14.417	0.177	17.001	0.257	0.021
Depression[c]	46.570	43.160	9.118	8.328	− 0.039	10.385	0.468	0.018
Pain Interference[c]	45.200	46.336	10.706	11.132	0.332	11.860	0.522	0.015

SD standard deviation, *SRM* standardized response mean, BF_{10} Bayes factor favouring the alternative hypothesis over the null hypothesis of no change, *%error* percent error

[a]The mean and SD values from week 1 were used instead of the baseline visit for METs and MVPA

[b]Measured on a 10-cm visual analog scale

[c]Measured using the Patient Reported Outcomes Measurement Information System

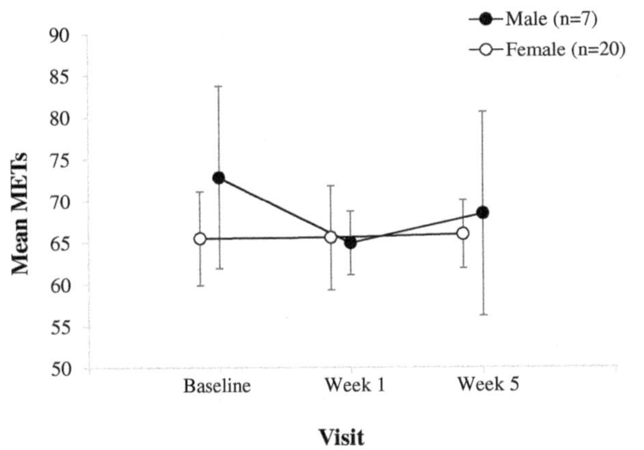

Fig. 1 Sex differences of the change in mean METs from baseline visit to week 5. Line graph shows the mean METs/day and 95% confidence intervals (95% CIs) corresponding to each visit time

participants that were able to synchronize the FitBit® and complete the study measurements. The superior wear time reported in their study (i.e., 92% vs. 72% of days) may be explained by the shorter intervention period. In contrast to our study, they did not report any FitBit® malfunction. This could also be related to the shorter intervention period or differences in device quality. The FitBit® devices are much more expensive than the comparable Misfit™ models, which may explain differences in malfunction rates but is an important factor in determining their utility in clinical and research settings.

Despite high malfunction rates, we received positive feedback from the participants during their study exit interviews. Almost all participants reported that they enjoyed wearing the tracker and the majority expressed interest in purchasing a tracker at the completion of the study. This positive feedback and interest in continued use demonstrates that activity trackers are well accepted in this population and supports the need for further research to determine their effectiveness in increasing physical activity levels. Piloting the feasibility questionnaire with adolescents beforehand could provide additional insight to improve the quality of feedback obtained from the participants in future studies.

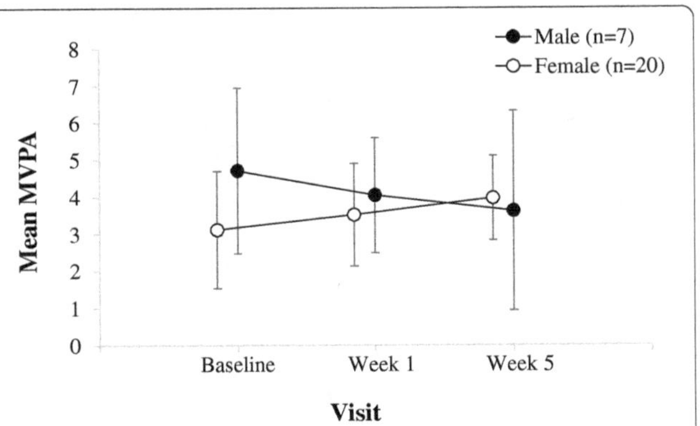

Fig. 2 Sex differences of the change in mean MVPA values from baseline visit to week 5. Line graph shows the mean MVPA blocks/day and 95% confidence intervals (95% CIs) corresponding to each visit time

The device return rate (55%) was low in our study. As many of the unreturned devices had malfunction, we did not make any additional attempts to have them returned if participants did not bring them to the final visit. Implementing better controls over returning the devices and removing barriers to returning them (e.g, postage paid return envelopes, reminder calls prior to the final study visit, etc.) would help address this issue in future studies.

The mean number of MVPA blocks per day and mean total METs per day for our sample were similar to those previously reported in healthy adolescent samples [4, 5]. Given that children and adolescents with JIA are less active than age-matched controls [8–10], there may have been a selection bias towards participants that are more physically active at baseline than the average JIA patient. Our result is even more surprising when we consider that female adolescents are less active than males [7] and 74% of our sample was female. Obtaining more detailed recruitment data including the reasons participants declined could help address this issue in future research. Alternatively, participants may have over-reported activity levels as a result of a social desirability bias. Finally, we tried to minimize the influence of the Hawthorne effect on the self-reported pre- and post-intervention PA levels by using the 3DPAR completed 1-week after study enrollment (but prior to using the activity tracker) as a baseline so that participants knew they were being observed for both the pre- and post-intervention measures of PA. While including more motivated patients could skew our feasibility results, we don't anticipate an effect on our measures of variability in the change of physical activity parameters as a result.

While there was no difference in pre- and post-intervention physical activity levels in our study, Hooke et al. report a trend towards increased steps per day from week 1 and week 2 with their FitBit® intervention [24]. Participant steps per day as a measure is more sensitive to change than blocks MVPA per day and total METs per day. Their intervention also incorporated daily coaching emails from a study nurse which may have an independent effect on participant activity levels. Future studies that assess these interventions separately may be needed to tease out the independent effect of the activity tracker on activity levels. Ideally, further research would also examine the sustainability of an effect with a study design that includes long-term follow up.

Although there was no significant difference in their 3DPAR scores, most participants reported a subjective increase in their activity level as a result of wearing the activity tracker. Since participants only wore the trackers while they were functional, we hypothesize that the high malfunction rates limited the effect of the intervention on physical activity levels.

There was no significant difference in participants PROMIS® scores or clinical parameters with our intervention. While there were few studies to compare with, Hook et al. also report no change in self-reported fatigue with their 2-week FitBit® intervention.

As there is no current evidence to support an effect of exercise intervention on JIA disease activity from previous studies, it is not surprising that this short intervention found no significant difference in clinical parameters. Based on our reported variability of change in physical activity parameters, our study was likely too small to have detected a difference should one exist.

Finally, the device we chose, primarily due to funding constraints, may have contributed to high malfunction rates. This issue should be considered in future research.

Conclusion

Overall, mobile activity trackers are feasible to employ and study and are well-tolerated and enjoyable for adolescents with JIA. We have estimated the variability in activity and response to wearing the tracker that will allow for the planning of a definitive intervention trial.

Abbreviations

3DPAR: 3-Day Physical Activity Recall; BF_{10}: Bayes factor favouring the alternative hypothesis over the null hypothesis of no change; CHAQ: Child Health Assessment Questionnaire; JIA: Juvenile idiopathic arthritis; METs: Metabolic equivalents; MVPA: Moderate-to-vigorous physical activity; RF: Rheumatoid factor

Authors' contributions

LDH contributed to the conception and design of the study, acquisition of data, interpretation of data, and drafted the manuscript. SD contributed to the design of the data collection tool, acquisition and interpretation of data and revised the manuscript critically for important intellectual content. YIG contributed to the design of the study, acquisition and analysis of data and revised the manuscript critically for important intellectual content. VAM contributed to acquisition of data and drafting the manuscript. GDW contributed to the conception and design of the study and revised the manuscript critically for important intellectual content. BMF contributed to the conception and design of the study, analysis and interpretation of data and revised the manuscript critically for important intellectual content. All authors read and approved the final manuscript.

Consent for publication

Not applicable.

Competing interests

The authors declare that they have no competing interests.

Author details

[1]Division of Rheumatology, The Hospital for Sick Children, 555 University Ave, Toronto, ON M5G 1X8, Canada. [2]Child Health Evaluative Sciences, The Hospital for Sick Children Research Institute, 686 Bay St, Toronto, ON M5G 0A4, Canada. [3]Department of Pediatrics and the Dalla Lana School of Public Health, University of Toronto, 155 College St., Toronto, ON M5T 3M7, Canada.

References

1. Kim Y, Barreira TV, Kang M. Concurrent associations of physical activity and screen-based sedentary behavior on obesity among US adolescents: a latent class analysis. J Epidemiol. 2016;26:137–44.
2. Pan Y, Pratt CA. Metabolic syndrome and its association with diet and physical activity in US adolescents. J Am Diet Assoc. 2008;108:276–86.
3. Christoffersen T, Winther A, Nilsen OA, Ahmed LA, Furberg AS, Grimnes G, et al. Does the frequency and intensity of physical activity in adolescence have an impact on bone? The Troms study, fit futures. BMC Sports Sci Med Rehabil. 2015;7:26.
4. Janssen I, Leblanc AG. Systematic review of the health benefits of physical activity and fitness in school-aged children and youth. Int J Behav Nutr Phys Act. 2010;7:40.
5. Andersen LB, Froberg K. Advancing the understanding of physical activity and cardiovascular risk factors in children: the European youth heart study (EYHS). Br J Sports Med. 2013;49:67–8.
6. Biddle SJ, Asare M. Physical activity and mental health in children and adolescents: a review of reviews. Br J Sports Med. 2011;45:886–95.
7. Colley RC, Garriguet D, Janssen I, Craig CL, Clarke J, Tremblay MS. Physical activity of Canadian children and youth: accelerometer results from the 2007 to 2009 Canadian health measures survey. Health Rep. 2011;22:15–23.
8. Troiano RP, Berrigan D, Dodd KW, Masse LC, Tilert T, McDowell M. Physical activity in the United States measured by accelerometer. Med Sci Sports Exerc. 2008;40:181–8.
9. Fakhouri TH, Hughes JP, Burt VL, Song M, Fulton JE, Ogden CL. Physical activity in US youth aged 12-15 years, 2012. NCHS Data Brief. 2014;141:1–8.
10. Hallal PC, Andersen LB, Bull FC, Guthold R, Haskell W, Ekelund U, et al. Global physical activity levels: surveillance progress, pitfalls, and prospects. Lancet. 2012;380:247–57.
11. Canadian Society for Exercise Physiology. Canadian physical activity guidelines and Canadian sedentary behaviour guidelines. 2018 http://csepguidelines.ca/children-and-youth-5-17/. Accessed 6 Mar 2018.
12. World Health Organization. Global recommendations on physical activity for health. 2018. http://www.who.int/dietphysicalactivity/factsheet_young_people/en/. Accessed 6 Mar 2018.
13. Bohr AH, Nielsen S, Muller K, Karup Pedersen F, Andersen LB. Reduced physical activity in children and adolescents with juvenile idiopathic arthritis despite satisfactory control of inflammation. Pediatr Rheumatol Online J. 2015;13:57.
14. Norgaard M, Twilt M, Andersen LB, Herlin T. Accelerometry-based monitoring of daily physical activity in children with juvenile idiopathic arthritis. Scand J Rheumatol. 2016;45:179–87.
15. Lelieveld OT, Armbrust W, van Leeuwen MA, Duppen N, Geertzen JH, Sauer PJ, et al. Physical activity in adolescents with juvenile idiopathic arthritis. Arthritis Rheum. 2008;59:1379–84.
16. Klepper SE. Exercise and fitness in children with arthritis: evidence of benefits for exercise and physical activity. Arthritis Rheum. 2003;49:435–43.
17. Tang T, Tang X, Xu L, Huang Y, Zeng J, Li Q. Evaluation of bone mass in children and young adults with juvenile idiopathic arthritis. Clin Exp Rheumatol. 2015;33:758–64.
18. Gueddari S, Amine B, Rostom S, Badri D, Mawani N, Ezzahri M, et al. Physical activity, functional ability, and disease activity in children and adolescents with juvenile idiopathic arthritis. Clin Rheumatol. 2014;33:1289–94.
19. Limenis E, Grosbein HA, Feldman BM. The relationship between physical activity levels and pain in children with juvenile idiopathic arthritis. J Rheumatol. 2014;41:345–51.
20. Singh-Grewal D, Schneiderman-Walker J, Wright V, Bar-Or O, Beyene J, Selvadurai H, et al. The effects of vigorous exercise training on physical function in children with arthritis: a randomized, controlled, single-blinded trial. Arthritis Rheum. 2007;57:1202–10.
21. Long AR, Rouster-Stevens KA. The role of exercise therapy in the management of juvenile idiopathic arthritis. Curr Opin Rheumatol. 2010;22:213–7.

22. Allison KR, Adlaf EM, Dwyer JJ, Lysy DC, Irving HM. The decline in physical activity among adolescent students: a cross-national comparison. Can J Public Health. 2007;98:97–100.
23. Ridgers ND, McNarry MA, Mackintosh KA. Feasibility and effectiveness of using wearable activity trackers in youth: a systematic review. JMIR Mhealth Uhealth. 2016;4(4):e129.
24. Hooke MC, Gilchrist L, Tanner L, Hart N, Withycombe JS. Use of a fitness tracker to promote physical activity in children with acute lymphoblastic leukemia. Pediatr Blood Cancer. 2016;63:684–9.
25. Mendoza JA, Baker KS, Moreno MA, Whitlock K, Abbey-Lambertz M, Waite A, et al. A Fitbit and Facebook mHealth intervention for promoting physical activity among adolescent and young adult childhood cancer survivors: a pilot study. Pediatr Blood Cancer. 2017;64(12):e26660.
26. Petty RE, Southwood TR, Manners P, Baum J, Glass DN, Goldenberg J, et al. International league of associations for rheumatology classification of juvenile idiopathic arthritis: second revision, Edmonton, 2001. J Rheumatol. 2004;31:390–2.
27. Beukelman T, Patkar NM, Saag KG, Tolleson-Rinehart S, Cron RQ, DeWitt EM, et al. 2011 American College of Rheumatology recommendations for the treatment of juvenile idiopathic arthritis: initiation and safety monitoring of therapeutic agents for the treatment of arthritis and systemic features. Arthritis Care Res (Hoboken). 2011;63:465–82.
28. Lee KS, Trost SG. Validity and reliability of the 3-day physical activity recall in Singaporean adolescents. Res Q Exerc Sport. 2005;76:101–6.
29. Pate RR, Ross R, Dowda M, Trost SG, Sirard JR. Validation of a 3-day physical activity recall instrument in female youth. Pediatr Exerc Sci. 2003;15:257–65.
30. Ainsworth BE, Haskell WL, Herrmann SD, Meckes N, Bassett DR Jr, Tudor-Locke C, et al. 2011 compendium of physical activities: a second update of codes and MET values. Med Sci Sports Exerc. 2011;43:1575–81.
31. Singh G, Athreya BH, Fries JF, Goldsmith DP. Measurement of health status in children with juvenile rheumatoid arthritis. Arthritis Rheum. 1994;37:1761–9.

Feasibility and safety of a 6-month exercise program to increase bone and muscle strength in children with juvenile idiopathic arthritis

Kristin M. Houghton[1,2*], Heather M. Macdonald[3,4], Heather A. McKay[3,4,5], Jaime Guzman[1,2], Ciarán Duffy[6], Lori Tucker[1,2] and on behalf of the LEAP Study Investigators

Abstract

Background: Arthritis in childhood can be associated with muscle weakness around affected joints, low bone mass and low bone strength. Exercise is recognized as an important part of management of children with juvenile idiopathic arthritis (JIA) but the exercise prescription to best promote bone and muscle health is unknown. We therefore aimed to: 1. assess feasibility and safety of a 6-month home- and group-based exercise program for children with JIA; 2. estimate the effect of program participation on bone mass and strength, muscle function and clinical outcomes and 3. determine if any positive changes in bone and muscle outcomes are maintained 6 months later.

Methods: We recruited 24 children with JIA who were part of the Linking Exercise, Physical Activity and Pathophysiology in Childhood Arthritis (LEAP) study to participate in a 6-month home-based exercise program involving jumping and handgrip exercises, resistance training and one group exercise session per month. We assessed lumbar spine bone mass (dual energy X-ray absorptiometry), distal tibia and radius bone microarchitecture and strength (high-resolution peripheral quantitative computed tomography), muscle function (jumping mechanography, dynamometry) and clinical outcomes (joint assessment, function, health-related quality of life) at baseline, 6- and 12-months. Adherence was assessed using weekly activity logs.

Results: Thirteen children completed the 6-month intervention. Participants reported 9 adverse events and post-exercise pain was rare (0.4%). Fatigue improved, but there were no other sustained improvements in muscle, bone or clinical outcomes. Adherence to the exercise program was low (47%) and decreased over time.

Conclusion: Children with JIA safely participated in a home-based exercise program designed to enhance muscle and bone strength. Fatigue improved, which may in turn facilitate physical activity participation. Prescribed exercise posed adherence challenges and efforts are needed to address facilitators and barriers to participation in and adherence to exercise programs among children with JIA.

Keywords: Exercise, Physical activity, Juvenile arthritis, Muscle, Bone

* Correspondence: khoughton@cw.bc.ca
[1]Division of Rheumatology, K4-123 ACB, British Columbia Children's Hospital, 4480 Oak Street, Vancouver, BC V6H 3V4, Canada
[2]Department of Pediatrics, University of British Columbia, Vancouver, BC, Canada

Background

Physical activity (PA) during childhood and adolescence is essential for optimal growth and development. However, compared with their healthy peers, children with juvenile idiopathic arthritis (JIA) are less physically fit, spend less time engaged in moderate to vigorous physical activity (MVPA) [1–4], and more often choose sedentary pursuits [5]. Physical inactivity may in turn exacerbate JIA symptoms and prevent children with JIA from achieving recommended levels of physical activity [6]. In keeping with an 'exercise is medicine' approach, PA is considered an important non-pharmacological therapy for children with JIA [7, 8].

A variety of exercise programs have been evaluated in children with JIA (reviewed in [9–11]) but it is unclear what specific exercise prescription best promotes bone and muscle health. Weight-bearing PA and muscle strengthening exercises are essential for optimal bone mass and strength accrual [12]. In children with JIA, bone accrual may be hindered by the combined effects of inflammatory cytokines, glucocorticoid therapy, low muscle mass and physical inactivity [13]. As a result, children with JIA are twice as likely to have low areal bone mineral density (aBMD by dual energy X-ray absorptiometry, DXA) as compared with their healthy peers [14, 15] as well as deficits in bone structure and strength as estimated with three-dimensional imaging tools [16, 17]. In turn, these bone deficits are associated with a 1.5–3 times higher risk of fracture among children with JIA [18]. Thus, strategies are needed to target musculoskeletal health in children with JIA. To date, only one study investigated the effects of a home-based exercise program on bone mass in children with JIA [8, 19]. However, this exercise program lasted only 12 weeks, which is likely insufficient to assess true benefits in bone accrual [20].

DXA is the current clinical gold standard for monitoring bone health; however, a two-dimensional scan cannot assess bone structural adaptations to exercise that influence bone strength. Three-dimensional imaging tools such as high-resolution peripheral quantitative computed tomography (HR-pQCT) have evolved to demonstrate compartment- (compact and trabecular bone) and strength-specific adaptations of growing bone. To our knowledge, this instrument has never been used to assess bone's response to exercise in children with JIA.

Our study in children with JIA had three objectives: 1. to evaluate safety and feasibility of a targeted 6-month home-based exercise program, 2. to estimate effect of the exercise program on bone mass (by DXA), structure and strength (by HR-pQCT), muscle function and clinical outcomes, 3. to assess stability of bone and muscle outcomes 6 months after the intervention. Results will be used to inform design and implementation of larger randomized controlled trials.

Methods

We conducted a pre-post exercise intervention trial with children and youth with JIA in Vancouver, Canada. This sub-study was part of a large multisite, longitudinal, observational cohort study of children with JIA (LEAP; Linking Exercise, Physical Activity and Pathophysiology in Childhood Arthritis). LEAP aims to investigate the relationships between JIA, PA and bone and muscle development (http://www.leapjia.com/).

Recruitment

Between September 2014 and February 2015, we recruited children aged 8 to 16 years with a diagnosis of JIA [21] who were willing and able to participate, irrespective of their subtype of JIA or disease activity status, and who lived in the Metro Vancouver area and could attend monthly group exercise sessions. Exclusion criteria were: 1. receiving bisphosphonate treatment (past or planned), 2. participation in high performance sports, training or competition >3 h/week, 3. participation >1 resistance training session per week for the past 4 months, and 4. pregnant or planning pregnancy. The Clinical Research Ethics Boards at the University of British Columbia approved all procedures (certificate H14–01572). Parents or guardians provided written informed consent and children provided assent.

Measurement

Following recruitment, participants attended baseline measurement at the Centre for Hip Health and Mobility in Vancouver. To account for rolling recruitment the intervention was conducted in three waves (February, March and April, 2015). Participants had follow-up assessments 3, 6 and 12 months after their baseline visit. At each assessment participants completed questionnaires, muscle testing and clinical assessment by a pediatric rheumatologist. Bone outcomes were assessed at baseline, 6- and 12-months.

Clinical assessment included count of joint and enthesitis sites with active inflammation by a pediatric rheumatologist, standing and sitting height using stretch stature (Seca Model 242, Hanover, MD) to the nearest 0.1 cm, body weight calibrated electronic scale (Seca Model 840, Hanover, MD) to the nearest 0.1 kg and arm (ulna) and lower leg (tibia) length (cm) to the nearest millimeter using a standard steel anthropometric tape. All measures were performed in duplicate by trained research assistants.

We estimated age at peak height velocity (APHV) as an indicator of somatic maturation using the Moore equation [22], and subsequently calculated maturity offset as a continuous measure of years from APHV. Self-report questionnaires included pain intensity in last week (10 mm visual analog scale where higher scores indicate more pain), function (Child Health Activity Questionnaire (CHAQ), 0–3 where higher scores indicate greater functional disability) [23], physical activity questionnaire for children (PAQ-C) and adolescents (PAQ-A) (score 1–5 with higher scores indicating higher PA) [24, 25], fatigue (PedsQL Multidimensional Fatigue Scale, 0–100 where higher scores indicate less fatigue) [26], Juvenile Arthritis Quality of Life Questionnaire (JAQQ, scores 1–7 with lower scores indicated better quality of life) [27], Child and Youth Physical Self-perception Profile (CYPSP, 4 sub-domains of sport competence, body attractiveness, physical condition, and physical strength as well as general physical self-worth; score 0–4 with 2.5 midpoint and higher scores indicating higher self-perception) [28], current medications, fracture history, dietary calcium intake [29] and self-assessed stage of sexual maturation as per the method of Tanner [30].

We used both DXA and HR-pQCT to assess bone outcomes at baseline, 6- and 12-months. Image acquisition and analysis protocols are described in detail elsewhere [31]. Lumbar spine bone mineral content (BMC, g) and areal bone mineral density (aBMD, g/cm^2) were assessed using DXA (Hologic QDR 4500 W) with standard positioning. A trained technician acquired and analyzed all scans and performed daily quality control procedures. We calculated lumbar spine BMC z-scores using published reference data [32]. Second, we used HR-pQCT (XtremeCT; Scanco Medical AG, Brüttisellen, Switzerland) to assess BMD, bone microarchitecture and bone strength at the non-dominant distal radius (7% site) and distal tibia (8% site). Outcomes of interest included total BMD (Tt. BMD, mg HA/cm^3), trabecular bone volume ratio (BV/TV), cortical thickness (Ct.Th, mm; mean cortical volume divided by the outer bone surface) and failure load (F.Load, N). We calculated age-, sex- and ethnicity-specific z-scores for each HR-pQCT outcome using published centile values [31].

Muscle testing included grip strength, peak power (single two-legged countermovement vertical jump) and force (multiple one-legged hopping) on Leonardo Mechanograph® Ground Reaction Force Plate, (GRFP; Novotec Medical GmbH, Germany), and isokinetic strength of non-dominant elbow flexors / extensors, knee flexors / extensors, hip abductors/ adductors using a Biodex dynamometer (System 4). We highlight grip strength, peak power, knee extensor peak torque, average power and total joint work per participant as clinically significant muscle measures.

Exercise intervention

The home-based exercise program included: jumping exercises (3 sessions/week, jumps associated with ground reaction forces of between 3 and 5 times body weight [33, 34]); handgrip exercises (3 sessions/week completed with hand grippers) and resistance training (2 sessions/week completed with Therabands® without handles). Before starting the program, our kinesiologist (KD) conducted a home visit to individually tailor the program to each participant's abilities. The kinesiologist provided each participant with pictures of their exercises, a schedule for exercise progression, Therabands® (color coded for resistance) and hand grippers. She also demonstrated modified exercises should specific exercises cause joint pain and recommended one rest day between resistance and jumping exercises.

The progressive exercise program was implemented over 26 weeks. Participants completed six 4-week blocks of jumping exercises (exercise load increased from 1 set of 5 jumps to 3 sets of 10 jumps; jumping difficulty progressed from simple jumping movements (e.g., tuck jumps/'motorcycle jumps') to hopping, skipping and multidirectional plyometric movements (e.g. jumping lunge/'leaping lizards') Additional file 1: Figure S1). We estimated ground reaction forces associated with these exercises were approximately 3 to 5 times body weight [35]. For resistance exercises the load increased from 1 set of 8 repetitions for 4 exercises to 3 sets of 15 repetitions for 7 exercises. Difficulty increased from simple single-joint exercise (e.g. biceps curl) to complex multiple- exercises (e.g. lunges). Participants were instructed to take a 20-s rest break between sets and exercises. Resistance exercises included upper extremity, core and lower extremity muscle groups. Handgrip exercises progressed from 2 sets of 5 repetitions to 3 sets of 12 repetitions. Children were instructed to squeeze a rubber cylinder with either 5 short, hard squeezes or hold a moderate to maximal squeeze for 5 s. We implemented a 2-week program of exercise maintenance at the end of the six 4-week blocks. The resistance training exercises required 10–30 min per session; jumping and handgrip exercises required 2–10 min per session.

Participants also attended one group-based exercise session each month. These kinesiologist-led sessions were held at three locations in Metro Vancouver as per the geographic distribution of participants. At each session, the kinesiologist reviewed participants' progress, introduced new exercises, conducted interactive strength and agility activities and provided children with the opportunity to meet fellow participants. The kinesiologist modified the exercise program for participants who reported pain during or after completion of prescribed exercises.

Participants received usual medical care throughout the study and had regular rheumatology clinic visits every three to 4 months. If clinically indicated, clinic visits included assessment by a physiotherapist who could prescribe additional exercises to target specific problem areas.

Monitoring / adherence

Participants completed a weekly exercise log, in print or online. (Additional file 1: Figure S2). Parents/guardians were asked to assist with scheduling and monitoring home exercise sessions, as needed. The kinesiologist contacted the family every 2 weeks to address questions about exercises and to monitor compliance. We recorded the proportion of prescribed exercise completed (total repetitions reported / total repetitions prescribed) and the proportion of group exercise sessions attended (sessions attended/total sessions). We also asked participants to use their log book to record completion of any additional exercises.

Safety and feasibility

Adverse events included JIA flare (defined as any increase in active joint count or Physician Global Assessment of disease activity that resulted in a change in treatment), post-exercise pain lasting > 24 h, and falls or injuries that occurred during exercise. To determine feasibility, we recorded participant recruitment, adherence to exercises, attendance at group exercise sessions, completion of questionnaires and attendance at measurement session. As a companion study, we conducted one-on-one interviews with child-caregiver dyads to identify facilitator and barriers to adherence [36].

Sample size

We recruited a convenience sample of 24 participants as this allowed 8 subjects per group for each recruitment wave.

Statistical analysis

We performed all analyses using Stata, version 10.1 (StataCorp, College Station, TX). We report means and standard deviations for anthropometry, clinical, bone and muscle outcomes. We report median and interquartile range (IQR) for categorical outcomes, including active joint count. We calculated the average (and range of) adherence for each 4-week exercise block and the proportion of participants attaining at least 80% adherence for each 4-week block. We used repeated-measures analysis of variance to compare clinical outcomes over time. To examine change in bone and muscle outcomes while accounting for the time-varying covariate change in height, we fit mixed effects models (*xtmixed* in Stata) with time as a fixed effect and maturity offset at baseline as an additional covariate. We used the *margins* command in Stata for pairwise comparisons between time points. We considered p values < 0.05 as statistically significant.

Results

We summarize flow of participants through the trial in Fig. 1. Twenty-four participants volunteered to participate out of 54 approached (44%). Those declining

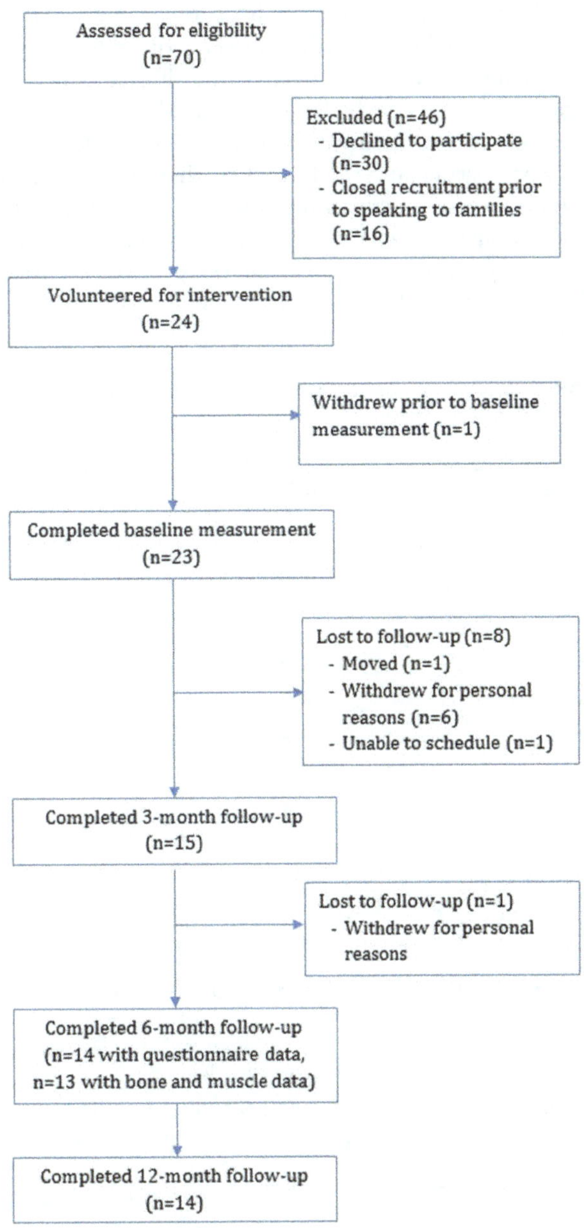

Fig. 1 Flow of participants through the trial

participation expressed no interest or lack of time. Twenty-three participants completed baseline assessment. Thirteen participants (56%) completed baseline, 6- and 12-month measures. Participants who withdrew were similar in age, height, weight and clinical characteristics to participants who completed the study (Additional file 2: Table S1).

In Table 1, we summarize descriptive characteristics at baseline for those who completed the study. Most children (62%) were Caucasian and pre- or early pubertal. Most participants had a healthy BMI ($n = 9$, 6 girls), 1 boy was underweight, 1 girl andl boy were overweight and 1 boy was obese, as per WHO criteria [37]. Most participants (77%) had oligoarticular disease; enthesitis-related arthritis was the most common JIA subtype in boys ($n = 3$, 50%). At baseline, 7 children were on non-steroidal anti-inflammatory drugs, 9 were on disease modifying therapy and 4 were on biologic therapy. Medication details for each participant are provided in Additional file 2: Table S2. Most participants had inactive disease at baseline; however, function, as measured by the CHAQ, was impaired in 6 participants (46%) (Table 2). Average PA score was low to average in girls and boys; general physical self-worth was higher than the midpoint score of 2.5 in both sexes.

Adherence

Participants completed a median of 46.9% (5.4, 66.7 IQR) of prescribed exercises. Adherence was highest during the first 4-week block of exercises (median 72.3%). It decreased but remained stable over the next 16 weeks (approximately 50%) and decreased during the final 4 weeks (median 38%). Attendance at monthly group sessions was variable across the intervention period, with a median of 66.7% (16.7, 100 IQR) sessions attended. Only 2 participants (15.4%) achieved the goal of 80% adherence, 3 (23.1%) achieved 60% adherence and 5 (38.5%) achieved 50% adherence. Completion of logbooks (paper or online) was 53.8% (19.2, 91.7 IQR) and declined across 24-weeks.

Pain, injury and flare

Pain scores were variable and generally low (27 ± 26 points) on 100-point scale (Table 2, Additional file 2: Table S2). Ten incidents of pain lasting > 24 h were reported by 8 participants. The incremental change in pain from pre- to post-exercise sessions was small (5.0, 0–20 Median, IQR on 100-point scale). Two participants reported falls or injuries; one participant 'rolled their ankle' during the jumping exercises and one participant reported a knee injury in two consecutive jumping

Table 1 Descriptive characteristics at baseline of participants who completed the study (n =!3). Values are mean (standard deviation) unless otherwise indicated

Variable	All participants (n = 13)	Girls (n = 7)	Boys (11 = 6)
Age (years)	13.0(2.0)	13.5 (2.3)	12.4(1.6)
Ethnicity (tt Asian/Caucasian/ Other)	3/8/2	1/5/1	2/3/ 1
Tanner stage (# 1/2/3/4/5)	3/3/4/2/1	1 /2/3/1/0	2/ 1/1/ 1/1
Maturity offset (years)	0.07(1.8)	1.0 (1.9)	−1.0 (1.0)
Height (cm)	149.7(8.3)	150.0(9.6)	149.4 (7.4)
Height z-score	−0.61 (0.83)	−0.80(0.%)	−0.39 (0.66)
Weight (kg)	42.6(7.0)	41.1 (43.9)	41.1 (5.0)
Weight z-score	−0.39 (1.26)	−0.48(1.21)	− 0.28 (1.42)
BMI (kg/m^2)	18.8(2.6)	19.4 (2.2)	18.5(3.1)
BMI z-score	−0.07 (1.26)	0.02(0.87)	−0.19 (1.69)
Clinical outcomes			
Time since diagnosis (months)	57 (47)	78 (23)	34 (49)
JIA subtvpes - polyarticular course	4 (2 poly RF negative, 2 oligo extended)	3 (2 poly RF negative, 1 oligo extended)	1 (oligo extended)
JIA subtypes - oligoarticular course	9 (2 oligo persistent. 3 ERA. 2 psoriatic, 2 undi fterentiated)	4 (2 psoriatic, 1 oligo persistent, 1 undifferentiated)	5 (3 ERA, 1 oligo persistent, 1 undifferentiated)
Medications (n)	7 NSAIDS,9 DMARDs, 4 Biologies	5 NSAIDS, 6 DMARDs, 3 biologies	2 NSAIDS, 3 DMARDs, 1 biologic
Fracture history	4	1 distal radius, 1 nasal	1 distal radius, 1 distal tibia
Dietary calcium intake (mg)	740 (410)	468 (196)	1058 (364)

NSAIDs non-steroidal anti-inflammatory medications including Naproxen. Ibuprofen. DMARDs, Disease modifying anti-rheumatic drugs including Methotrexate, Leflunomide, Sulfasalazine. Biologies - including Etanercept. Infliximab, Humira

Table 2 Clinical measures for group at baseline, 3- and 6- and 12-months. Values are mean (standard deviation) unless otherwise indicated. *P*-value indicates the main effect of time from the repeated measures analysis of variance

Clinical measure	Baseline	3-months	6-months	12-months	p-value
Median active joint count[a]	0 (0, 0) range 0–1	0 (0,0.5) range 0–7	0 (0, 0) range 0–1	0 (0,0) range 0–2	
Median restricted joint count	0 (0, 0) range 0–3	0 (0,0) range 0–13	0 (0, 0) range 0–3	0 (0,0) range 0–1	
Median active enlhesitis count	1.0 (1.5)	0 (0.0) range 0–3	0 (0.0) range 0–0	0 (0.0.5) range 0–4	
Functional ability (CHAQ, range 0–3)	0.20 (0.42)	0.38 (0.54)	0.46 (0.53)	0.33 (0.48)	0.216
Pain (VAS, range 0–100)	26.0 (26.6)	15.5 (20.8)	25.4 (20.4)	18.0(22.5)	0.334
JAQQ score (range 1–7)	2.6 (1.0)	2.3 (1.2)	2.3 (1.0)	2.4 (1.2)	0.384
PA Score (range 1–5)	2.3 (0.6)	2.6 (0.72)	2.2 (0.5)	2.3 (0.9)	0.469
Fatigue (PedsQL. range 0–100)	57.0 (18.2)	66.0 (18.0)	69.9 (18.9)	67.3 (17.2)	0.034b
Physical self-worth (CYPSPP. range 0–4)	3.3 (0.6)	3.2 (.6)	3.3 (0.7)	3.4 (0.6)	0.966

CHAQ Child Health Assessment Questionnaire, *VAS* visual analog scale, *JAQQ* Juvenile Arthritis Quality of Life Questionnaire, *PA* physical activity score from the Physical Activity Questionnaire for Children (8–14 y) and Adolescents (14–18 y), *PedsQL* Pediatric Quality of Life Inventory, *CYPSPP* Child and Youth Physical Self-perception Profile

[a]Most participants had 0 active joints. At baseline 1 participant had 1 active joint. At 3 months, 1 patient had 7 active joints. At 6 months, one participant had 2 active joints and 1 had 3 active joints. At 12 months, 1 participant had 1 active joint and 1 had 2 active joints. b $p < 0.05$

exercises sessions. Seven participants had their exercise programs modified for pain, injury or flare, and 3 withdrew because of pain. There were 4 JIA flares during the intervention (3 mild, 1 moderate). Of those participants with mild flares, one participant (#16) was previously in clinical remission and started NSAID therapy and two participants (#9, #19) were previously in clinical remission on stable DMARD therapy but started NSAID therapy during the intervention. One participant (#8) had a moderate flare that required addition of prednisone and biologic therapy to stable DMARD therapy.

Clinical outcomes

Total fatigue scores were low at baseline (mean 57.9, SD 18.2) and improved by 8.1 points and 12.0 points, on average, at 3 and 6 months, respectively, with some improvement maintained at 12 months (9.4 points) (Table 2, Fig. 2). Total fatigue scores were lower than previously reported scores of a general pediatric rheumatology population aged 2 to 18 years (mean 73.8, SD 21.9) [26]. We did not observe improvements in any other clinical outcomes.

Bone outcomes

We provide bone outcomes at baseline, 6- and 12-months in Table 3. We excluded one participant's baseline radius HR-QCT scan because of significant motion artifact (motion grade of 5 on a 5-point scale). We identified one potential outlier for HR-pQCT outcomes at 12-months. Distal radius Z-scores for this participant at 12-months were more than 2 standard deviations higher than their z-scores at baseline or 6-months and review of the participant's scan revealed callus formation of unknown origin (no history of fracture). We removed the 12-month HR-pQCT scan for this participant from our analysis.

At baseline, all participants had a LS BMC z-score within the normal range as compared with international reference data [32]. In contrast, 4 participants had z-scores < −2 for HR-pQCT outcomes at the distal tibia (Tt.BMD, BV/TV, Ct.Th and F.Load). Three of these participants also had z-scores < −2 for F.Load and BV/TV at the distal radius.

LS BMC z-score did not change over the course of the intervention or follow-up period (Table 3, Fig. 2). At the distal tibia, Ct.Th z-score appeared to decrease during the intervention; however, this trend was not maintained after 12-months. Total BMD at the distal tibia increased by 5% after 12 months, but Tt.BMD z-score did not change significantly. Z-scores for distal tibia BV/TV and F.Load did not change significantly. At the distal radius, Tt.BMD z-score decreased during follow-up after adjusting for change in height and maturity. Z-scores for other bone outcomes at the distal radius did not change significantly over time.

Muscle outcomes

We provide key muscle outcomes at baseline, 3-, 6- and 12-months in Table 4. Briefly, after adjusting for height and maturity offset, grip strength and knee extensor peak torque, average power and total joint work did not improve over the course of the intervention (Table 4, Fig. 2). Absolute values for peak force of the right and left legs increased between baseline and 12-months, but z-scores for mechanography outcomes did not change significantly during the intervention.

Discussion

We address an important knowledge gap in the area of exercise therapy for children with JIA and extend the current literature in five ways. First, results of our intervention trial suggest it is safe to engage children with

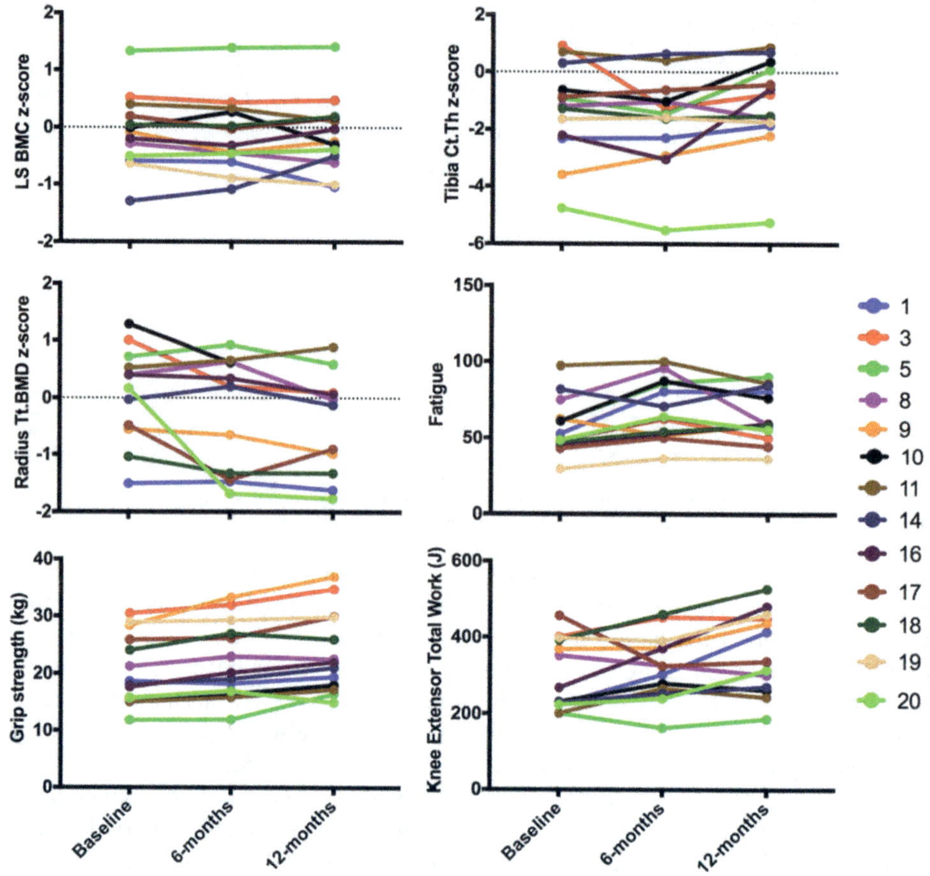

Fig. 2 Individual time series plots for the 13 participants that completed the 6-month intervention and 6-month follow-up. The plot for total bone mineral density (Tt.BMD) z-score at the distal radius does not include data for participant 19 due to significant motion artifact present in the baseline scan

JIA in a home-based exercise program, designed to enhance muscle and bone strength. Second, participation and adherence were low, suggesting the exercise program was not feasible to extend to the larger JIA population. Third, fatigue improved among those participants who completed the study, and was sustained 6 months after cessation of the intervention. Fourth, we used standard clinical DXA to assess change in bone mass and an advanced imaging tool, HR-pQCT to assess change in bone microstructure, BMD and estimated bone strength. Fifth, and finally, we used several techniques to assess muscle function that were feasible for children with JIA to perform.

Safety and feasibility

Our exercise program is the first to include impact exercise and resistance training in both home- and group-based sessions. As noted by others [6], a 'one size fits all' approach to exercise prescription is likely not appropriate for children with JIA. Thus, our kinesiologist tailored the program to each participant's abilities and modified the program when necessary. Modifications were made for pain, injury or flare in seven participants. Adverse events and post-exercise pain were rare, which suggests the exercise program is safe for children with JIA.

The six-month intervention was necessarily longer (to promote osteogenesis) than previous studies that employed resistance training and weight-bearing exercise to promote bone strength [19, 38]. The longer duration may have contributed to high participant attrition and relatively low adherence. Some participants expressed lack of motivation, which also emerged as a recurring theme in our companion study where we used qualitative methods to better understand barriers to participating in exercise among children with JIA [36]. Previous studies also reported low adherence to exercise programs and physical therapy among children with JIA [39–41]. However, even partial adherence to treatment plans may significantly decrease pain and improve function and quality of life [39].

Our study demonstrates a clear need to better understand barriers and facilitators to participation in and adherence to exercise programs in children with JIA. In

Table 3 Bone outcomes at baseline, 6- and 12-months of those participants who completed the study ($n = 13$). Values are mean (standard deviation) at baseline and 6- and 12-months and adjusted mean change (95% confidence interval) from baseline to 6-months and 12-months

Variable	Baseline	6-months	12-months	Baseline – 6-months change[d]	Baseline – 12-months change[d]
LS BMC (g)	32.6 (8.4)	35.0 (8.3)	37.0 (9.1)	0.3 (− 0.9, 1.6)	1.2 (− 0.5, 2.8)
LS BMC z-score	−0.09 (0.64)	− 0.14 (0.65)	− 0.14 (0.65)	− 0.04 (− 0.24, 0.16)	−0.02 (− 0.28, 0.23)
Distal tibia Tt.BMD (mg/cm^3)	223.1 (34.1)	223.8 (28.7)	234.9 (29.5)	2.7 (−5.0, 10.5)	15.0 (5.0, 25.0)[a]
z-score	− 0.98 (1.73)	− 1.10 (1.47)	− 0.86 (1.60)	− 0.15 (− 0.44, 0.13)	0.06 (− 0.30, 0.43)
# with z-score < − 2	3	2	3		
Distal tibia BV/TV	0.141 (0.026)	0.141 (0.022)	0.144 (0.026)	−0.001 (− 0.006, 0.004)	0.001 (− 0.005, 0.007)
z-score	− 0.74 (1.48)	− 0.79 (1.30)	− 0.69 (1.46)	− 0.08 (− 0.31, 0.15)	0.01 (− 0.29, 0.30)
# with z-score < − 2	4	3	3		
Distal tibia Ct.Th (mm)	0.69 (0.15)	0.69 (0.17)	0.77 (0.14)	−0.002 (− 0.054, 0.050)	0.075 (0.009, 0.142)[b]
z-score	−1.35 (1.62)	− 1.65 (1.59)	− 1.08 (1.62)	− 0.62 (− 1.14, − 0.10)[d]	−0.23 (− 0.91, 0.44)
# with z-score < − 2	4	4	2		
Distal tibia F.Load (N)	3628 (845)	3825 (771)	4121 (878)	4.8 (− 204.9, 214.6)	190.2 (−81.1, 461.5)
z-score	−1.57 (1.58)	− 1.58 (1.14)	− 1.33 (1.39)	−0.08 (− 0.40, 0.25)	0.13 (− 0.29, 0.55)
# with z-score < − 2	4	4	4		
Distal radius Tt.BMD (mg/cm^3)[c]	251.3 (37.7)	245.5 (29.4)	242.3 (33.8)	−0.5 (− 14.2, 13.1)	1.5 (− 16.6, 19.6)
z-score	0.07 (0.83)	−0.26 (0.99)	− 0.47 (0.90)	− 0.42 (− 0.80, − 0.03)[d]	−0.60 (− 1.11, − 0.09)[b]
# with z-score < − 2	0	0	0		
Distal radius BV/TV[c]	0.136 (0.022)	0.139 (0.023)	0.135 (0.027)	0.002 (−0.004, 0.007)	− 0.004 (− 0.011, 0.004)
z-score	−0.50 (0.97)	− 0.42 (1.01)	−0.67 (1.32)	0.01 (− 0.27, 0.30)	−0.27 (− 0.64, 0.10)
# with z-score < − 2	1	1	1		
Distal radius Ct.Th (mm)[c]	0.62 (0.15)	0.60 (0.13)	0.60 (0.16)	0.03 (−0.03, 0.10)	0.08 (− 0.01, 0.16)
z-score	−0.21 (1.01)	− 0.61 (0.98)	−0.77 (0.83)	− 0.36 (− 0.97, 0.24)	−0.39 (− 1.18, 0.40)
# with z-score < − 2	0	1	0		
Distal radius F.Load (N)[c]	1217 (392)	1297 (393)	1301 (375)	27.6 (−43.7, 99.0)	− 10.2 (− 105.3, 84.8)
z-score	−0.93 (1.47)	− 1.02 (1.32)	−1.25 (1.37)	− 0.22 (− 0.55, 0.12)	−0.38 (− 0.83, 0.06)
# with z-score < − 2	3	2	3		

BMC bone mineral content, *Tt.BMD* total bone mineral density, *BV/TV* trabecular bone volume ratio, *Ct.Th* cortical thickness, *F.Load* failure load

[a] $p < 0.01$; [b] $p < 0.05$

[c] $n = 12$ at baseline and 6-months and $n = 11$ at 12-months

[d] Adjusted for change in height and maturity offset at baseline

Table 4 Muscle outcomes assessed by dynamometry and mechanography in those participants that completed the study ($n = 13$). Values are mean (standard deviation) at baseline, 3-, 6- and 12-months and adjusted mean change (95% confidence interval) for change from baseline to 3-, 6- and 12-months

Variable	Baseline	3-months	6-months	12-months	Baseline-3 months[c]	Baseline-6 months[c]	Baseline-12 months[c]
Grip strength, left (kg)	19.5 (6.3)	19.6 (6.1)	19.8 (6.8)	21.6 (6.1)	−0.8 (−2.2, 0.6)	−1.5 (−3.2, 0.2)	−0.7 (2.9, 1.5)
Grip strength, right (kg)	20.9 (6.0)	22.3 (7.5)	22.0 (6.6)	23.7 (.1)	0.6 (−0.6, 1.9)	−0.4 (−1.9, 1.0)	0.5 (−1.4, 2.4)
Peak power (W/kg)	37.8 (5.5)	39.3 (7.3)	38.2 (5.5)	39.3 (5.9)	0.8 (−1.1, 2.7)	−0.9 (−3.3, 1.4)	− 0.7 (− 3.6, 2.3)
Peak power z-score	− 0.79 (0.95)	−0.58 (0.98)	− 0.84 (0.94)	−0.70 (0.91)	0.13 (− 0.21, 0.47)	−0.20 (− 0.61, 0.21)	−0.15 (− 0.67, 0.37)
Peak force, right leg (F_{max}/BW)	2.84 (0.40)	2.82 (0.39)	2.80 (0.33)	2.90 (0.33)	−0.00 (− 0.01, 0.01)	−0.01 (− 0.02, 0.00)	0.21 (0.19, 0.22)[a]
Peak force, right leg z-score	−0.82 (1.18)	− 0.52 (1.30)	−0.95 (1.16)	− 0.63 (1.07)	0.31 (− 0.14, 0.75)	−0.12 (− 0.66, 0.41)	0.21 (− 0.48, 0.89)
Peak force, left leg	2.75 (0.42)	2.94 (0.41)	2.74 (0.31)	2.80 (0.36)	−0.01 (− 0.02, 0.00)	−0.02 (− 0.03, − 0.003)[b]	0.19 (0.17, 0.21)[a]
Peak force, left leg z-score	− 1.15 (1.36)	−0.88 (1.25)	−1.16 (1.06)	− 1.02 (1.28)	0.15 (− 0.29, 0.59)	−0.23 (− 0.78, 0.30)	−0.23 (− 0.91, 0.45)
KE Peak torque (N-m)							
60 °·s 1	182.0 (29.4)	192.5 (38.9)	203.4 (53.1)	219.7 (65.5)	−3.4 (−21.9, 15.0)	−8.6 (− 31.3, 14.0)	− 5.8 (− 33.9, 22.3)
180 °·s 1	145.1 (27.3)	160.9 (29.5)	167.7 (34.7)	181.3 (49.5)	7.3 (− 4.5, 19.0)	4.5 (−9.9, 19.0)	9.6 (−8.4, 27.6)
KE Average power (W)							
60 °·s 1	44.1 (11.2)	50.3 (15.2)	53.1 (17.4)	56.3 (22.7)	0.1 (−6.5, 6.7)	−3.5 (−11.6, 4.6)	− 6.7 (− 16.8, 3.3)
180 °·s 1	91.5 (24.6)	105.6 (25.7)	107.4 (27.1)	112.0 (31.6)	7.0 (−2.4, 16.4)	2.1 (−9.4, 13.6)	−1.4 (− 15.7, 12.9)
KE Total joint work (J)							
60 °·s 1	303.5 (91.8)	318.0 (76.6)	322.5 (89.1)	360.7 (107.3)	−4.8 (−38.6, 29.0)	− 18.8 (− 60.3, 22.6)	−2.9 (− 54.3, 48.4)
180 °·s 1	571.5 (162.1)	635.8 (154.1)	639.9 (156.7)	667.8 (170.2)	31.0 (−26.4, 88.5)	4.2 (−66.2, 74.7)	−7.3 (− 94.8, 80.1)

KE knee extensor; [a]$p < 0.001$; [b] $p < 0.05$; [c] adjusted for change in height and maturity offset at baseline

future, the exercise intervention could be adapted to include more group- or in person-contact with the exercise instructor, incentives for participation, or incorporate interactive technologies (e.g. Fitbits), social media (e.g. Strava) or internet-based interventions to monitor and encourage adherence, particularly when participants are not in close geographic proximity [42–44]. Armbrust and colleagues recently reported promising results for their internet-based PA intervention, "Rheumates @ Work" (R@W) [45]. In contrast to the present study, R@W did not include a prescriptive exercise component. Instead, each week of the interactive, cognitive-behavioral program targeted a different theme such as health education and barriers and benefits of being physically active through online films, animations, puzzles and/or assignments. Acceptance and satisfaction with R@W were very high (93.8% and 85%, respectively) among children aged 8 to 13 years [44] and this translated into improvements in children's PA and exercise capacity [45]. Further, low program costs suggest this might be a feasible program for others to implement, perhaps in combination with recommended activities to promote muscle and bone strength, rather than a prescriptive exercise component.

Clinical outcomes

Participants had low disease activity for the duration of the study, but almost half reported some functional difficulties (CHAQ above 0). PA levels were low to average and did not change during the study. Fatigue was common but diminished after 6 months of exercise; this decrease was sustained at 12 months. This is promising as fatigue may be a barrier to participation in PA and organized sport among children with JIA [46]. We did not observe any other improvements in clinical outcomes, which may in part relate to low adherence.

Bone and muscle outcomes

Ours is the first study to utilize HR-pQCT to examine bone structure and strength in children with JIA. Of note, whereas DXA-derived lumbar spine BMC z-scores were within the normal range for all participants, several participants had z-scores for bone strength, structure and density lower than two standard deviations at both the distal tibia and radius. Similar to previous studies that employed pQCT imaging [15–17], this finding suggests that bone strength and structure may be compromised in children with JIA. We aim to investigate this further in the larger LEAP study.

The intervention did not positively influence children's bone mass, structure or strength z-scores. Although short bouts of jumping activity are known to benefit bone structure at the weight-bearing tibia in school-aged children without JIA [34, 47], low adherence and attrition (implementation factors) likely contributed to our inability to adequately assess effect of the intervention itself (design factors) on bone mass, structure and strength in children with JIA. Further, 6 months may have been insufficient to accurately assess exercise-related adaptations in these bone outcomes. The decline in Tt.BMD z-score at the distal radius may also suggest that modifications to the exercise program are required to provide a more osteogenic stimulus (e.g., dynamic loads of greater magnitude) to the upper limbs.

We extend previous studies of children with JIA that measured strength for single muscle groups, by incorporating jumping mechanography to assess peak force and peak power [48]. Muscle function measured by mechanography is not well described in children with arthritis. However, these measures may be more relevant to children's daily activities than traditional single muscle or muscle group strength testing. Children with JIA performed jumping mechanography without difficulty and demonstrated modest improvements in muscle function over the course of the study. However, changes in z-scores for mechanography outcomes as well as grip strength and knee extensor torque, power and total work were likely a function of normal growth and development as the increases over 3-, 6- and 12-months were no longer significant after we accounted for height and maturity.

We acknowledge several limitations of our study. Intervention efficacy was hampered by relatively high attrition and low adherence. It will be important in future to identify factors that negatively impact implementation and overcome them, where possible. Also, we did not have a control group with which to compare change in outcomes and accurately tease out the distinct influences of growth and maturation separate from the intervention on bone and muscle outcomes. Finally, we did not assess serum levels of vitamin D nor did we provide participants with calcium (or vitamin D) supplements despite the fact that most participants did not meet the dietary reference intake for calcium of 1300 mg/day [49]. Supplementation may be warranted in future exercise trials. Further, the influence of dietary calcium intake on bone outcomes in children with JIA will be explored in the larger LEAP study.

Conclusions

Children with JIA safely participated in a 6-month targeted home- and group-exercise program that incorporated short bouts of high-impact exercise and resistance training to increase bone and muscle strength. We highlight key challenges of exercise interventions in this population including high attrition and low adherence. There is a sensitive balance between designing an effective exercise program to promote children's muscle and bone health and implementing it effectively in children with JIA.

Future studies should devise strategies that mitigate pain and barriers to implementation, including novel approaches to enhance compliance and minimize attrition. Examples may include innovative program delivery via web-based online platforms and more effective participation incentives using customized apps and wearable technology. Promotion of physical literacy and age appropriate physical activity, including recommendations of activities that strengthen muscle and bone at least 3 days per week, may be more effective than precise exercise prescription. Continued efforts are needed to encourage a physically active lifestyle as a means to promote overall health and well-being in children with JIA.

Abbreviations

APHV: Age at peak height velocity; BMC: Bone Mineral Content; BMD: Bone Mineral Density; BV/TV: Trabecular bone volume ratio; CHAQ: Child Health Activity Questionnaire; Ct.Th: Cortical thickness; CYPSP: Child and Youth Physical Self-perception Profile; DXA: Dual energy X-ray absorptiometry; F.Load: Failure load; HR-pQCT: High-resolution peripheral quantitative computed tomography; JAQQ : Juvenile Arthritis Quality of Life Questionnaire; JIA: Juvenile idiopathic arthritis; LEAP: Linking Exercise, Physical Activity and Pathophysiology in Childhood Arthritis; MVPA: Moderate to vigorous physical activity; PA: Physical activity; PAQ-A: Physical activity questionnaire - adolescents; PAQ-C: Physical activity questionnaire – child

Acknowledgements

We gratefully acknowledge the participants and their families whose commitment and contributions to the LEAP study are invaluable. We also acknowledge the dedication of the LEAP research team, particularly the efforts of our kinesiologist Kara Delaney, research coordinators Felice Mizan and Douglas Race, summer research student Adam Mitha and the supervision of image acquisition and processing from Dr. Danmei Liu (Centre for Hip Health and Mobility, Vancouver Coastal Health Research Institute). We are also grateful to Dr. Leigh Gabel (University of Calgary) for her assistance with the statistical analysis. We acknowledge members of the LEAP investigator team including: Roberta Berard, Gilles Boire, Alessandra Bruns, Sarah Campillo, Gaëlle Chédeville, Paul Dancey, Janet Ellsworth, Debbie Feldman, Adam Huber, Nicole Johnson, Roman Jurencak, Claire LeBlanc, Deborah Levy, Paivi Miettunen, Kimberly Morishita, Suzanne Ramsey, Alan Rosenberg, Johannes Roth, Dax Rumsey, Heinrike Schmeling, Rosie Scuccimarri, Natalie Shiff, Elizabeth Stringer, Shirley Tse and Leanne Ward.

Funding

We received funding from the Canadian Institutes of Health Research (CIHR; GRANT# 107535).

Authors' contributions

All authors made substantial contributions to conception and design, analysis and interpretation of data. KH and LT performed all clinical assessments. KH and

HMac drafted the manuscript and all authors critically revised the manuscript for important intellectual content. All authors read and approved the final manuscript.

Consent for publication

Parents or guardians provided written informed consent and children provided assent.

Competing interests

The authors declare that they have no competing interests.

Author details

[1]Division of Rheumatology, K4-123 ACB, British Columbia Children's Hospital, 4480 Oak Street, Vancouver, BC V6H 3V4, Canada. [2]Department of Pediatrics, University of British Columbia, Vancouver, BC, Canada. [3]Department of Family Practice, University of British Columbia, Vancouver, BC, Canada. [4]Centre for Hip Health and Mobility, Vancouver Coastal Health Research Institute, Vancouver, BC, Canada. [5]Department of Orthopaedics, University of British Columbia, Vancouver, BC, Canada. [6]Division of Rheumatology, Department of Pediatrics, Children's Hospital of Eastern Ontario and University of Ottawa, Ottawa, Canada.

References

1. Bos GJFJ, Lelieveld OTHM, Armbrust W, Sauer PJJ, Geertzen JHB, Dijkstra PU. Physical activity in children with juvenile idiopathic arthritis compared to controls. Pediatr Rheumatol Online J. 2016;14:42.
2. Lelieveld OTHM, Armbrust W, van Leeuwen MA, Duppen N, Geertzen JHB, Sauer PJJ, et al. Physical activity in adolescents with juvenile idiopathic arthritis. Arthritis Rheum. 2008;59:1379–84.
3. van Brussel M, Lelieveld OTHM, van der Net J, Engelbert RHH, Helders PJM, Takken T. Aerobic and anaerobic exercise capacity in children with juvenile idiopathic arthritis. Arthritis Rheum. 2007;57:891–7.
4. Cavallo S, April KT, Grandpierre V, Majnemer A, Feldman DE. Leisure in children and adolescents with juvenile idiopathic arthritis: a systematic review. PLoS One. 2014;9:e104642.
5. Cavallo S, Majnemer A, Duffy CM, Feldman DE. Participation in leisure activities by children and adolescents with juvenile idiopathic arthritis. J Rheumatol. 2015;42:1708–15.
6. Gualano B, Bonfa E, Pereira RMR, Silva CA. Physical activity for paediatric rheumatic diseases: standing up against old paradigms. Nat Rev Rheumatol. 2017;13:368–79.
7. Philpott J, Houghton K, Luke A. Physical activity recommendations for children with specific chronic health conditions: juvenile idiopathic arthritis, hemophilia, asthma and cystic fibrosis. Paediatr Child Health. 2010;15:213–25.
8. Cavallo S, Brosseau L, Toupin-April K, Wells GA, Smith CA, Pugh AG, et al. Ottawa panel evidence-based clinical practice guidelines for structured physical activity in the management of juvenile idiopathic arthritis. Arch Phys Med Rehabil. 2017;98:1018–41.
9. Kuntze G, Nesbitt C, Whittaker JL, Nettel-Aguirre A, Toomey C, Esau S, et al. Exercise therapy in juvenile idiopathic arthritis: a systematic review and meta-analysis. Arch Phys Med Rehabil. 2018;99:178–193.e1.
10. Takken T, van Brussel M, Engelbert RH, van der Net JJ, Kuis W, Helders PP. Exercise therapy in juvenile idiopathic arthritis: a Cochrane Review. Eur J Phys Rehabil Med. 2008;44:287–97.
11. Catania H, Fortini V, Cimaz R. Physical exercise and physical activity for children and adolescents with juvenile idiopathic arthritis: a literature review. Pediatr Phys Ther. 2017;29:256–60.
12. Tan VPS, Macdonald HM, Kim S, Nettlefold L, Gabel L, Ashe MC, et al. Influence of physical activity on bone strength in children and adolescents: a systematic review and narrative synthesis. J Bone Miner Res. 2014;29: 2161–81.
13. Lien G, Selvaag AM, Flato B, Haugen M, Vinje O, Sorskaar D, et al. A two-year prospective controlled study of bone mass and bone turnover in children with early juvenile idiopathic arthritis. Arthritis Rheum. 2005;52:833–40.
14. Burnham JM, Leonard MB. Bone disease in pediatric rheumatologic disorders. Curr Rheumatol Rep. 2004;6:70–8.
15. Stagi S, Cavalli L, Signorini C, Bertini F, Cerinic MM, Brandi ML, et al. Bone mass and quality in patients with juvenile idiopathic arthritis: longitudinal evaluation of bone-mass determinants by using dual-energy x-ray absorptiometry, peripheral quantitative computed tomography, and quantitative ultrasonography. Arthritis Res Ther. 2014;16:R83.
16. Burnham JM, Shults J, Dubner SE, Sembhi H, Zemel BS, Leonard MB. Bone density, structure, and strength in juvenile idiopathic arthritis: importance of disease severity and muscle deficits. Arthritis Rheum. 2008;58:2518–27.

17. Roth J, Palm C, Scheunemann I, Ranke MB, Schweizer R, Dannecker GE. Musculoskeletal abnormalities of the forearm in patients with juvenile idiopathic arthritis relate mainly to bone geometry. Arthritis Rheum. 2004;50: 1277–85.
18. Burnham JM, Shults J, Weinstein R, Lewis JD, Leonard MB. Childhood onset arthritis is associated with an increased risk of fracture: a population based study using the general practice research database. Ann Rheum Dis. 2006; 65:1074–9.
19. Sandstedt E, Fasth A, Fors H, Beckung E. Bone health in children and adolescents with juvenile idiopathic arthritis and the influence of short-term physical exercise. Pediatr Phys Ther. 2012;24:155-61–discussion162.
20. Heaney RP. The bone-remodeling transient: implications for the interpretation of clinical studies of bone mass change. J Bone Miner Res. 1994;9:1515–23.
21. Petty RE, Southwood TR, Manners P, Baum J, Glass DN, Goldenberg J, et al. International league of associations for rheumatology classification of juvenile idiopathic arthritis: second revision, Edmonton, 2001. J Rheumatol. 2004;31:390–2.
22. Moore SA, McKay HA, Macdonald H, Nettlefold L, Baxter-Jones ADG, Cameron N, et al. Enhancing a somatic maturity prediction model. Med Sci Sports Exerc. 2015;47:1755–64.
23. Singh G, Athreya BH, Fries JF, Goldsmith DP. Measurement of health status in children with juvenile rheumatoid arthritis. Arthritis Rheumatol. 1994;37: 1761–9.
24. Crocker PR, Bailey DA, Faulkner RA, Kowalski KC, McGrath R. Measuring general levels of physical activity: preliminary evidence for the physical activity questionnaire for older children. Med Sci Sports Exerc. 1997;29: 1344–9.
25. Kowalski KC, Crocker P, Faulkner RA. Validation of the physical activity questionnaire for older children. Pediatr Exerc Sci. 1997;9:174–86.
26. Varni JW, Burwinkle TM, Szer IS. The PedsQL multidimensional fatigue scale in pediatric rheumatology: reliability and validity. J Rheumatol. 2004;31: 2494–500.
27. Duffy CM, Arsenault L, Duffy KN, Paquin JD, Strawczynski H. The juvenile arthritis quality of life questionnaire--development of a new responsive index for juvenile rheumatoid arthritis and juvenile spondyloarthritides. J Rheumatol. 1997;24:738–46.
28. Whitehead JR. A study of children's physical self-perceptions using an adapted physical self-perception profile questionnaire. Pediatr Exerc Sci. 1995;7:132–51.
29. Barr SI. Associations of social and demographic variables with calcium intakes of high school students. J Am Diet Assoc. 1994;94:260–6.
30. Tanner JM. Foetus into man. Cambridge: Harvard University Press; 1978.
31. Gabel L, Nettlefold LA, Macdonald HM, McKay HA. Sex-, ethnic- and age-specific centile curves for pQCT- and HR-pQCT-derived measures of bone structure and strength in adolescents and young adults. J Bone Miner Res. 2018;33:987–1000.
32. Baxter-Jones ADG, Burrows M, Bachrach LK, Lloyd T, Petit M, Macdonald H, et al. International longitudinal pediatric reference standards for bone mineral content. Bone. 2010;46:208–16.
33. McKay HA, MacLean L, Petit M, MacKelvie-O'Brien K, Janssen P, Beck T, et al. "Bounce at the bell": a novel program of short bouts of exercise improves proximal femur bone mass in early pubertal children. Br J Sports Med. 2005; 39:521–6.
34. Macdonald HM, Kontulainen SA, Khan KM, McKay HA. Is a school-based physical activity intervention effective for increasing tibial bone strength in boys and girls? J Bone Miner Res. 2007;22:434–46.
35. McKay H, Tsang G, Heinonen A, MacKelvie K, Sanderson D, Khan KM. Ground reaction forces associated with an effective elementary school based jumping intervention. Br J Sports Med. 2005;39:10–4.
36. Sims-Gould J, Race DL, Macdonald H, Houghton KM, Duffy CM, Tucker LB, McKay HA. "I just want to get better": experiences of children and youth with juvenile idiopathic arthritis in a home-based exercise intervention. Pediatr Rheumatol Online J. 2018;16:59.
37. de Onis M, Onyango AW, Borghi E, Siyam A, Nishida C, Siekmann J. Development of a WHO growth reference for school-aged children and adolescents. Bull World Health Organ. 2007;85:660–7.
38. Sandstedt E, Fasth A, Eek MN, Beckung E. Muscle strength, physical fitness and well-being in children and adolescents with juvenile idiopathic arthritis and the effect of an exercise programme: a randomized controlled trial. Pediatr Rheumatol Online J. 2013;11:7.
39. Feldman DE, De Civita M, Dobkin PL, Malleson PN, Meshefedjian G, Duffy CM. Effects of adherence to treatment on short-term outcomes in children with juvenile idiopathic arthritis. Arthritis Rheum. 2007;57:905–12.
40. Singh-Grewal D, Schneiderman-Walker J, Wright V, Bar-Or O, Beyene J, Selvadurai H, et al. The effects of vigorous exercise training on physical function in children with arthritis: a randomized, controlled, single-blinded trial. Arthritis Rheum. 2007;57:1202–10.
41. Rapoff MA. Compliance with treatment regimens for pediatric rheumatic diseases. Arthritis Care Res. 1989;2:S40–7.
42. Coda A, Sculley D, Santos D, Girones X, Brosseau L, Smith DR, et al. Harnessing interactive technologies to improve health outcomes in juvenile idiopathic arthritis. Pediatr Rheumatol Online J. 2017;15:40.
43. Lelieveld OTHM, Armbrust W, Geertzen JHB, de Graaf I, van Leeuwen MA, Sauer PJJ, et al. Promoting physical activity in children with juvenile idiopathic arthritis through an internet-based program: results of a pilot randomized controlled trial. Arthritis Care Res. 2010;62:697–703.
44. Armbrust W, Bos JJFJ, Cappon J, van Rossum MAJJ, Sauer PJJ, Wulffraat N, et al. Design and acceptance of Rheumates@work, a combined internet-based and in person instruction model, an interactive, educational, and cognitive behavioral program for children with juvenile idiopathic arthritis. Pediatr Rheumatol Online J. 2015;13:31.
45. Armbrust W, Bos GJFJ, Wulffraat NM, van Brussel M, Cappon J, Dijkstra PU, et al. Internet program for physical activity and exercise capacity in children with juvenile idiopathic arthritis: a multicenter randomized controlled trial. Arthritis Care Res. 2017;69:1040–9.
46. Armbrust W, Lelieveld OHTM, Tuinstra J, Wulffraat NM, Bos GJFJ, Cappon J, et al. Fatigue in patients with juvenile idiopathic arthritis: relationship to perceived health, physical health, self-efficacy, and participation. Pediatr Rheumatol Online J. 2016;14:65.
47. MacKelvie KJ, Petit MA, Khan KM, Beck TJ, McKay HA. Bone mass and structure are enhanced following a 2-year randomized controlled trial of exercise in prepubertal boys. Bone. 2004;34:755–64.
48. Fricke O, Weidler J, Tutlewski B, Schoenau E. Mechanography–a new device for the assessment of muscle function in pediatrics. Pediatr Res. 2006;59:46–9.
49. Institute of Medicine. Dietary Reference Intakes for Calcium and Vitamin D. Washington, DC: Institute of Medicine; 2010. Available from: http://www.nationalacademies.org/hmd/Reports/2010/Dietary-Reference-Intakes-for-Calcium-and-Vitamin-D.aspx

Self-management needs of Irish adolescents with Juvenile Idiopathic Arthritis (JIA): how can a Canadian web-based programme meet these needs?

Grace O'Sullivan[1], Siobhán O'Higgins[1], Line Caes[2*], Sophia Saetes[1], Brian E. McGuire[1] and Jennifer Stinson[3,4,5]

Abstract

Background: *Juvenile Idiopathic Arthritis* (JIA) affects over 1000 children and adolescents in Ireland, potentially impacting health-related quality-of-life. Accessible self-management strategies, including Internet-based interventions, can support adolescents in Ireland where specialist rheumatology care is geographically-centralised within the capital city. This study interviewed adolescents with JIA, their parents, and healthcare professionals to (i) explore the self-management needs of Irish adolescents; and (ii) evaluate the acceptability of an adapted version of a Canadian JIA self-management programme (*Teens Taking Charge: Managing Arthritis Online,* or *TTC*) for Irish users.

Methods: Focus groups and interviews were conducted with Irish adolescents with JIA ($N = 16$), their parents ($N = 13$), and Irish paediatric healthcare professionals (HCPs; $N = 22$). Adolescents were aged 12–18 ($M_{age} = 14.19$ years), and predominantly female (62.5%). Participants identified the needs of adolescents with JIA and evaluated the usefulness of the TTC programme. Data were analysed using a thematic analysis approach.

Results: Five themes emerged: *independent self-management; acquiring skills and knowledge to manage JIA; unique challenges of JIA in Ireland; views on web-based interventions;* and *understanding through social support*. Adolescents acknowledged the need for independent self-management and gradually took additional responsibilities to achieve this goal. However, they felt they lacked information to manage their condition independently. Parents and adolescents emphasised the need for social support and felt a peer-support scheme could provide additional benefit to adolescents if integrated within the *TTC* programme. All participants endorsed the *TTC* programme to gain knowledge about JIA and offered suggestions to make the programme relevant to Irish users.

Conclusions: There is scope for providing easily-accessible, accurate information to Irish families with JIA. The acceptability of adapting an existing JIA self-management intervention for Irish users was confirmed.

Keywords: Juvenile arthritis, Adolescence, Self-management, Online intervention, Needs assessment

Introduction

Juvenile Idiopathic Arthritis (JIA) describes a cluster of exclusionary rheumatic diagnoses "*...that begin before the age of 16 years, persist for more than six weeks, and are of unknown origin*" [1–4]. JIA is the most common childhood rheumatic disease; in the Republic of Ireland, approximately 1200 children have JIA and over 100 children are diagnosed annually [5]. Symptoms include joint pain, swelling, inflammation, stiffness and fatigue, leaving children in significant pain and making school attendance or daily tasks difficult [6]. Physical and emotional symptoms restrict social interactions for these adolescents, isolating them from their peers, and has the potential to negatively impact health-related quality-of-life (HRQL) [7–11]. Compared to healthy peers, adolescents with JIA often report decreased HRQL and scores deteriorate with increased disease severity, pain, and degree of disability [8, 9, 12]. However,

* Correspondence: line.caes@stir.ac.uk
[2]Division of Psychology; Faculty of Natural Sciences, University of Stirling, Stirling, Scotland, UK

children with newly-diagnosed JIA can achieve HRQL similar to healthy children [13, 14], provided intervention begins at diagnosis.

Treatment for JIA is often multidisciplinary and includes pharmacological treatments, physiotherapy and psychological support. In the absence of a cure, treatments prioritise secondary prevention of complications and improving HRQL through disease self-management of *"physical or psychological consequences, and lifestyle changes"* [15]. Greater awareness and self-management among adolescents reduces associated adverse health outcomes [16]. Adolescence is a crucial life-stage for young people to gain independence from parents and take responsibility for their own needs. This applies to every adolescent, and particularly to those with chronic diseases, who must gradually learn independent disease self-management, and navigating the healthcare system. However, many adolescents with JIA do not receive comprehensive JIA self-management guidance [17–20], and feel unprepared to transfer from paediatric to adult care [8, 19, 21]. Additional barriers for effective self-management are perceived within the Irish health-care context, and raised by the participants of this study: long wait-times for appointments, inconsistent access to services outside of urban areas, and limited availability of child and adolescent rheumatology professionals; the latter becoming common across Europe, with many countries failing to supply satisfactory training in adolescent health and medicine [22, 23]. Accessible interventions to assist adolescents with self-management strategies can reduce these barriers [24–28].

Tailored online interventions can improve behavioural outcomes [28–30], and a Canadian study of adolescents with JIA, their parents and healthcare professionals revealed that adolescents wanted to manage JIA to maintain a 'normal' lifestyle with peers [22]. This prompted the development, usability and feasibility-testing of '*Teens Taking Charge*' (TTC), a self-management website for adolescents with JIA [22]. *TTC* contains twelve weekly modules with themed lessons and videos for adolescents, including skills-training, communication, advocacy, information on treatments, and service availability (e.g., school assistance). A parent site contains the same information without the twelve-week structure, and two additional modules on promoting their child's independence. Studies implementing *TTC* reported improvements in disease-related knowledge, decreased pain, and increased exercise adherence [12, 27, 29]. Before implementing programmes in other health-care contexts, it is imperative to evaluate their cultural appropriateness in the target population, who may experience different issues to adolescents elsewhere [30]. As a result, hypotheses were not specified at the outset. The primary aims were to (i) conduct a qualitative exploration of the self-management needs of Irish adolescents living with JIA, from their own perspective, and of their parents and healthcare professionals; and (ii) evaluate whether the *TTC* self-management website could be successfully adapted to meet the needs of Irish users.

To achieve this, qualitative interviews and focus groups were conducted with Irish adolescents with JIA, their parents, and paediatric health-care professionals.

Methods

Participants

All potential participants were identified through partnership with [1] the paediatric rheumatology departments of two large specialist children's hospitals in Dublin, Ireland, and [2] Irish arthritis organisations, *iCAN (Irish Children's Arthritis Network)* and *Arthritis Ireland,* who identified local primary care physicians, and families which met the eligibility criteria. This ensured the involvement of healthcare professionals (HCPs) from the core rheumatology teams within the children's hospitals and from primary care centres across Ireland. For adolescents and parents, eligibility screening was completed via telephone, using a pre-defined script. Eligibility criteria were: (i) adolescent is 12–18 years old, (ii) has diagnosis of a JIA subtype classified by the International League of Associations of Rheumatology (ILAR) [31], and (iii) has no comorbid conditions. Following inclusion criteria from similar studies, we used convenience sampling [22]. We did not differentiate between JIA subtypes, in line with the study's primary aim to qualitatively explore the self-management needs for adolescents with JIA.

Procedure

Once participation was agreed, dates for the adolescent and parent focus groups were arranged in three Irish cities closest to participating families, to allow participants to attend a conveniently-located focus group. Those unable to attend any focus group were offered an individual interview (in person, or via telephone; Table 1).

Adolescents, parents, and HCPs were interviewed in their respective groups by an interviewer and assistant. Focus groups lasted 60–75 min; individual interviews lasted 35–50 min. All interviews explored the challenges of living with (or treating those with) JIA, knowledge of medication or other therapies, how adolescents manage their condition, and sources of information [interview guides were adapted from previous needs assessments [22]]. The final section focused on the features and usability of the *TTC* programme for Irish families. This generally lasted 10–20 min, with adolescents spending more time in discussion than parents or HCPs. To facilitate this, all participants received access to the *TTC* website two weeks beforehand, and the website was also displayed on-screen during the interview.

Table 1 – Participant breakdown by group, location, and type of participation

	Focus group			Individual interview		Total
	Galway	Cork	Dublin	In person	Phone interview	
Adolescents	4	2	4	1	1	16[a]
Parents	4	3	4	1	1	13
HCPs	5	–	12	5	–	22

[a]16 adolescents were involved, as two parents participated without their children (1 in Cork; 1 phone interview)

Data analysis

Demographic data were analysed using descriptive tests in SPSS 22.0. Interviews were digitally-recorded and transcribed verbatim (GOS; SS). Transcriptions were analysed independently by two of the authors (GOS; SOH), using NVivo.11 [32], to compare to previously-identified themes [22] and identify potential new themes on the impact of JIA on daily life and on the future. New themes were agreed by both authors, who analysed transcriptions a second time against new and existing themes for confirmation.

Results

Fifty-three parents and adolescents were approached to participate (25 adolescents; 28 parents), with 43 meeting eligibility requirements. However, 14 of these eligible respondents (7 parent-adolescent pairs) did not attend their focus group, leaving 29 participants who met eligibility requirements (16 adolescents, 13 parents) (Fig. 1).

The participating adolescents were mostly in early (11–14 years, $N = 8$) or mid adolescence (15–16 years, $N = 7$), with one late-stage adolescent (17–18 years; $N = 1$) ($M = 14.19$ years; $SD = 2.07$). Most were female ($N = 10$; 62.5%) and of Irish nationality ($N = 15$; 93.7%). Mean time since diagnosis was 3.6 years ($SD = 3.28$ years; range = 0.58–13.83 years) and the most frequent subtype was psoriatic arthritis ($N = 5$; 31.3%) (Table 2).

Of the thirteen parents, most were biological mothers ($N = 12$; 92.3%), Irish ($N = 12$; 92.3%), and the typical age-range was 40–49 years ($N = 10$; 76.9%). Most were married ($N = 10$; 76.9%), had a university degree ($N = 7$; 53.9%), and were employed full-time or part-time ($N = 8$; 61.5%). Two were full-time carers for their child ($N = 2$; 15.4%).

Eligibility for HCPs included minimum one year of experience in working with JIA. All but two of the approached HCPs participated in the study. The 22 HCPs had an average of 8.45 years of experience working with chronic pain and were representative of most disciplines involved in treating adolescents with JIA (Table 3).

Thematic clusters

Across all participant groups (parents, adolescents, HCPs), four main themes emerged: [1] *independent self-management (*including the sub-theme *"the impact of JIA on the future"* for parents and adolescents only); [2] *acquiring JIA knowledge and skills;* [3] *the unique challenges of JIA in Ireland;* [4] *web-based approaches to self-management.* A fifth theme appeared from parent and adolescent accounts: *experiencing understanding through social support.* Each theme and subtheme are discussed in detail below.

1. Independent self-management

Most adolescents wanted to become more self-sufficient before transferring to adult care. Some adolescents started this process by attending appointments alone:

> *Mam takes care of hospital appointments and bloods. I take care of my injections...She tries not to remind me anymore, I have to learn one day* (Adolescent 7)

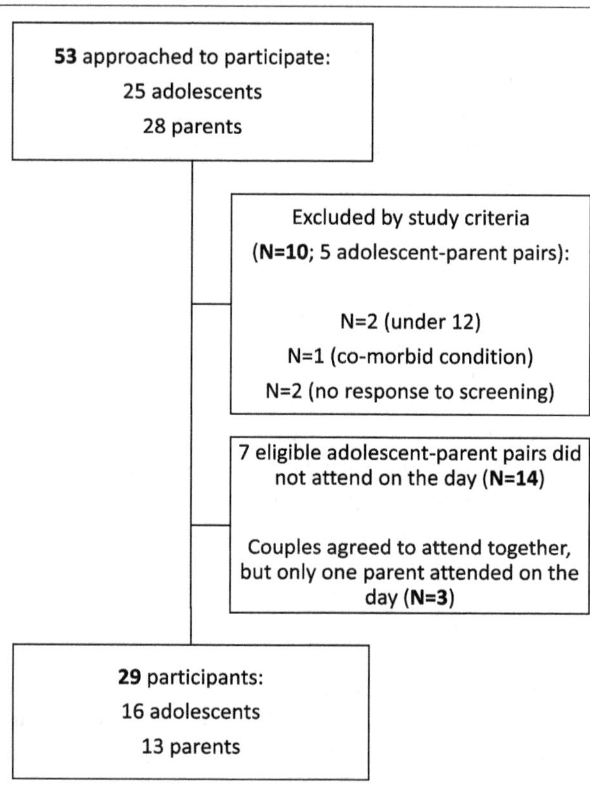

Fig. 1 – Screening process for parent and adolescent participants

Table 2 – JIA subtypes within the adolescent group

Arthritis subtype	Number in sample
Systemic	2
Polyarticular (RF Negative)	1
Polyarticular (RF Positive)	2
Psoriatic	5
Enthesitis-related	4
Other	2 (1 Poly/systemic overlapping; 1 undifferentiated)
Oligoarticular	0
Extended oligo-articular	0

Parents of younger adolescents encouraged responsibility over a gradual period:

> *She's twelve, but I get her into some OT [occupational therapy] appointments on her own, and I meet up with them after* (Parent 4)

> *She does her injections all the time now. We'd be there with her though* (Parent 13)

Medication presented a major barrier to gaining independence for adolescents, with parents often reminding them or administering it for them:

> *I take two injections every week and I always forget. I'll be in bed and Mum will shout up to me 'Have you taken your medications?' And I'm like 'Oh!'* (Adolescent 16).

One HCP felt that overprotective parental attitudes prevented adolescents from becoming self-sufficient:

> *A lot of it is breaking away from their parents and accepting the responsibility. Teenagers think 'Oh Mum or Dad will do that'. It's difficult for the parents to trust them* (HCP 20)

The HCPs suggested building trust gradually, through increasing the responsibilities handled by the adolescents, and offering support during that transition:

> *It's giving them responsibility and saying, 'You can do it, and if you need support or resources, here they are'* (HCP 20)

Impact of JIA on the future

Adolescents had not considered a future with JIA beyond career concerns (understandable given the younger age of this cohort). Parents had weighed the impact of JIA on their child's future:

> *I've always wanted to do teaching...But I'm worried I'm not going to be able to stand for six hours* (Adolescent 17)

> *You just want them to go out and do the same things as their peers. Get the job, go to college. You want them to be normal, to be like everyone else* (Parent 19)

Table 3 – Overview of the HCP group

Profession	Frequency	Percentage (%)
Physician	5	22.7
Nurse	5	22.7
Physiotherapist	5	22.7
Psychologist	1	4.5
Physical Therapist	1	4.5
Occupational Therapist	5	22.7
Demographics		
Mean age range	30–39 years (N = 10; 45.5%)	
Gender	Female (N = 16; 72.7%); Male (N = 6; 27.3%)	
Highest educational level	Bachelor's degree (N = 8; 36.4%) Master's degree (N = 5; 22.7%) PhD or Medical degree (N = 6; 27.2%) Other (N = 3; 13.6%)	
Mean years of clinical experience	16.8 years (SD = 9.79 years; range = 3–46)	
Mean years of experience with chronic pain	8.45 years (SD = 5.47 years; range = 0–16)	
Work in a multi-disciplinary pain team?	Yes = 10 (45.5%)	

Generally, parents and adolescents prioritised managing JIA day-to-day, rather than planning for the future.

2. Acquiring knowledge and skills to manage JIA

a) ***Acquiring arthritis knowledge and awareness***

Adolescents gained most of their information on JIA from parents, which was limited as parents struggled to find accurate information themselves. Sources of information included medical pamphlets, websites and other parents, who often 'crowdsourced' their knowledge:

> *I was quite young when I got it, so the doctors told my parents and my parents told me* (Adolescent 8)

> *[Daughter] was getting more pains, and [another parent] said to me 'If you're not getting Omega-3's, she'll end up with more pains in her muscles'* (Parent 14)

Parents often used Google or Facebook pages of arthritis support organisations; however, such information was considered insufficient:

> *When you're online in American or Canadian stuff, they're [medications] different names! They don't know what we take, and they'll be taking different things. You have to Google what it is...* (Parent 15)

Parents of newly-diagnosed children relied heavily on more experienced parents:

> *I'm at such an early stage, I don't know where to turn. If she's having a flare, what do I do? I'm learning by the other parents* (Parent 18)

> *This is something I've been going on about, there's no information pack, you're thrown into this... It's like getting hit by a bus* (Parent 3)

However, HCPs emphasised that literature was readily available:

> *When they come to physio they get a lot of paperwork about activity, lifestyle, balance, sleep, hygiene, and exercise programs* (HCP 22)

Though parents and HCPs disagreed over the availability of information, each agreed that a comprehensive source was needed for Irish families to learn JIA self-management skills.

b) ***Managing pain and discomfort***

All adolescents followed pharmacological treatment plans at the time of interview and many attended physiotherapists for joint pains. For most, managing pain and discomfort was achieved by reducing or switching activities:

> *I'm very sporty. I did Irish dancing, boxing and hurling. But I had to give up all of them, I was too sore* (Adolescent 13).

For most adolescents, the primary motivation for managing pain and discomfort was to join in activities and appear 'normal' with friends:

> *It can affect your friendships. If they're going out and you come too, you can't keep up. Or if you try, you need physio for the next three days* (Adolescent 35).

Parents and HCPs did not discuss pain and discomfort.

c) ***Managing emotions***

The language describing emotional struggles varied greatly between participant groups. Adolescents and HCPs discussed issues matter-of-factly, while parents used emotive language, highlighting the strain they felt:

> *I would say fight, fight, fight for everything you can* (Parent 14)

> *My daughter takes an injection every day. And the battle we have is every evening. It's a huge battle* (Parent 19)

Formal emotional support for JIA diagnoses was hardly discussed, as only a few adolescents had attended appointments with a psychologist:

> *I was in psychology for a bit, which I didn't feel was needed. Even when I was doing it. It was good that even if I didn't need it...it was available* (Adolescent 15).

Parents found day-to-day management of JIA stressful. They appreciated that psychological assessment could help their child, but accessibility issues were prevalent, confirmed by HCPs:

> *The service is disjointed. [Area] have a physio unit and OT, but mental health services are in a different area. It's difficult for people to get to* (Parent 34)

> *We have no psychologist in the paediatric department and the only psychological help is from referring it*

through Child and Adolescent Mental Health Services and there's waiting lists... (HCP 11)

Adolescents and parents preferred informal support from peers instead of psychological services (see *Section 5: Gaining Understanding through Social Support*). HCPs theorised this came from negative attitudes in Ireland towards seeking psychological services:

It's seen that if you need psychology, you aren't able to cope. It's 'What's wrong with you?' (HCP 26)

If you see psychology as a treatment for pain, they automatically think 'It's in my head' or 'We don't believe you' (HCP 32)

Frustrated by the stigma and accessibility issues for psychologists, HCPs encouraged their adolescent patients to seek support from informal sources:

I suppose the advice is to talk to a peer or a friend and maybe link into counselling, until they can get them in (HCP 24)

3. Unique challenges of a JIA diagnosis in Ireland

While elements of JIA diagnosis are similar worldwide, all participant groups perceived that Ireland had unique challenges, including lack of infrastructure, disproportionate division of services across the country, and cultural differences.

a) ***Long wait times for diagnosis***

The primary challenge for Irish families was receiving a diagnosis. With only three paediatric rheumatologists (all located in the capital city), there were significant delays in initial appointments. All participant groups mentioned lengthy wait times for services:

They wanted us to see [a psychologist] when I got diagnosed, which is nearly three years ago, and we're still waiting to see one (Adolescent 3)

We opted to go privately. The wait time for Rheumatology was two years or more going the public route... (Parent 34)

b) ***Unequal access to services***

This geographically-centralised care system involved long journeys for families outside Dublin, who missed work or school to travel for appointments. Some scheduled multiple appointments for one date, to reduce frequent cross-country trips, at the cost of long days:

Yeah, early start. We'd get up at five in the morning, to be there for 8:30. And we wouldn't get home until 7pm (Adolescent 4)

All participant groups agreed that the geographical concentration disadvantaged families outside the capital:

Our patients can be five hours from Dublin. We have a paediatrician who has an interest in rheumatology. He'll give infusions so they don't have to travel up and down (HCP 20)

I'm still struggling to get OT. I'd say if you were in Dublin it would be easier, but in [area] it's very hard (Parent 34)

c) ***High expenditure associated with the disease***

JIA placed a heavy financial burden on Irish families. Government-funded medical treatment is not guaranteed, and parents struggled with spiralling prescription and appointment costs:

I have to apply for the long-term illness payment. [Son's] medication bills were €200 a month. It's supposed to be about €140, that's a lot of money every month... (Parent 34)

Parents can take 'Carer's Leave' for up to two years (an employment break to care for relatives, with a small financial stipend). Some parents felt they had no other choice:

I gave up working. She was diagnosed at three and I never went back... (Parent 7)

HCPs asserted that high costs deterred treatment, as parents struggled to pay for everything:

You might say 'Oh, the dietitian might also be good'. But they pay extra or pay separately, so they pick and choose what they think is important (HCP 1)

Adolescents did not discuss the costs of JIA treatment.

d) ***Issues with Methotrexate***

Adherence issues were discussed specifically for Methotrexate, a disease-modifying anti-rheumatic drug

(DMARD). For adolescents, the unpleasant side-effects made them reluctant:

I'm tired every day. I'm not a morning person as it is, but the methotrexate makes it ten times worse (Adolescent 18)

Parents felt that long-term concerns also factored into this reluctance:

She had a flare a while back; they had to increase the methotrexate and she was devastated. She said to me, "How am I ever going to get pregnant?" (Parent 19)

Adolescent reluctance may also be related to alcohol consumption, which is contra-indicated while Methotrexate is prescribed. Irish adolescents commonly drink alcohol at social gatherings, so those with JIA would feel "different" from peers, according to parents and HCPs:

That group between fourteen and sixteen, we have the biggest issues with... Maybe they can't drink and have Methotrexate... There's pressure on teenagers to drink (HCP 9)

While avoiding Methotrexate is not exclusive to Irish adolescents, participants felt that avoidance in Irish adolescents may have been based on alcohol due to cultural practices around celebrating milestones; e.g., the 'Junior Certificate' (state exams taken midway through high school) are completed aged 14–15, and celebrations often include parties and alcohol, which may exacerbate feeling "different" in those taking Methotrexate.

4. Views on web-based approach to self-management

The adolescents were overwhelmingly positive about the *TTC* website:

I've never seen anything like it before. I've never seen a website that has all the information that you could think of (Adolescent 7)

Parents felt it would be particularly useful when families were first diagnosed:

For newly-diagnosed parents, who are finding their way in the first year, who don't know what an appointment with an OT or a physio is... (Parent 7)

They also praised the fact that the website could reassure adolescents on topics deemed too sensitive to discuss with parents:

It's good because 17A recently brought up about a tattoo when she's older. There's going to be something else that she wants to do that she won't ask her mother... But now there's a website where she can look (Parent 17)

HCPs appreciated the availability of a trusted site with accurate information:

It's very comprehensive, but simplistic enough to follow. I was pretty impressed. I learned loads of stuff myself, because it's a one-stop shop! (HCP 2)

However, they worried that the website would replace traditional medical advice:

My concern with that is they'll go to the website before they go to the GP (HCP 23)

Each participant group offered suggestions to make the *TTC* programme relevant for Irish users. Adolescents suggested Irish content: e.g., changing the names of medications and treatments (if trade names differed); replacing Canadian sports references with Irish sports; and adding video-clips featuring Irish adolescents:

It would be good to have a mix of videos from different places, because people would know that it happens everywhere (Adolescent 8)

As parents mainly used Google and North American websites for information, they proposed adding curated information suitable for Irish parents. Parents also wanted practical information regarding service access and entitlements:

What you're entitled to from the government... Links of where to go and how to apply. Services in their areas, walking groups and stuff (Parent 15)

One HCP suggested that the instructional videos could link to existing videos online:

You could have links to YouTube stretching programmes or how to perform certain exercises Then they could YouTube 'hamstring stretches' or 'back stretches' (HCP 20)

5. Gaining understanding through social support

Adolescents spoke positively about JIA support organisations and meeting each other at events:

I went on [organisation's] road trip and met loads of new friends...I talk to [14A] all the time because she understands what I'm going through... (Adolescent 16)

However, they avoided discussing their condition with non-JIA friends to not appear 'different':

I'm sure I could talk to them, but I don't. I stick to myself (Adolescent 15)

This was confirmed by parents:

I don't think [19A] was talking about her condition with her friends. I'm not sure that she shares with them how she's feeling every day (Parent 19)

Parents saw arthritis organisations as vital sources of social support:

That's why I joined iCAN. I could interact on my own terms (Parent 10)

It's tough going, if I wasn't with these [other parents], I wouldn't be sane (Parent 3)

Support from school teachers varied. Some adolescents experienced understanding from teachers, while others felt singled out, making them feel different from classmates:

[14A] and I go to the same school, so our teachers are pretty understanding. If I miss a day, I can catch up on work and print off the sheets and turn them in (Adolescent 16)

It's things like [17A]'s school tour. The teacher makes her sit at the front, and she's like 'No! Everyone will know there's something wrong with me!' (Parent 17)

Parents and adolescents agreed that teachers are not fully equipped to understand JIA:

The teacher said "Oh, [8A] is great, but he's a bit slower than the others". I said, '[8A] has arthritis'. And she said, 'Does he? You'd never know it to look at him'. (Parent 8)

Throughout the interviews, adolescents and parents highlighted social support from others living with JIA, and the idea was raised of integrating a peer-mentoring scheme, *iPeer2Peer,* into the *TTC* self-management program [26]. Adolescents liked discussing their condition with someone who understood:

It's harder to talk to someone who doesn't have [JIA] than someone who's gone through what you've gone through, who knows what mind-set you have (Adolescent 8)

Put [iPeer2Peer] on the front of the website so people will see it every time they log on. If they didn't pick it the first time, they might a few weeks later (Adolescent 14)

Parents were enthusiastic about their child linking up with older adolescents with JIA:

I do think it's a great idea! (Parent 19)

HCPs spoke positively of peer-to-peer mentoring, but worried about the spread of misinformation:

I would worry about life experiences they might share. If they had negative experiences with a staff member that would impact the mentee. (HCP 33)

Discussion

The identified themes match other countries, including the UK, US, and Canada [6, 22, 33], reinforcing that adolescents with JIA need information and support for their condition, to develop effective strategies to improve HRQL [6, 7, 10, 25]. Participants from all stakeholder groups agreed that Irish adolescents with JIA needed to become self-sufficient and take responsibility in managing their condition while transferring to adult care [17, 19, 34]. However, this independence can backfire when adolescents fail to adopt good self-care practices such as physiotherapy exercises or self-administering medications [35]. Methotrexate is often a contentious issue, partly due to contra-indications with alcohol, as previously mentioned by older adolescents in the UK [20]. Irish adolescents taking methotrexate may have felt hesitant to 'stand out' from their peers, according to parents and HCPs. Though underage drinking is declining across Europe, including Ireland, participants perceived that cultural practices involving alcohol meant Irish adolescents still drink more excessively than counterparts; this is partly corroborated by recent data [36]. Conversely, Canadian research found that adolescents sometimes used their JIA as a convenient means to avoid peer-pressure for risky behaviours such as underage drinking or unsafe sex [22].

Irish adolescents experienced lengthy wait-times for paediatric rheumatology consultations, despite guidelines stating that delays in diagnosis adversely impact disease prognosis, and should not exceed 10 weeks from symptom onset [37], as early diagnosis is crucial for interventions to successfully improve or maintain high levels of HRQL [13, 14] Almost 900 Irish children and adolescents are awaiting rheumatology services, and nearly 60% have been waiting for over one year [38, 39]. Several adolescents in this study quoted waiting two years for initial appointments and waiting times are increasing annually [39–41].

Regarding self-management, parents prioritised emotional and financial struggles, while adolescents focused on pain-management. The adolescents paced themselves to avoid injury or gave up cherished hobbies to reduce pain and discomfort. This resourcefulness has featured in previous qualitative studies on living with JIA, as adolescents 'strive for normality' [6, 20, 34], and persevere through pain to keep up with peers, rather than avoiding activities and being 'different' [6]. Adolescents may need to adjust coping strategies, and accept limitations as part of managing their condition [15]. Managing JIA was also difficult for parents, who struggled to support and advocate for their child; this struggle to 'master' their child's chronic pain has been previously reported [35]. Arguably the most striking finding was the combative parental language when describing difficulties in accessing supports (*'fight'; 'battle'*). Similar language was used by parents of children with complex regional pain syndrome [35], but to our knowledge, has not emerged in arthritis research before. Such *'fighting'* exhausted parents, who relied on support from each other rather than seek formal psychological support for the emotional strain of JIA. The HCPs felt that stigma surrounding psychological services in Ireland deterred many families, echoed by the families themselves.

It is notable that families were wary of psychological services. A study of healthy Irish adults reported more favourable attitudes towards seeking psychological help than similar European counterparts [42]. However, as our study asked adolescents and adults with personal or professional experience of pain and associated emotional strains, their perspectives may differ. Indeed, interviews with Irish adults living with psychological illnesses revealed strong stigma and discrimination towards them, and a preference for disclosing to family and friends rather than health professionals [43], which reflects our findings. Future online interventions should address the emotional strain of living with chronic illness, to equip families with coping strategies, especially if reluctant to seek formal support.

In acquiring information, a clear discrepancy in perspectives emerged. Families often struggle for knowledge about JIA [6, 34], and while adolescents in this study had found information on JIA, others relied on their parents who felt the information from HCPs was inadequate. This conflicted with HCP perspectives, who were adamant that families received information at diagnosis and when new medications or treatments were introduced. Disagreements about knowledge-sharing were found previously in JIA research [44], and these discrepancies emphasise the need for accessible sources of information on JIA that are relevant for Irish families and allow them to share with HCPs.

The *TTC* website was accepted by all participant groups as a promising means of providing information. Adolescents and parents unanimously supported a centralised website to learn about JIA, reflecting previous findings [22, 29, 30], and future studies could compare the Irish experience of using self-management websites with different countries including UK and Canada. The HCPs appreciated that the website offers current information to adolescents between visits. However, one HCP was concerned that the website would replace GP visits. This could be addressed by incorporating messaging to refer families to their GP with concerns, as learning to navigate primary care is a key self-management skill during transfer to adult services. The HSE (Health Service Executive) in Ireland offers an interactive map of local services [45]; this could be embedded within the *TTC* website or linked to externally.

The adolescents revealed strong desires to "fit in". Adolescents struggled with peers not understanding the restrictions of JIA, finding support instead from others with JIA with whom they identified more easily [20, 22]. Irish JIA adolescents often met through arthritis organisations and connected through social media. Internet-based initiatives are a promising means to promote 'normality' amongst adolescents with JIA [6, 21, 29], and this group strongly endorsed online peer-mentoring programmes like *iPeer2Peer* [26] to discuss their experiences with like-minded peers. In a systematic review of peer relationships in adolescents with chronic pain, parents reported their children were less socially-active and had fewer 'close' friends than healthy peers [11]. While this was not expressed here, the parents praised *iPeer2Peer* for allowing their child to socialise with similar adolescents. One HCP was concerned that adolescents would share bad experiences with each other; while this is possible, the benefits of online support groups outweigh the downsides [22, 46]. Ultimately, *iPeer2Peer* was regarded as a positive addition to the tailored self-management offered by *TTC*.

Strengths

This study presents diverse viewpoints from adolescents with JIA across Ireland, their parents and their healthcare providers. Parents were exceptionally keen to participate, as some mentioned being 'desperate' for assistance. HCPs agreed to share their experience of treating adolescents with JIA in Ireland, despite busy schedules. A higher-than-average proportion of HCPs worked within a multi-disciplinary team as paediatric rheumatology services are geographically-centralised in Dublin and specialists worked together to treat young people with JIA. While this may be atypical, it produced a rich variety of viewpoints which we feel benefitted this study.

Limitations

As with any qualitative study, the findings may apply only to that population and may not be generalisable. The distribution of JIA subtypes was skewed in our sample; as each subtype has different symptoms, treatment needs and their experiences with JIA may vary. Larger samples (with a better distribution of subtypes) would offer stronger conclusions. Of further note is the lack of participation by male adolescents and parents: our sample was predominantly female, and the views shared may not apply equally to boys with JIA and their fathers. All participating families were affiliated with national arthritis organisations, but families outside of this network may have different experiences with JIA, and these perspectives should be included. Finally, the busy schedules of the paediatric rheumatology consultants limited interviews to brief discussions, where in-depth discussions would have provided stronger insight.

Conclusion

Discrepancies in the availability and quality of arthritis information demonstrate the need for a concise source of information on JIA self-management [20, 24]. While general information is available on developing self-management skills, there is scope for providing easily-accessible, accurate information on JIA to Irish families. The TTC website was well-received by Irish participants, with generally positive reaction for combining the online self-management program with Skype-based peer-mentoring [26] for JIA adolescents to share their experiences. In short, the acceptability of adapting an existing self-management intervention for Irish users has been confirmed.

Abbreviations

HCP: Healthcare professional; HRQL: Health-related quality-of-life; HSE: Health Service Executive; JIA: Juvenile idiopathic arthritis; TTC: "Teens Taking Charge"

Acknowledgements

We would like to thank the families and HCPs who participated in this study. We wish to acknowledge *Arthritis Ireland* and *iCAN (Irish Children's Arthritis Network)*, for their assistance with identifying and recruiting suitable families, and the help given by the paediatric rheumatology teams at *Our Lady's Children's Hospital, Crumlin, Temple Street Children's Hospital*, and *St. Vincent's Hospital*.

Funding

This research project was funded by a Small Grant from the Wellcome Trust - Humanities and Social Sciences (reference number: 201709/Z/16/Z) awarded to Dr. Line Caes (Principal Investigator), Prof Jennifer Stinson (Co-investigator) and Prof Brian McGuire (Co-investigator). The James Flaherty Research Scholarship from the Ireland Canada University Foundation was awarded to Prof Jennifer Stinson to facilitate a research visit to Ireland, to collaborate with the Irish-based researchers and lead the interview programme.

Authors' contributions

Recruitment and eligibility screening for the parents and adolescents was conducted by GOS. LC conducted recruitment of eligible HCPs. LC, SOH, and JS conducted the interviews. GOS and SS acted as interview assistants. GOS and SS transcribed the interviews. GOS and SOH analysed the qualitative data from the interviews, and GOS analysed the demographic data. All authors contributed to the editing of the manuscript. All authors read and approved the final manuscript.

Authors' information

None.

Consent for publication

Not applicable as no personal information is being reported in the article.

Competing interests

The authors declare that they have no competing interests.

Author details

[1]Centre for Pain Research; School of Psychology, College of Arts, Social Sciences & Celtic Studies, Galway, NUI, Ireland. [2]Division of Psychology; Faculty of Natural Sciences, University of Stirling, Stirling, Scotland, UK. [3]The Hospital for Sick Children, Toronto, Canada. [4]Child Health Evaluative Sciences, The Hospital for Sick Children, Toronto, Canada. [5]Lawrence S. Bloomberg Faculty of Nursing, University of Toronto, Toronto, Canada.

References

1. Ravelli A, Martini A. Juvenile idiopathic arthritis. Lancet. 2007;369(9563):767–78.
2. Martini A, Lovell DJ. Juvenile idiopathic arthritis: state of the art and future perspectives. Ann Rheum Dis. 2010;69(7):1260–3.
3. Martini A. It is time to rethink juvenile idiopathic arthritis classification and nomenclature. Ann Rheum Dis. 2012;71(9):1437–9.
4. Prakken B, Albani S, Martini A. Juvenile idiopathic arthritis. Lancet. 2011; 377(9783):2138–49.
5. Arthritis Ireland. JIA Facts 2017 [Available from: http://www.juvenilearthritis.ie/Parents/About-JIA/JIA-Facts/.
6. Tong A, Jones J, Craig JC, Singh-Grewal D. Children's experiences of living with juvenile idiopathic arthritis: a thematic synthesis of qualitative studies. Arthritis Care & Research. 2012;64(9):1392–404.
7. Lundberg V, Eriksson C. Health-related quality of life among Swedish children with juvenile idiopathic arthritis: parent-child discrepancies, gender differences and comparison with a European cohort. Pediatr Rheumatol. 2017;15(1):26.
8. Dzhus M. Influence of juvenile idiopathic arthritis on the quality of life of young adults in the transition period to adult rheumatologic care. Psychosom Med Gen Pract. 2017;2(4):e020478.
9. Gutierrez-Suarez R, Pistorio A, Cespedes Cruz A, Norambuena X, Flato B, Rumba I, et al. Health-related quality of life of patients with juvenile idiopathic arthritis coming from 3 different geographic areas. The PRINTO multinational quality of life cohort study. Rheumatology. 2006;46(2):314–20.
10. Haverman L, Grootenhuis MA, van den Berg JM, van Veenendaal M, Dolman KM, Swart JF, et al. Predictors of health-related quality of life in children and adolescents with juvenile idiopathic arthritis: results from a web-based survey. Arthritis Care & Research. 2012;64(5):694–703.
11. Forgeron PA, King S, Stinson JN, McGrath PJ, MacDonald AJ, Chambers CT. Social functioning and peer relationships in children and adolescents with chronic pain: a systematic review. Pain Res Manag. 2010;15(1):27–41.

12. Stinson J, Ahola Kohut S, Forgeron P, Amaria K, Bell M, Kaufman M, et al. The iPeer2Peer program: a pilot randomized controlled trial in adolescents with juvenile idiopathic arthritis. Pediatr Rheumatol. 2016;14(1):48.
13. Listing M, Mönkemöller K, Liedmann I, Niewerth M, Sengler C, Listing J, et al. The majority of patients with newly diagnosed juvenile idiopathic arthritis achieve a health-related quality of life that is similar to that of healthy peers: results of the German multicenter inception cohort (ICON). Arthritis research & therapy. 2018;20(1):106–17.
14. Oen K, Guzman J, Dufault B, Tucker LB, Shiff NJ, Duffy KW, et al. Health-related quality of life in an inception cohort of children with juvenile idiopathic arthritis: a longitudinal analysis. Arthritis care & research. 2018;70(1):134–44.
15. Barlow J, Wright C, Sheasby J, Turner A, Hainsworth J. Self-management approaches for people with chronic conditions: a review. Patient Educ Couns. 2002;48(2):177–87.
16. Sansom-Daly UM, Peate M, Wakefield CE, Bryant RA, Cohn RJ. A systematic review of psychological interventions for adolescents and young adults living with chronic illness. Health Psychol. 2012;31(3):380–93.
17. Hilderson D, Eyckmans L, Van der Elst K, Westhovens R, Wouters C, Moons P. Transfer from paediatric rheumatology to the adult rheumatology setting: experiences and expectations of young adults with juvenile idiopathic arthritis. Clin Rheumatol. 2012;32(5):575–83.
18. Guzman J, Gomez-Ramirez O, Jurencak R, Shiff NJ, Berard RA, Duffy CM, et al. What matters most for patients, parents, and clinicians in the course of juvenile idiopathic arthritis? A qualitative study. J Rheumatol. 2014;41(11):2260–9.
19. van Staa AL, Jedeloo S, van Meeteren J, Latour JM. Crossing the transition chasm: experiences and recommendations for improving transitional care of young adults, parents and providers. Child Care Health Dev. 2011;37(6):821–32.
20. Cartwright T, Fraser E, Edmunds S, Wilkinson N, Jacobs K. Journeys of adjustment: the experiences of adolescents living with juvenile idiopathic arthritis. Child Care Health Dev. 2015;41(5):734–43.
21. Tuchman LK, Slap GB, Britto MT. Transition to adult care: experiences and expectations of adolescents with a chronic illness. Child Care Health Dev. 2008;34(5):557–63.
22. Stinson JN, Toomey PC, Stevens BJ, Kagan S, Duffy CM, Huber A, et al. Asking the experts: exploring the self-management needs of adolescents with arthritis. Arthritis Rheum. 2008;59(1):65–72.
23. Michaud PA, Schrier L, Ross-Russel R, van der Heijden L, Dossche L, Copley S, et al. Paediatric departments need to improve residents' training in adolescent medicine and health: a position paper of the European academy of Paediatrics. Eur J Pediatr. 2018;177(4):479–87.
24. Coda A, Sculley D, Santos D, Girones X, Brosseau L, Smith DR, et al. Harnessing interactive technologies to improve health outcomes in juvenile idiopathic arthritis. Pediatr Rheumatol. 2017;15(1):40–4.
25. Connelly M, Schanberg LE, Ardoin S, Blakley M, Carrasco R, Chira P, et al. Multisite randomized clinical trial evaluating an online self-management program for adolescents with juvenile idiopathic arthritis. J Pediatr Psychol. 2018.
26. Kohut SA, Stinson JN, Ruskin D, Forgeron P, Harris L, van Wyk M, et al. iPeer2Peer program. Pain. 2016;157(5):1146–55.
27. Stinson JN, McGrath PJ, Hodnett ED, Feldman BM, Duffy CM, Huber AM, et al. An internet-based self-management program with telephone support for adolescents with arthritis: a pilot randomized controlled trial. J Rheumatol. 2010;37(9):1944–52.
28. Ritterband LM, Thorndike FP, Cox DJ, Kovatchev BP, Gonder-Frederick LA. A behavior change model for internet interventions. Ann Behav Med. 2009; 38(1):18–27.
29. Stinson J, McGrath P, Hodnett E, Feldman B, Duffy C, Huber A, et al. Usability testing of an online self-management program for adolescents with juvenile idiopathic arthritis. J Med Internet Res. 2010;12(3):e30.
30. Wu YP, Steele RG, Connelly MA, Palermo TM, Ritterband LM. Commentary: pediatric eHealth interventions: common challenges during development, implementation, and dissemination. J Pediatr Psychol. 2014;39(6):612–23.
31. Petty RE, Southwood TR, Manners P, Baum J, Glass DN, Goldenberg J, et al. International league of associations for rheumatology classification of juvenile idiopathic arthritis: second revision (Edmonton). J Rheumatol. 2004; 31(2):390–2.
32. Sandelowski M, Voils CI, Leeman J, Crandell JL. Mapping the mixed methods–mixed research synthesis terrain. J Mixed Methods Res. 2012;6(4):317–31.
33. Livermore P, Eleftheriou D, Wedderburn L. The lived experience of juvenile idiopathic arthritis in young people receiving etanercept. Pediatr Rheumatol. 2016;14(1):1–6.
34. Eyckmans L, Hilderson D, Westhovens R, Wouters C, Moons P. What does it mean to grow up with juvenile idiopathic arthritis? A qualitative study on the perspectives of patients. Clin Rheumatol. 2010;30(4):459–65.
35. Jordan AL, Eccleston C, Osborn M. Being a parent of the adolescent with complex chronic pain: an interpretative phenomenological analysis. Eur J Pain. 2007;11(1):49.
36. (HBSC) HBiSC. Adolescent alcohol-related behaviours: trends and inequalities in the WHO European Region, 2002–2014. Copenhagen, Denmark; 2018. http://www.euro.who.int/__data/assets/pdf_file/0007/382840/WH15-alcohol-report-eng.pdf.
37. Davies K, Cleary G, Foster H, Hutchinson E, Baildam E. BSPAR standards of care for children and young people with juvenile idiopathic arthritis. Rheumatology. 2010;49(7):1406–8.
38. National Treatment Purchase Fund. Inpatient/Day Case Specialty by Hospital, as at 30/08/2018. Dublin, Ireland.2018 [Available from: http://www.ntpf.ie/home/pdf//2018/08/specialities/in-patient/2500.pdf.
39. McDonagh M. Juvenile idiopathic arthritis: the invisible disease 1,200 Irish children live with. Irish Times; 2018.
40. Arthritis Ireland. Urgent investment required in paediatric rheumatology Dublin, Ireland2018 [Available from: http://www.arthritisireland.ie/go/about_us/news/urgent_investment_required_in_paediatric_rheumatology.
41. National Treatment Purchase Fund. Comparison between outpatient waiting lists, speciality rheumatology, in January 2017 and January 2018. Dublin, Ireland: National Treatment Purchase Fund; 2018 [Available from: http://www.ntpf.ie/home/pdf//2018/01/specialities/out-patient/2500.pdf.
42. Coppens E, Van Audenhove C, Scheerder G, Arensman E, Coffey C, Costa S, et al. Public attitudes toward depression and help-seeking in four European countries baseline survey prior to the OSPI-Europe intervention. J Affect Disord. 2013;150(2):320–9.
43. Lakeman R, McGowan P, MacGabhann L, Parkinson M, Redmond M, Sibitz I, et al. A qualitative study exploring experiences of discrimination associated with mental-health problems in Ireland. Epidemiol Psychiatr Sci. 2012;21(3):271–9.
44. Sztajnbok F, Coronel-Martinez DL, Diaz-Maldonado A, Novarini C, Pistorio A, Viola S, et al. Discordance between physician's and parent's global assessments in juvenile idiopathic arthritis. Rheumatology. 2007;46(1):141–5.
45. Health Service Executive. Find your nearest hospital health centre, GP and more 2017 [Available from: http://hse.ie/eng/services/maps/.
46. Barak A, Boniel-Nissim M, Suler J. Fostering empowerment in online support groups. Comput Hum Behav. 2008;24(5):1867–83.

Juvenile idiopathic arthritis managed in the new millennium: one year outcomes of an inception cohort of Australian children

Georgina Tiller[1*], Joanne Buckle[1,2], Roger Allen[1], Jane Munro[1,2], Peter Gowdie[1], Angela Cox[1] and Jonathan Akikusa[1,2]

Abstract

Background: The advent of new treatments for Juvenile Idiopathic Arthritis (JIA) has prompted interest in systematically studying the outcomes of patients treated in the 'modern era'. Such data provide both benchmarks for assessing local outcomes and important information for use in counselling families of newly diagnosed patients. While data are available for cohorts in Europe and North America, no such data exist for Australian patients.
The aim was to examine the demographics, treatment and outcomes at 12 months of an inception cohort of newly diagnosed patients with JIA at a single tertiary referral paediatric rheumatology centre in Australia.

Methods: Retrospective review of prospectively collected data from patients newly diagnosed with JIA between 2010 and 2014 at the Royal Children's Hospital in Melbourne.

Results: One hundred thirty four patients were included (62% female). Oligoarthritis was the single largest category of JIA (36%) and rheumatoid factor positive polyarthritis the least common (2%). Undifferentiated JIA accounted for 13% of patients and was the third largest category. Across the cohort 94% received NSAIDs, 53% oral steroids, 62% methotrexate and 15% a biologic DMARD. Intra-articular steroids were used in 62%, most commonly in the oligoarticular subtype (94%). 95% of patients achieved a joint count of zero at a median of 4.1 months, however flares occurred in 42%. At 12 months 65% had no active joint disease, though more than half remained on medication.

Conclusion: Australian children with JIA managed in the modern era have similar characteristics and achieve short term outcomes comparable to cohorts in Europe and North America, with high rates of joint remission in the first 12 months of follow-up but with a significant relapse rate and requirement for ongoing medication.

Keywords: Juvenile idiopathic arthritis, Cohort, Outcomes

Introduction

Juvenile idiopathic arthritis (JIA) is a heterogeneous group of conditions, characterized by the onset of persistent arthritis before the 16th birthday for which no cause can be identified [1]. It is the most common inflammatory rheumatic disease in childhood [2]. Recent reports of large prospective cohorts of patients with JIA from North America and Europe have led to an improved understanding of the early disease course, contemporary management and short-term outcomes of this condition [3–6]. In addition, these and other studies have contributed to the understanding that early disease course and response to treatment may predict outcome more accurately than disease category, making studies focused on the early disease period in the era of contemporary treatments increasingly important [7, 8].

In Australia, the estimated overall prevalence of JIA is 1–4 per 1000 children although national statistics and publications are limited [9, 10]. Despite its importance and relative frequency, there are no studies describing the outcome of children with JIA in Australia managed with current treatments. The aim of this study was to describe the clinical features, management, course and

* Correspondence: georgina.tiller@rch.org.au
[1]Department of Rheumatology, The Royal Children's Hospital, 50 Flemington Rd, Parkville, Melbourne, VIC 3052, Australia

outcomes during the first 12 months of follow up, for an inception cohort of Australian children with JIA.

Patients and methods

We conducted a retrospective review of data from an inception cohort of children with JIA diagnosed between October 2010 and October 2014 at The Royal Children's Hospital (RCH), Melbourne, Australia. All children newly diagnosed with JIA during the relevant period and whose subsequent follow-up had been at the RCH were eligible for inclusion. All data had been prospectively documented in the Rheumatology Department database, a comprehensive clinical tool coded in Microsoft Access™ in which patient demographic details, diagnoses, clinic visits, medications, elective admissions for procedures and communications are recorded. At our institution, patients with a new diagnosis of JIA are followed routinely at least every three months for the first 12–18 months of their arthritis course. For the purposes of this study, patients followed less frequently than this over the relevant period were considered to have incomplete follow-up and were excluded. Acute hospital admissions between scheduled appointments were not included in this analysis.

For ease of analysis, data from the Rheumatology database were exported into an Excel ™ workbook. Exported data fields included patient demographics, assigned JIA category, medications, procedures, clinic visit dates and active joint count at each visit. The JIA category assigned by the treating rheumatologist was confirmed by the primary investigator (GT) using the International League of Associations for Rheumatology (ILAR) classification criteria. For the systemic category, where the ILAR classification was not met due to absence of active arthritis, the diagnosis was made by the treating paediatric rheumatologist. For the purposes of analysis, the two oligoarthritis categories (i.e. persistent and extended) were combined due to a small number of patients in the extended category.

The first visit was defined as the date of diagnosis of JIA. The 12-month visit was the date closest to 12 months from the date of first visit within a 2-month window. The time to zero joint count was calculated as the interval between the first visit and the date on which the treating rheumatologist recorded an active joint count of 0, which for the purposes of this study was considered to represent inactive arthritis. The date of first arthritis flare was the visit date at which a joint count was recorded as > 0 following the first visit at which the joint count had been 0. Uveitis at diagnosis was defined as uveitis detected prior to, or within one month of the diagnosis of JIA. The date of a first episode of uveitis was the visit at which uveitis was first documented by an ophthalmologist. Uveitis was recorded if present at any time during the 12 months of follow up and at the 12-month visit. For patients who did not reach examined outcomes in the first year of follow-up, additional data were collected up to the time at which the relevant outcome occurred or 36 months, whichever came first.

Medications were grouped as non-steroidal anti-inflammatories (NSAIDS), conventional disease modifying agents (cDMARDS) (ie. methotrexate, sulfasalazine, leflunomide), biologic disease modifying agents (bDMARDS) (ie. adalimumab, etanercept, infliximab, tocilizumab, anakinra), oral, intravenous (IV) and ophthalmic steroids. Medications were recorded as ever used in the 12 month follow up period, and in use at the 12 month visit. For cDMARDS and bDMARDS the time from first visit to commencement was calculated in months. Intra-articular steroid (IAS) injections were recorded as the number of visits for joint injections in the 12-month period of follow up. The time to first joint injection was calculated in months. Analysis was performed using descriptive statistics. Survival curves were used to examine medication exposure across the cohort.

The Royal Children's Hospital (RCH) Human Research Ethics Committee approved the study.

Results

One hundred sixty one patients were identified, of whom, 27 were excluded because of incomplete follow-up. Demographic and disease details of the 161 patients are given in Table 1. Of the 17 undifferentiated patients: 7 were males > 6 years, HLAB27 positive with a family history of psoriasis; 8 were oligo or poly arthritis with a family history of psoriasis with no other features; 2 were oligoarthritis with B27 and rheumatoid factor (RF) positivity. There were no statistically significant differences in age at diagnosis, gender and proportion of patients when comparing included and excluded patients.

Disease course

Details of the disease course of the cohort over the study period are provided in Table 2. In the 12 months following diagnosis, 127 (95%) of patients achieved an active joint count of zero on at least one occasion. The median time to achieve this outcome within the first 12 months was 3.1 months (Range 0.4–13.1 months) (Table 2). For the 7 (5%) who did not reach a joint count of zero, the median time to a joint count of zero was 18.5 months (range 15.2–32.0 months). Of this group, 4 (57%) were in the polyarticular RF negative JIA category. One patient, in the undifferentiated category, a 14 year old female with ANA and RF positive oligoarthritis, treated with two joint injections and methotrexate in the first 12 months, did not attain a zero-joint count during the 36 months of available follow up data.

Fifty six subjects (42%) had at least one arthritis flare from a joint count of zero. The median number of flares was 1 and the median time to flare was 3.6 months

Table 1 Demographics of the excluded patients and cohort presented in decreasing order of frequency of JIA category

	Number of excluded patients n (%)	Mean age excluded patients at diagnosis (years)	Female excluded patients n (%)	Number of included patients n (%)	Median age included patients at diagnosis (years)	Female included patients n (%)	Pre-diagnosis symptom period average months (range)	Median joint count baseline (range)	ANA positive n/n done (%)
Oligoarticular	12 (44)	7.5	7 (58)	48 (36)	3.4	34 (71)	3.9 (0.3–24.0)	2 (1–4)	36/47 (77)
Polyarticular RF-	1(4)	9.9	0 (0)	34 (25)	9.0	26 (76)	5.3 (0.5–24.0)	8 (1–42)	21/33 (64)
Undifferentiated	8 (30)	8.4	4 (50)	17 (13)	12.3	7 (41)	7.4 (0.5–24.0)	5 (1–43)	8/16 (50)
Enthesitis related arthritis	2(7)	10.8	0 (0)	13 (10)	13.9	1 (8)	11.2 (0.5–48.0)	2 (1–18)	0/7 (0)
Systemic	1(4)	3.2	0 (0)	10 (7)	8.4	7 (70)	1.4 (0.3–4.0)	5 (0–22)	3/8 (38)
Psoriatic arthritis	3(11)	11	1 (33)	9 (7)	9.3	5 (56)	9.9 (1.5–24.0)	5 (1–36)	2/7 (29)
Polyarticular RF +	0(0)	n/a	n/a	3 (2)	15.6	3 (100)	7.5 (3.8–12.1)	10 (7–44)	2/3 (67)
Overall	27	9.2	12 (44)	134	8.3	83 (62)	5.7 (0.3–48.0)	2 (0–44)	72/121 (60)

Table 2 Metrics of arthritis and uveitis activity of the cohort by JIA category for outcomes attained in the first twelve months

	Reached zero joint count in first year n (% of subtype)	Median time to zero joint count in the first twelve months (range)	Median joint count at 12 months (range)	Flared ever during first 12 months n (%)	Mdn time to flare from zero joint count (months)	Uveitis during first 12 months n (%)	Active uveitis at 12 months n (%)
Oligoarticular	48 (100)	2.8 (1.0–12.6)	0 (0–4)	15 (31)	3.2	8 (17)	5 (10)
Polyarticular RF -	30 (88)	5.3 (1.1–12.8)	0 (0–14)	16 (47)	3.5	0 (0)	0 (0)
Undifferentiated	16 (94)	3.9 (0.6–13.1)	0 (0–7)	11 (65)	3.9	0 (0)	0 (0)
Enthesitis related arthritis	11 (85)	6.6 (1.4–12.0)	1 (0–15)	5 (38)	5.5	0 (0)	0 (0)
Systemic	10 (100)	1.7 (0.4–8.1)	0 (0–8)	5 (50)	1.2	0 (0)	0 (0)
Psoriatic arthritis	9 (100)	7.6 (1.2–12.2)	0 (0–24)	4 (44)	3.1	1 (11)	1 (11)
Polyarticular RF +	3 (100)	5.9 (3.7–7.0)	0 (0–0)	0 (0)	n/a	0 (0)	0 (0)
Overall	127 (95)	3.1 (0.4–13.1)	0 (0–24)	56 (42)	3.6	9 (7)	6 (4)

(range 1.2–5.5 months). Of those patients that flared within the first 12 months, 30 (54%) were on a disease modifying medication at the time of the flare, most commonly methotrexate, 26 (50%).The JIA category with the highest proportion of arthritis flares was the undifferentiated group with 65% of patients flaring over the first 12 months. Where patients had first arthritis flares after the first 12 months of follow up, the median time to flare from zero joint count was 13.5 months and from first visit was 20.5 months. All the RF positive polyarthritis patients had arthritis flares, although none within the first 12 months of follow up. In this group, the median time to arthritis flare from a joint count of zero was 17.0 months (range 11.0–25.5 months). Of the 45 (34%) patients who never had an arthritis flare, 53% were in the oligoarthritis category. The proportion of oligoarthritis patients who had no arthritis flares in the first 12 months was 69%.

Uveitis occurred in 2 (1%) patients at diagnosis, 9 (7%) patients in the first 12 months of follow up. 89% of these patients were in the oligoarticular category. 100% of the patients with uveitis were ANA positive.

Medications

Table 3 details the exposure of the cohort to medications over the study period. Non-steroidal anti-inflammatory drugs were almost universally used (94%). Seventy-one patients (53%) were treated with oral corticosteroids at least once and 10 (7%) were treated with intravenous steroids. The median initial dose of oral steroids was 1 mg/kg/day (range 0.2–2) and the median duration of oral steroids, including the completed taper was 4 months (range 0.25–12 months). Eighty-three (62%) were treated with methotrexate, by far the most common cDMARD. Two patients were treated with sulfasalazine in the first 12 months, both of whom had also been treated with methotrexate. Across the whole cohort the median time to commencement of methotrexate was 0.9 months (Table 3). It was shortest in the RF positive polyarthritis category (median 0 months) and longest in patients with enthesitis related arthritis (ERA) (median 3.1 months) (Table 3, Fig. 1). Twenty patients (15%) were commenced on a bDMARD at a median of 5.5 months (Table 3). The patients with the highest rate of bDMARD commencement were in the polyarticular RF positive (33%), ERA (31%) and systemic (sJIA) (30%) categories. All patients with uveitis were treated with ophthalmic steroids during the first 12 months of follow up. Five (56%) were additionally commenced on methotrexate, either for arthritis or uveitis or both. None required addition of a bDMARD within that timeframe.

Sixty two percent of patients underwent at least one joint injection in the first year of follow up; the median time to first joint injection was 0.9 months (Range 0–11 months). Fifty four percent of patients undergoing intra-articular steroid therapy were in the oligoarticular category, 94% of whom had at least one joint injection in the year following diagnosis (Fig. 2). Ten patients (7%) required their first joint injection after the first 12 months of follow up. The median time to joint injection for this group was 21 months. Seven of these 10 patients were in the RF negative polyarthritis JIA category.

Outcome at twelve months

Seventy three percent of the cohort were on at least one medication at 12 months, with the two most common being methotrexate (79%) and NSAIDS (62%). Twenty-three (17%) were on oral corticosteroids. The JIA categories with the highest oral steroid use at 12 months were ERA (31%), sJIA(30%), and undifferentiated (29%). All but one patient (with systemic disease) commenced on a bDMARD remained on a bDMARD at 12 months.

Figure 3 outlines arthritis activity status according to medication use for each JIA category at the 12 month visit. Eighty-eight (66%) of patients had inactive arthritis. Thirty-six (41%) of these patients were of the oligoarticular subtype, of whom 75% had inactive arthritis at this time point. Of the 88 patients with inactive arthritis, 61% were on medications and 39% were off medication. All the RF factor positive polyarticular patients had inactive arthritis on medication at 12 months. Four patients (7%) with inactive arthritis at 12 months had active uveitis.

Of the 46 patients with active arthritis at 12 months, 96% were on medication. The two patients not on medication were awaiting intra-articular therapy. The categories with the highest proportion of patients with active arthritis at 12 months were, polyarticular RF negative (47%) and ERA (46%).

Six patients (4%) had active uveitis at 12 months: 2 had concurrent active arthritis on medication and 4 had inactive arthritis on medications.

Discussion

This study is the first report of early outcomes for Australian children newly diagnosed with JIA managed in the modern era of arthritis therapy. It demonstrates that Australian children with JIA have similar demographic features, disease course and medication exposure to those reported in large cohorts from Europe and North America [2–5] .

The sex distribution, proportion of patients within each JIA category and prevalence of ANA positivity concur with previously published cohorts [2, 4, 5]. Consistent with previous cohorts, the shortest and longest times from symptom onset to diagnosis were in the sJIA and ERA categories respectively [3, 11]. This likely reflects

Table 3 Medication exposure during first 12 months and at 12 months by JIA category

	Any	NSAIDS		Oral steroids		IV steroids	Methotrexate			bDMARD			Ocular steroids		Steroid joint injections	
	Ever n (%)	Ever n (%)	At 12 m n (%)	Ever n (%)	At 12 m n (%)	Number given IV steroids n(%)	Ever n (%)	Med. time to (m)	At 12 m n (%)	Ever n (%)	Med. time to (m)	At 12 m n (%)	Ever n (%)	At 12 m n (%)	Ever n (%)	Med joint injections per patient[a] (range)
Oligoarticular	43(90)	43 (90)	13 (27)	7 (15)	4 (8)	0 (0)	9 (19)	2.1	9 (19)	1 (2)	12.2	1 (2)	8(17)	4(8)	45 (94)	1 (0–3)
Polyarticular RF -	34 (100)	33 (97)	17 (50)	21 (62)	5 (15)	2 (6)	32 (94)	0.8	32 (94)	6 (18)	5.4	6 (18)	0 (0)	0 (0)	16 (47)	0 (0–4)
Undifferentiated	17 (100)	17 (100)	12 (71)	13 (76)	5 (29)	1 (6)	13 (76)	0	12 (71)	3 (18)	5.5	3 (18)	0 (0)	0 (0)	10 (59)	1 (0–2)
Enthesitis related arthritis	13 (100)	13 (100)	7 (54)	10 (76)	4 (31)	0 (0)	12 (92)	3.1	8 (62)	4 (31)	5.8	4 (31)	0 (0)	0 (0)	5 (38)	0 (0–3)
Systemic	10 (100)	9 (90)	5 (50)	10 (100)	3 (30)	6 (60)	7 (70)	0.5	6 (60)	3 (30)	2.4	2 (20)	0 (0)	0 (0)	2 (20)	0 (0–1)
Psoriatic arthritis	9 (100)	8 (89)	5 (56)	7 (78)	2 (22)	0 (0)	7 (78)	1.1	7 (78)	2 (22)	6.0	2 (22)	1 (11)	1 (11)	5 (56)	1 (0–1)
Polyarticular RF +	3 (100)	3 (100)	1 (33)	3 (100)	0 (0)	1 (33)	3 (100)	0	3 (100)	1 (33)	4.7	1 (33)	0 (0)	0 (0)	0 (0)	0 (0–0)
Overall	129 (96)	126 (94)	60 (45)	71 (53)	23 (17)	10 (7)	83 (62)	0.9	77 (57)	20 (15)	5.5	19 (14)	9 (7)	5 (4)	83 (62)	0 (0–4)

Key: *Med.* median; *NSAIDS* non-steroidal anti-inflammatory drugs; *bDMARD* biologic disease modifying anti-rheumatic drug

[a]Median number of elective admissions for joint injections per patient

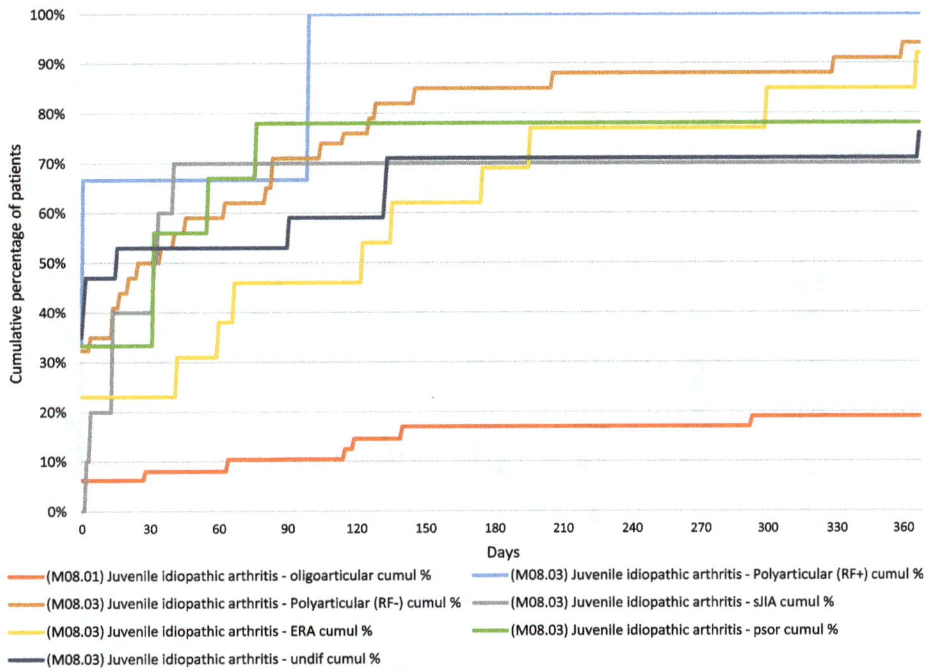

Fig. 1 Time to methotrexate commencement by JIA category

the common presentation of sJIA as an acute febrile illness, in contrast to the less dramatic symptoms of ERA, typically in adolescent boys, which may be incorrectly interpreted as non-inflammatory musculoskeletal pain or even ignored by the patients themselves. As expected, the systemic category was the only JIA category in which some patients had a zero joint count at diagnosis. It is well recognized that systemic features may precede joint disease in sJIA [12].

Most patients (95%) in our cohort achieved a joint count of zero in the first 12 months of follow up. This outcome was achieved relatively early, at a median time from

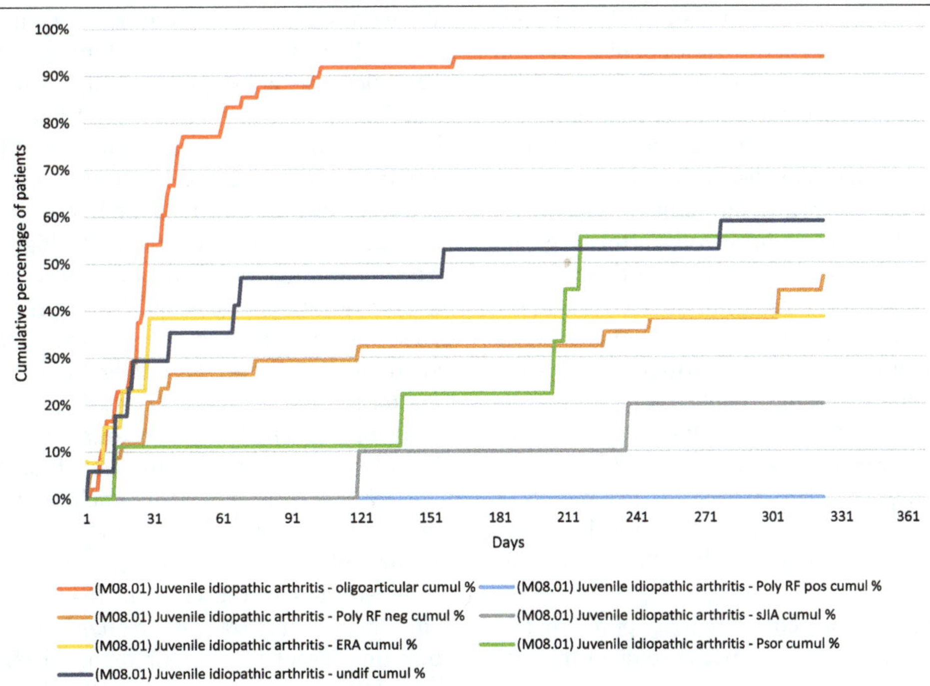

Fig. 2 Time to first intra-articular corticosteroid injection by JIA category

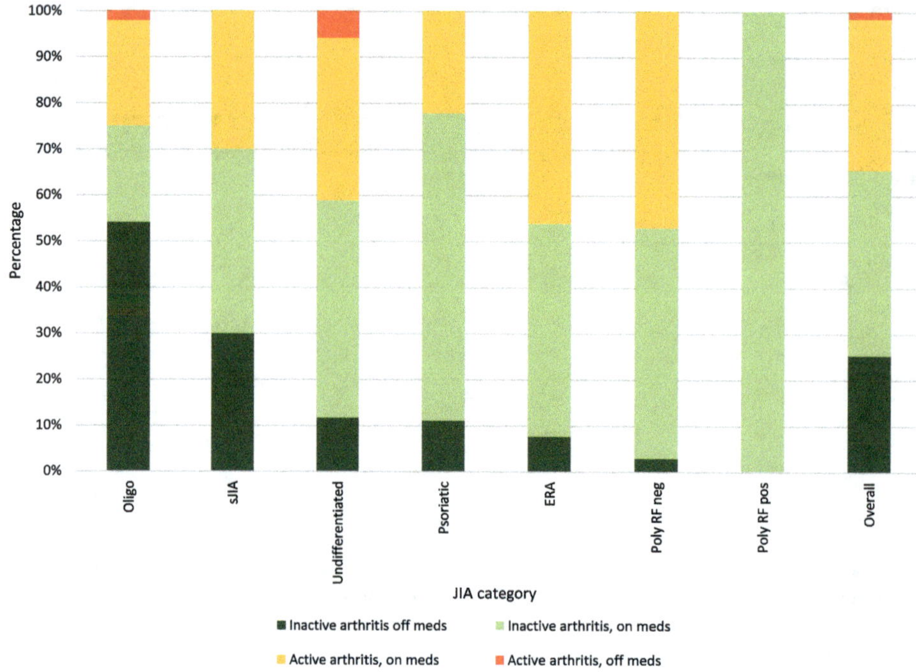

Fig. 3 Arthritis activity status by medication use at 1 year according to JIA category

diagnosis of 4.1 months. These figures are broadly comparable to those in the ReACCh-Out cohort in which ~ 91% of children achieved a zero joint count at a median of 7 months [5]. The slightly greater median time to zero joint count in that cohort may in part relate to the longer period over which this outcome was potentially captured [5]. The time to zero joint count was shortest in the sJIA and oligoarthritis categories (1.7 and 2.8 months, respectively). Early attainment of an active joint count of zero in ssJIA relative to the other categories was also found in the ReACCh-Out cohort [5]. In our patients, this likely reflects the early use of corticosteroids to control systemic disease in patients whose joint disease would not otherwise warrant their use (median joint count at baseline 0, range 0–8). The early response in the oligoarthritis group likely relates to the early use of intra-articular therapy with ~ 90% being injected within three months of diagnosis. This proportion is higher than reported in other cohorts in which rates of intra-articular corticosteroid use were just ~ 50–78% in the first year of follow-up [4, 5]. The higher rate of use of intra-articular steroid use in our patients may relate to ease of access - with 3 scheduled sedation lists and 1 general anaesthetic list per month at our centre - and physician preference. Our results would argue in favour of the early use of this therapy for this group of patients.

A surprising finding in our cohort is that approximately half of all patients received oral corticosteroids in the first year of follow up. This exposure is greater than reported in other cohorts, where oral corticosteroid use in the first year has ranged between 20 and 33% [4, 5, 13]. In our study oral steroids use was captured when an initial dosage was commenced and the date of the completed taper was then recorded. This gives an indication of exposure but makes accurate inferences regarding the cumulative exposure difficult. As expected, steroids were used most commonly in the sJIA and ERA categories and intravenous steroid use was most common in systemic disease. Oral steroids were used in significantly symptomatic patients as a 'bridging' measure while awaiting onset of action of DMARDS, or for joint injections. There were clear variations in practice relating to their use between clinicians, with rates of exposure per clinician patient group ranging between 25 and 50% (data not shown). Interestingly, despite the relatively high 'ever used' oral steroid exposure found in our cohort, the proportion of patients on oral steroids at 12 months (17%) was similar to the 14% reported in the German JIA cohort [4] and would be consistent with their short-term rather than long-term use.

The use of cDMARDS in our cohort was common; 63% of patients were commenced on a cDMARD in their first year of follow-up including 84% percent of non-oligoarticular and 25% of oligoarticular patients. The overall rate of cDMARDs use was broadly similar to those reported in the German (64.7% on methotrexate) and Canadian (47.6% on first DMARD) cohorts at the same time point [4, 5]. Our reported cDMARD use was higher than reported in the Childhood Arthritis and Rheumatology Research Alliance registry (CARRA), although the 30% cDMARD use in this study was in patients with less than 6 months of disease duration [13]. As in other cohorts, methotrexate was the cDMARD most commonly used and was started at a median of 0.7 months in non-oligoarticular disease and 2.1 months in oligoarticular disease, the latter consistent with its introduction following failure to achieve remission post early intra-articular steroid therapy. Fifteen percent of patients were commenced on biologic therapy; this is substantially more than the ~ 5% at 12 months reported in the ReACCH-Out cohort, and lower than the 38% of any biologic use in the newly diagnosed group in the CARRA cohort, but in line with the experience in the German cohort (22%) [4, 5, 13]. The median time to commencement of a bDMARD was 5.5 months, consistent with adherence to the requirements for accessing government-funded bDMARDS in Australia, which requires demonstration of failure to respond to a minimum of 3 months' methotrexate therapy [14]. 30% of the systemic arthritis group were commenced on a biologic agent, fewer than would be expected in the era of consensus treatment plans for systemic arthritis [13, 15]. This is likely multifactorial, reflecting a changing practice pattern as new guidelines and data emerge on the first line use of biologics in sJIA, and restrictions of access to biologic treatments for sJIA in Australia particularly at the start of data collection for this study [16]. Taken together these data are consistent with early aggressive treatment of JIA in the modern era, an approach based on predominantly adult data suggesting that early disease control improves long term outcomes in arthritis [17–19]. While the majority of our cohort achieved a zero joint count in the first year of follow-up, a significant minority (42%) subsequently flared. Despite this, across the cohort 65% of patients had inactive joint disease at 12 months although more than half remained on medication. Inactive joint disease off medication was uncommon (25%) except in patients with oligoarthritis (50%) and sJIA (30%), which were the two JIA categories most likely to experience a period of inactive disease in the German cohort [4]. These data suggest modern therapies in JIA are effective in controlling active joint disease in the majority of patients but that the underlying tendency to relapse - and therefore need for ongoing treatment - remains high.

The findings of this study should be interpreted taking into consideration several limitations. Compared to the cohorts in Germany and Canada our sample size is relatively small and from a single centre. Patient related outcomes, such as pain and quality of life, were not included as these data were not available. Similarly, disease remission as per the widely used 'Wallace criteria' [20] was not used as an outcome, because components of these criteria (such as acute phase reactants and physician global assessment of disease activity) are not routinely collected in every patient at every visit at our centre. Instead we chose to focus on active joint count which is documented at every visit and which, pragmatically, at most centres is the primary variable that drives contemporaneous treatment decisions in the majority of patients [21, 22]. Using the Juvenile Arthritis Disease Activity Score (JADAS) as an outcome measure, as has been done in other cohorts, may have strengthened our findings, and, we suspect, would have led to lower reported rates of inactive disease in our cohort [6, 22].

Our study also has a number of strengths. It provides 'real world' outcome data from consecutively diagnosed patients with JIA managed in a general rheumatology clinic at the largest paediatric rheumatology centre in Australia. Data were prospectively collected in a dedicated database used to record patient encounters in the clinic and, for each patient, joint counts were conducted by the same clinicians over time, negating the risk of inter-observer variability. The paediatric rheumatology department includes five rheumatologists, majority trained in North America, with experience ranging from 5 to 30 years, along with one supervised fellow. Finally, the primary outcome examined - zero joint count- is a concept that is easy to convey when discussing likely outcomes at the start of treatment, making our outcome data directly relevant to patients and their families.

Conclusions

We have shown that Australian children with JIA managed in the modern era have similar characteristics and achieve short term outcomes comparable to cohorts in North America and Europe. Whether their longer-term outcomes are similar is unknown. While the majority of patients achieve a zero joint count at least once within the first year of follow-up, relapses are common such that one third have active arthritis and three quarters require ongoing medication at 12 months. Ongoing research is required to further understand determinants of disease course and optimum management strategies.

Abbreviations

ANA: Anti-nuclear antibody; DMARD: Disease-modifying anti-rheumatic drug; ERA: Enthesitis related arthritis; IAS: Intra-articular steroid; ILAR: International League of Associations for Rheumatology; JIA: Juvenile idiopathic arthritis; NSAID: Non-steroidal anti-inflammatory drug; RCH: The Royal Children's Hospital; RF: Rheumatoid factor; sJIA: Systemic juvenile idiopathic arthritis

Acknowledgements

None.

Funding

No funding source.

Authors' contributions
All authors were involved in clinical care and the recording of data via the rheumatology database. All authors were invited to participate in peer review of the manuscript. All authors read and approved the final manuscript.

Consent for publication
All authors have consented to publication of the manuscript. Individual person's data: not applicable.

Competing interests
None to declare.

Author details
[1]Department of Rheumatology, The Royal Children's Hospital, 50 Flemington Rd, Parkville, Melbourne, VIC 3052, Australia. [2]Murdoch Childrens Research Institute, Melbourne, Australia.

References
1. Ravelli A. Juvenile idiopathic arthritis. Lancet (North American ed.). 2007; 369(9563):767.
2. Petty RE. Epidemiology of juvenile rheumatoid arthritis World. Pediatr Child Care. 1987;3:205–10.
3. Oen K, et al. Early outcomes and improvement of patients with juvenile idiopathic arthritis enrolled in a Canadian multicenter inception cohort. Arthritis care & research. 2010;62(4):527–36.
4. Sengler C, et al. The majority of newly diagnosed patients with juvenile idiopathic arthritis reach an inactive disease state within the first year of specialised care: data from a German inception cohort. RMD Open. 2015; 1(1):e000074.
5. Guzman J, et al. The outcomes of juvenile idiopathic arthritis in children managed with contemporary treatments: results from the ReACCh-out cohort. Ann Rheum Dis. 2015;74(10):1854–60.
6. Nordal E, et al. Ongoing disease activity and changing categories in a long-term nordic cohort study of juvenile idiopathic arthritis. Arthritis & Rheumatism. 2011;63(9):2809–18.
7. Bartoli M, et al. The magnitude of early response to methotrexate therapy predicts long-term outcome of patients with juvenile idiopathic arthritis. Ann Rheum Dis. 2008;67(3):370–4.
8. Wallace CA, et al. Trial of early aggressive therapy in polyarticular juvenile idiopathic arthritis. Arthritis & Rheumatism. 2012;64(6):2012–21.
9. The Australian Institute of Health and Welfare. Juvenile arthritis in Australia. Arthritis series no. 7. Cat. no. PHE 101. 2008 [cited 2016 Aug 31]; Available from: http://www.aihw.gov.au/publication-detail/?id=6442468170.
10. Manners P, Bower C. Worldwide prevalence of juvenile arthritis—why does it vary so much? J Rheumatol. 2002;29(7):1520–30.
11. Bowyer SL, et al. Health status of patients with juvenile rheumatoid arthritis at 1 and 5 years after diagnosis. J Rheumatol. 2003;30(2):394–400.
12. Behrens EM, et al. Evaluation of the presentation of systemic onset juvenile rheumatoid arthritis: data from the Pennsylvania systemic onset juvenile arthritis registry (PASOJAR). J Rheumatol. 2008;35(2):343–8.
13. Ringold S K.Y, Schanberg LE, Natter MD, Xie F, Ilowite N, Jones J, Mieszkalski K, Beukelman T, Patterns of Medication Use in Children with Juvenile Idiopathic Arthritis: Results from the Childhood Arthritis & Rheumatology Research Alliance Registry [abstract]. 2016: Arthritis Rheumatol.
14. DHHS A.G. Juvenile idiopathic arthritis: Initial PBS authority application. 2017 [cited 2017 13/11/12017]; Available from: https://www.humanservices.gov.au/organisations/health-professionals/forms/pb060.
15. Kimura Y, et al. Pilot study comparing the Childhood Arthritis & Rheumatology Research Alliance (CARRA) systemic juvenile idiopathic arthritis consensus treatment plans. Pediatr Rheumatol. 2017;15(1):23.
16. Nigrovic PA, et al. Anakinra as first-line disease-modifying therapy in systemic juvenile idiopathic arthritis: report of forty-six patients from an international multicenter series. Arthritis & rheumatism. 2011;63(2):545–55.
17. Anink J, et al. Two-year outcome of juvenile idiopathic arthritis in current daily practice: what can we tell our patients? Clinical & Experimental Rheumatology. 2012;30(6):972–8.
18. Tynjala P, et al. Aggressive combination drug therapy in very early polyarticular juvenile idiopathic arthritis (ACUTE-JIA): a multicentre randomised open-label clinical trial. Ann Rheum Dis. 2011;70(9):1605–12.
19. Boers M. Understanding the window of opportunity concept in early rheumatoid arthritis. Arthritis & Rheumatology. 2003;48(7):1771–4.
20. Wallace CA, Ruperto N, Giannini E. Preliminary criteria for clinical remission for select categories of juvenile idiopathic arthritis. J Rheumatol. 2004;31(11):2290–4.
21. Van Mater HA, et al. Psychometric characteristics of outcome measures in juvenile idiopathic arthritis: a systematic review. Arthritis care & research. 2012;64(4):554–62.
22. Consolaro A, et al. Development and validation of a composite disease activity score for juvenile idiopathic arthritis. Arthritis & Rheumatism. 2009; 61(5):658–66.

17

Feasibility of a musculoskeletal ultrasound intervention to improve adherence in juvenile idiopathic arthritis

Leslie A. Favier[1,2*], Tracy V. Ting[1] and Avani C. Modi[2*]

Abstract

Background: Non-adherence is a prevalent and modifiable issue in juvenile idiopathic arthritis (JIA) that currently lacks provider-based intervention. Education surrounding disease status is one way in which families remain engaged in their care. Musculoskeletal ultrasound is one such form of demonstrative, real-time education that may impact the way patients and caregivers self-manage their disease. The aims of this study are to 1) assess the feasibility, acceptability and perceived usefulness of musculoskeletal ultrasound as a non-adherence intervention tool and 2) to examine changes in methotrexate adherence in adolescents with JIA following the ultrasound.

Methods: Eight adolescents with polyarticular or extended oligoarticular JIA and their caregivers completed this 12 week study. A within subject design was used to compare baseline and post-intervention adherence, quality of life and disease activity indices. Adherence measures included electronic measurement of methotrexate in addition to self-reported adherence questionnaires. The ultrasound intervention included a one-time, rheumatologist provided, educational examination of three or more currently or historically active joints.

Results: The ultrasound intervention was found to be both feasible and acceptable. One hundred percent of eligible participants completed the ultrasound intervention. The ultrasound was well received by patients and caregivers, with most believing this to be a helpful tool. Baseline adherence was 75.3% among participants, with half of the participants being classified as non-adherent. Electronically measured and self-reported adherence measures did not show significant changes during the post-intervention period. Two participants improved, four participants maintained, and two participants decreased adherence. On ultrasound, 18/27 (66.7%) of the examined joints displayed abnormalities, with 63% being discrepant and additive to the rheumatologist's physical examination.

Conclusions: While our intervention did not show any changes in adherence, quality of life or disease activity indices in this proof-of-concept trial, the intervention does show promise in acceptability measures and merits future study in a more robust trial design. An additional study benefit was that the musculoskeletal ultrasound intervention was able to demonstrate subclinical disease, leading to clinically impactful therapeutic changes in several participants.

Keywords: Adherence, Juvenile idiopathic arthritis, Musculoskeletal ultrasound

* Correspondence: Leslie.favier@gmail.com; Avani.modi@cchmc.org
[1]Cincinnati Children's Hospital Medical Center, Department of Pediatric Rheumatology, 3333 Burnet Ave, MLC 4010, Cincinnati, OH 45229, USA
[2]Cincinnati Children's Hospital Medical Center, Behavioral Medicine and Clinical Psychology, Center for Adherence and Self-Management, 3333 Burnet Ave, MLC 7039, Cincinnati, OH 45229, USA

Background

Juvenile Idiopathic Arthritis (JIA) is the most common rheumatic condition affecting children worldwide, with an estimated prevalence rate of 132 per 100,000 [1]. The disease spectrum includes classification into seven subtypes based on the number of joints affected and differences in symptom development and prognosis. Disease control is based on management of inflammation and progression of disease while limiting disability and deformity over time. The treatment regimen for JIA is multifaceted and includes oral and/or injectable medications, physical and occupational therapies, and some lifestyle modifications. Studies focused on patients with polyarticular JIA indicate that early and aggressive therapeutic approaches increased the likelihood of attainment and maintenance of disease remission [2, 3]. Nevertheless, even after remission is attained, the current risk of disease recurrence reaches approximately 40%, which in part may be due to waning treatment adherence [4].

Adherence is defined as the extent to which a person's behavior follows healthcare treatment recommendations [5]. Factors that contribute to poor adherence include delayed benefits in early treatment, need for consistency over a long period of time, and negative side effects [6]. Unfortunately, poor adherence in JIA impacts health-related quality of life [7] and rates of active disease control [8]. For example, prescription refills for adherence to disease modifying anti-rheumatic drugs (DMARD) and injectable anti-tumor necrosis-alpha drugs only occurred 46.9 and 65.7% of the time, respectively [9]. Our prior work studying adherence barriers in the current treatment landscape indicates that 70% of adolescents with JIA and 77% of their caregivers endorse at least one adherence barrier [10]. The most commonly reported barriers include worry about future consequences, pain, and forgetting, which are all amenable to intervention. In fact, recent meta-analyses have demonstrated that healthcare provider-based adherence interventions have greater effects on adherence compared to other multi-component interventions [11]. To date, there are no evidence-based adherence promotion interventions within standard clinical rheumatology practice and this current study sought to establish proof-of-concept for a rheumatologist-provided intervention.

Musculoskeletal ultrasound (MSKUS) is an emerging form of disease surveillance that an increasing number of rheumatology providers are utilizing in clinical practice. Symptoms of chronic arthritis due to synovial hypertrophy and fluid accumulation within the joint space can accurately be identified in real-time during routine clinic visits [12, 13]. Ultrasound studies are efficient in both time and cost expenditure, as compared to the imaging gold standard MRI, and are able to spare the use of radiation or intravenous (IV) contrast burden [12]. Some evidence has suggested that subclinical disease activity including synovitis can be identified by the use of MSKUS surveillance [14–16]. MSKUS provides a longitudinal, objective characterization of disease status that allows an important opportunity for patient inclusion via demonstrative real-time education. Specifically, visual demonstration modalities reduce limitations imposed by healthcare literacy variation and possibly may better equip patients with knowledge regarding their disease [17]. Additionally, MSKUS may foster increased patient-provider interaction through shared disease visualization and discussion. Studies assessing adults with rheumatoid arthritis (RA) revealed that those who underwent ultrasound evaluation had more confidence in their ability to complete treatment recommendations [18, 19].

As the routine use of ultrasound increases in pediatric rheumatology, our aim in this proof-of-concept study is to assess the impact of MSKUS on adherence in adolescents with polyarticular JIA. This pilot study serves to efficiently establish the merit for more rigorous testing of the intervention. Our hypothesis was that MSKUS would be rated as feasible and acceptable to patients and parents and that following receipt of an MSKUS intervention, participants would demonstrate improvement in electronically-monitored and patient-reported adherence measures.

Methods

Study population

Participants were recruited from a rheumatology clinic at a Midwestern children's hospital. Inclusion criteria were as follows: (1) adolescents, ages 10 to 17 years of age and their primary caregiver; (2) diagnosed with polyarticular or extended oligoarticular JIA and (3) taking methotrexate (oral or injectable) as part of their arthritis treatment regimen. Pertinent exclusion criteria included: (1) patients who were undergoing treatment for other chronic rheumatic conditions, (2) patients with other underlying chronic medical conditions involving daily prescribed therapy (i.e. Diabetes) and (3) patients with the diagnosis of significant developmental disorders impacting the ability to complete a questionnaires or understand a MSKUS intervention.

Study design

This proof-of-concept study used a within-subject design where subjects act as their own control in a pre-post intervention comparison. The study time-line consisted of three total visits. At enrollment, participants were given an electronic adherence monitor to use for the entire study period. At baseline, demographic screening, patient/parent reported adherence questionnaires and disease-specific chart review were collected. Two to three-months later, participants received the intervention (i.e. MSKUS) and completed questionnaires to ensure no significant changes in outcomes of interest prior to the intervention. An additional two to three-months following the intervention, electronic adherence was recorded and repeated outcome measures were collected in addition to a feasibility and acceptability questionnaire. Study visits were scheduled along with regularly scheduled rheumatology clinic appointments, so there was some natural variation in the three-visit study timeline between patients. While three adolescent-parent dyads completed the final study questionnaires remotely and returned via mailer, the remainder of the sample completed all materials face-to-face. The relative small scale of this study serves to test this novel intervention using both a convenient sample and study visit timeline, with the intention of performing a more rigorous trial design in the future.

Primary outcome measures

Primary outcome measures focused on the implementation of the intervention which included: 1) enrollment and retention rates, 2) proportion of completed questionnaires, 3) ability to utilize and return the electronic adherence monitoring device, and 4) acceptability of the ultrasound intervention as characterized by a written questionnaire. Caregivers and adolescents were asked to complete a study-specific questionnaire assessing feasibility and acceptability of the adherence intervention. Similar questionnaires have been used by adherence researchers and provide critical information on ways to improve upon the adherence intervention [20]. The measure included 9 items, demonstrated in Table 2. The questionnaire includes items related to the format, content, convenience, as well as perceived impact of the ultrasound intervention on outcomes. These items were scored on a 5-point Likert scale, with a score of 4 or 5 denoting a high degree of acceptability (i.e. agree or strongly agree).

Secondary outcome measures

Secondary outcomes were designed to assess effectiveness of the intervention as an adherence promoter. The *Medication Event Monitoring Systems (MEMS)*, made by AARDEX Corporation, is an electronic monitoring system that measures the dosing histories of patient prescribed oral medications. It has two components: a standard plastic bottle with a threaded opening and a closure for the vial that contains a micro-electronic circuit to register the dates and times the bottle is opened and closed. Based on its reputation as the most prevalent adherence tracking device, with strong correlations to both pharmacy refill data and serum assay adherence measures, it was used to monitor adherence to methotrexate for the current study [21, 22]. The bottles used accommodated both pill and injectable vial form of methotrexate and this represents the first time that adherence to an injectable DMARD has been quantitatively measured in JIA. The MEMS TrackCap stores times and dates and the data can be transferred to a Windows-based computer. Data from the MEMS TrackCap was downloaded during the intervention and post-intervention study visit. Adolescents and caregivers were asked at study visits if there are any situations or times that the cap was not used to account for intentional dosing breaks or illnesses that may have prohibited dosing, and the data were edited to reflect these changes. Notably, our baseline assessment was 2–3 months in length, giving sufficient time for typical reactivity (e.g. 2–3 weeks) to using the monitor [23].

Adherence questionnaires included the *Parent Adherence Report Questionnaire (PARQ) and Child Adherence Report Questionnaire (CARQ).* These JIA-specific tools measure beliefs and behaviors related to adherence to various prescribed JIA therapies. The tool is composed of parent and patient specific forms including 10 and 8 questions respectively, using a visual analog scale. Rasch analysis of the parent form demonstrated validity and reliability of the instrument [24, 25]. Currently, there are no scoring criteria for this tool and items are examined individually. For our study purpose, the item asking "how often do you follow your medication treatment" was used to ascertain self-reported adherence, for the parent and child separately.

Barriers to adherence were measured via a JIA-specific barriers assessment tool previously reported by our group, *Barriers to Adherence Tool (BAT)* [10]. This fourteen item checklist assesses logistical, social, psychological and knowledge-based adherence barriers in both patients and caregivers for all treatment modalities (medications, injections, infusions and physical/occupational therapy). While validation of this tool has not been formally undertaken in JIA, the themes represented by this measure have been systematically validated in other chronic pediatric conditions [26–28].

Baseline measures of current and historical disease activity, treatment regimens, and demographics were obtained at the time of study recruitment. Disease activity parameters extracted from the medical record included physical examination (including active joint counts), duration of disease, serologies and inflammatory indices (i.e. sedimentation rate and C-reactive protein) if available. Additionally, the patient and provider global assessment scores were used which include a visual analog log (VAS) score assessment of the patients overall well-being (Range 0–10, 10 being poor). These disease related measures were used to assess overall disease activity via the cJADAS (clinical juvenile disease activity score) scoring system [29]. The cJADAS is a validated for clinical and research use in JIA.

Pediatric Quality of Life Inventory (PedsQL™) Rheumatology Module is a disease-specific quality of life measure that assesses pain and hurt, daily activities, treatment, worry and communication. For the purpose of this study, the total score was used. Reliability for the total scale is 0.93 for the parent proxy report [30].

JIA-specific knowledge about disease and prescribed therapies was assessed by a tool designed for use in this study. This tool contains 11 items to measure baseline knowledge. All items were true/false for ease of completion for the adolescent. Themes addressed in the questionnaire included JIA comorbidities (i.e. eye disease), common therapies (i.e. immunosuppressants), aspects of JIA care (i.e. the need for physical therapy, lab testing and joint exams), and some items specific to methotrexate dosing (i.e. folic acid supplementation and nausea as an adverse effect). This tool is available upon request of corresponding author (LF).

Ultrasound intervention

The ultrasound intervention was designed to be succinct and complementary to standard rheumatology care. An introduction to joint anatomy, physical disease manifestations and a brief synopsis of ultrasound imaging was provided to each family. The ultrasound included assessment of three or more historically active or symptomatic joints as demonstrated via prior provider physical examination. The ultrasound assessed at minimum 2 views (in orthogonal planes) of every joint evaluated; via both grayscale and Power Doppler (PD) modes. Standardized guidelines for image acquisition in JIA are limited [31]; joint specific images were obtained using recommendations for the knee joint by Ting et al. and other joints by Collado et al. [32] Determination of abnormal effusion, synovial hypertrophy and Power Doppler enhancement was completed in accordance to consensus guidance for synovitis in pediatrics [33]. PD mode was chosen over color Doppler based on optimal performance of the machines used at our center. Patient and caregiver were provided with verbal review of the findings and they were encouraged to participate in direct visualization of the images in real-time. No other specifics of their care (i.e. treatments) were verbally discussed at the time of the ultrasound, except in the case of one patient who was treated by the ultrasound interventionist. Each intervention took on average 20 min. Ultrasounds were performed by clinicians (LF, TT) with training levels of 2–6 years in MSKUS. No ultrasonographer blinding was pursued in this study. Abnormal findings based on the ultrasound were communicated to the patient's primary rheumatologist.

Statistical analysis

Adherence was calculated as the number of doses taken/number of doses prescribed *100%. Adherence was capped at 100% for all analyses [20, 34]. Because this is a proof-of-concept study, we examined descriptive information and used basic statistical tests (e.g., paired t-tests) to examine pre-post changes in electronically-monitored and self/parent-reported adherence. We also assessed correlations between baseline JIA-specific knowledge, disease activity, and complexity of medication regimen in regard to adherence rates. Feasibility and acceptability of the intervention was analyzed via means and standard deviations and percentages of responses in the acceptable range.

Results

Study population and demographics

Figure 1 depicts our consort diagram of enrollment. Our patient sample included both polyarticular (80%) and extended oligoarticular (20%) subtypes. As noted in Table 1, the average patient age in years was 12.70 ± 2.06 with the majority being Caucasian (90%) females (80%). Parental marital status varied in our sample with 60% reporting being married. All patients were treated with methotrexate, with oral tablets being the most common formulation prescribed (55%). Most patients were on a concomitant biologic medication (63%), with 50% of those being infusion therapies.

Feasibility and acceptability

Feasibility of the study was based on full participation in the intervention and retention in the study until the final post-intervention visit. As seen in Fig. 1, of the 15 participants recruited, only one declined to participate. All of the eligible patients completed the intervention. Eight patients completed the entire study and were successful in returning the MEMS TrackCaps; however, two patients did not return their MEMS TrackCaps.

As noted in Table 2, based on a five point Likert Scale, the intervention was rated as comfortable (child M = 4.88 out of 5; parent M = 4.63) and a majority of patients felt that the ultrasound was helpful (child M = 4.25; parent M = 4.25), could benefit other children with arthritis (child M = 4.38; parent M = 4.75), and was explained in a clear way (child M = 4.63; parent M = 4.63). Lower acceptability ratings were noted in the ability of the intervention to change the way the family took their medications (child M = 2.63; parent M = 3.625) and change in their overall confidence in their care (child M = 3.5; parent M = 4.0). Most patients and parents were glad they participated in this study (child M = 4.5; parent M = 4.5).

Intervention preliminary efficacy

Mean adherence at baseline was 75.3%, of which three patients had 100% adherence. Using a traditional 80%

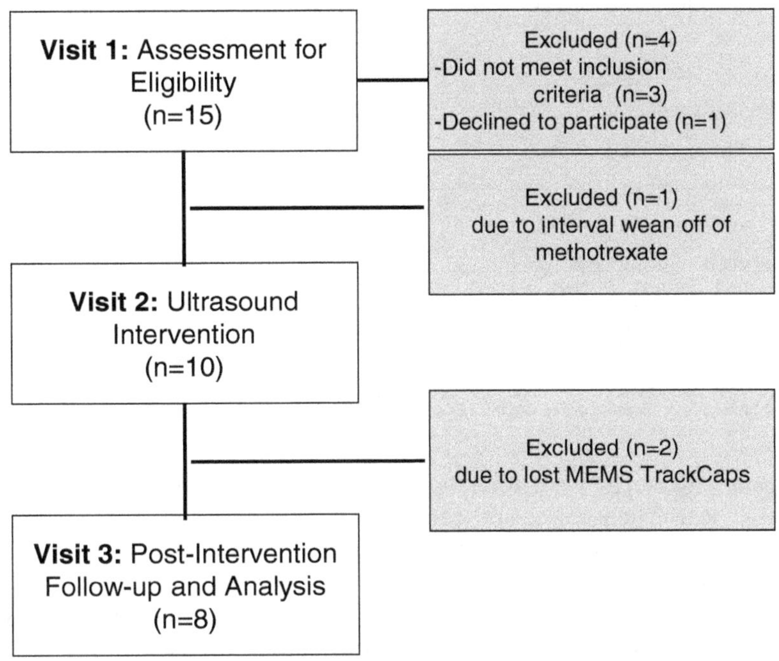

Fig. 1 CONSORT Diagram

Table 1 Descriptive Statistics of Participants

Characteristic	Total Sample ($n = 11$)	Completed Analysis ($n = 8$)
Patient Age (mean ± SD)	12.70 ± 2.06	12.75 ± 2.31
Gender (female %)	80	80
Race (white %)	90	87.5
Parental Marital Status (%)		
Single	20	25
Married	60	62.5
Divorced	10	12.5
Arthritis Type (%)		
Polyarticular RF-negative	80	75
Extended oligoarticular	20	25
Disease Duration (years)	3.9 ± 3.37	3.0 ± 3.05
Methotrexate route of administration (%)		
Oral	55	62.5
Subcutaneous	45	37.5
Concomitant Biologic (%)		
None	37	25
Etanercept	9	12.5
Adalimumab	9	12.5
Infliximab	27	37.5
Tocilizumab	18	12.5
Oral Steroids (%)	20	25

goal adherence level [33], 50% ($n = 4$ of 8) of patients were classified as "non-adherent" to methotrexate based on electronic monitoring at baseline. Each participant's adherence data from pre to post-intervention is shown in Fig. 2. Two participants improved, four maintained adherence over time, and two participants declined. No significant differences were found from pre to post intervention for the sample for electronically-monitored adherence (t (df) = – 0.45, $p = 0.67$), self-reported adherence (t (df) = 1.35, $p = 0.90$) or parent-reported adherence (t (df) = 1.75, $p = 0.12$); See Table 2.

The number of adherence barriers decreased slightly for adolescents but increased slightly for parents (see Table 3). Specific examination of individual barriers (i.e. forgetting, pain, embarrassment etc.) revealed no major changes based on type.

Intervention findings and clinical impact

At least three joints were examined per participant, with 27 joints examined overall for the sample. Eighteen (66.7%) of the examined joints displayed abnormalities on ultrasound examination (see Fig. 3 for specific findings). Of note, there was a 63% discrepancy between the documented rheumatologist's physical examination and the ultrasound exam, with the ultrasound picking up more joint pathology compared to physical examination. In total, four (50%) patients received a therapeutic change based on the ultrasound findings, including three new biologic starts.

Table 2 Descriptive Data of Feasibility and Acceptability Questionnaire ($N = 8$ Children and 8 Parents)

Title Items	Child N in the Ideal Range[a]	Parent N in the Ideal Range[a]
The ultrasound was not painful or uncomfortable.	7	8
The ultrasound provided me with new information.	5	7
The ultrasound provider explained the exam in a clear way.	6	8
The information that I learned from the ultrasound was helpful to me.	5	7
The ultrasound findings change the way we take medications.	2	4
I believe other children could benefit from ultrasounds in clinic.	5	8
The ultrasound made us feel more confident in our care.	4	4
I value the feedback I received from the MEMS TrackCaps.	6	6
Overall I am glad we participated.	7	7

[a]Based on a 4–5 score on a 5 point Likert Scale denoting agree or strongly agree. Assumption is made that a rating in this range notes a high rate of acceptability by respondents

No statistically significant differences were found on disease activity indices (i.e., active join count and provider and patient global assessment); however, trends in improvement were demonstrated (See Table 3). Further, no changes in HRQOL were found.

Post-hoc analyses indicated that the three patients that received a biologic treatment change had improvements in their disease activity scores, with average decreases ranging from high to moderate disease activity, which is clinically meaningful. Further patient-level comparative data is noted in Table 4.

Discussion

This proof-of-concept study was designed to test a MSKUS education-based adherence intervention amongst adolescents with JIA and their caregivers. Innovative aspects of the current study includes the novel multi-modal method used to demonstrate oral and injectable methotrexate adherence rates in this population, and the application of a rheumatology provider-based educational intervention for adolescents and their caregivers within the clinic setting.

Based on our retention rate of 80% and intervention completion rate of 100%, our study design and intervention methods appear to be feasible. The majority of participants found the ultrasound intervention to be clear, helpful and beneficial. Additionally, the MEMS TrackCap was an acceptable form of adherence measurement with no malfunctioning or missing data noted in the caps that were returned. Further, it was able to capture

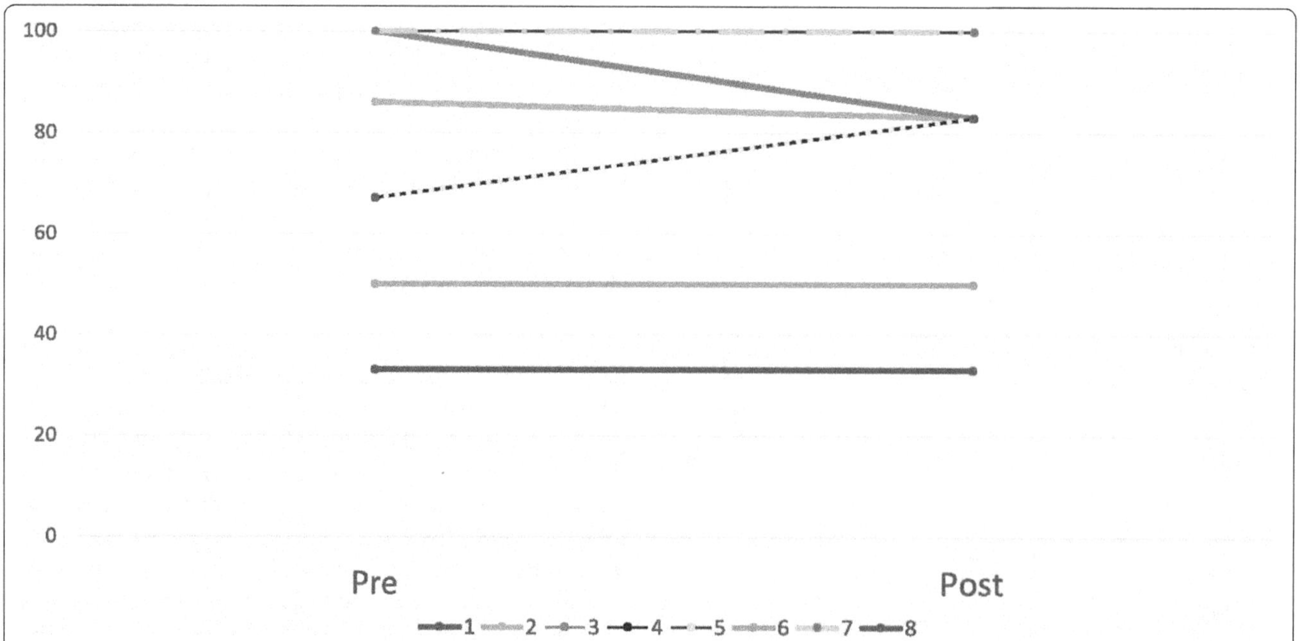

Fig. 2 Participant Adherence Trajectory. Legend: Adherence is represented as the percentage of methotrexate dosages administered via MEMs TrackCap over the total prescribed treatment regimen doses. Adherence goal range is classically above 80%. Dashed lines represent overlapping participant data

Table 3 Pre- and Post- Comparative Statistics

Measure	Pre	Post	Mean % Change	Significance
% Adherence	75.34	77.06	1.73 ± 10.78	0.665
JIA Knowledge Score %	74.1	86.5	12.38 ± 15.17	0.054
Self-Report Adherence (Child)[a]	86.5	87.2	0.07 ± 1.31	0.890
Self-Report Adherence (Parent)[a]	88.0	80.8	−0.76 ± 1.74	0.124
Adherence Barriers Count Child[b]	6.75	3.13	−3.63 ± 5.88	0.125
Adherence Barriers Count Parent [b]	4.88	5.38	0.50 ± 4.60	0.767
cJADAS[c]	12.13	6.13	−6.0 ± 10.00	0.133
Active Joint Count	7.38	2.50	−4.87 ± 6.10	0.058
Provider Global Assessment[d]	1.83	0.75	−1.06 ± 1.61	0.105
Patient Global Assessment[d]	3.19	2.88	−3.13 ± 2.25	0.706
PedsQL Parent Total Score (rg 0–100)[e]	76.98	76.28	−0.70 ± 17.72	0.934
Average Pain (VAS rg 0–10)	4.25	3.25	−1.00 ± 2.20	0.240

[a]PARQ/CARQ- Visual Analog Scale (VAS)– maximum 100 mm
[b]BAT- Represented as N out of a maximum 54 barriers
[c]cJADAS – Range 0–40, based on provider and patient global assessment and a 10 point joint exam
[d]Provider/Patient Global Assessment – VAS (0–10) with 0 being low disease activity
[e]PEdsQL scoring based on 5 point functional assessments. Range 0–100, with 100 being optimum functioning

medication-taking behavior of both formulations of methotrexate, which is a significant strength of the study. To our knowledge, this is the first time MEMS TrackCaps have been used to measure adherence to injectable arthritis medications in pediatric rheumatology. Although adherence rates were capped at 100% for analyses, it is important to note that one family was actually found to have administered more than the prescribed regimen based on the patient living in two households due to divorce. That particular family valued the use of the TrackCaps for added accountability.

While mean adherence did not change significantly from pre to post intervention and correlations cannot be made based on the study size and scope, maintenance and improvements in patient self-reported and electronically-monitored adherence were observed in some patients. Additionally, the percentage of patients with "good" adherence (> 80%) [35] rose from 50 to 75% percent. Given that adherence typically declines over time [36], improvements and/or maintenance when adherence is already high is considered successful. Notably, 50% of our patients were non-adherent at baseline, which is consistent with the larger literature [23, 34],

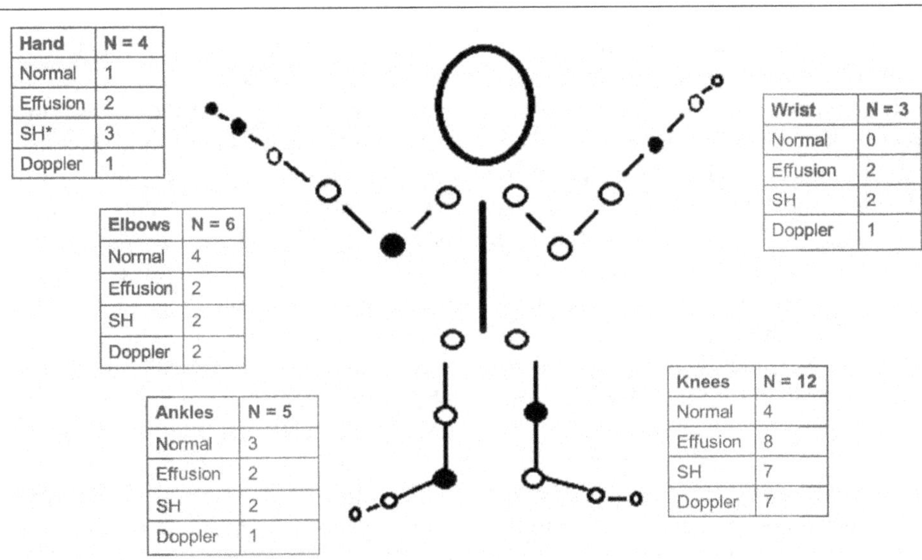

Fig. 3 Ultrasound Intervention Findings. Legend: This figure demonstrates the location and description of the ultrasound findings by joint. SH- Synovial Hypertrophy

Table 4 Patient-level Comparative Statistics

	Intervention			Characteristics						Outcomes			
	Abnormal U/S	Discrepant exams	New Biologic Started	MEMs Adherence (%)		Pt Self-reported Adherence[a]		Pt Number of Adherence Barriers		Joint Count		cJADAS	
				Pre	Post	Pre	Post	Pre	Post	Pre	Post	Pre	Post
1	Yes	Yes	No	33.3	33.3	52	79	10	4	0	0	3	3
2	Yes	Yes	Yes	86	83.3	92	97	4	6	6	0	8	6.5
3	Yes	Yes	Yes	100	83.3	93	94	10	7	7	3	28	11
4	Yes	Yes	Yes	66.7	83.3	93	87	18	2	8	3	15	7
5	No	No	No	100	100	100	100	0	1	0	0	3	3
6	Yes	Yes	No	50	50	80	77	2	3	12	5	3.5	6
7	Yes	No	No	100	100	87	88	2	0	0	1	0.5	1.5
8	Yes	No	No	66.7	83.3	95	75	8	2	26	8	20	11

Individual level data is demonstrated for intervention results, adherence pre and post comparisons and joint activity outcomes
[a]Based on CARQ responses on a 100 mm VAS

indicating that adherence is a significant issue for these patients.

Our data assessing self-reported and parent-reported adherence is consistent with prior studies suggesting inflation or over reporting. This may reflect response bias or pressure around social desirability. Prior data assessing self-reported adherence for adolescents with JIA (*N* = 116) on methotrexate found a median adherence of 98% [37]. Additionally, parent perceived adherence using the PARQ over a one year time period reported similarly high rates, varying between 86.1 and 92.0% [38]. In that study, the most highly correlated factor predicting higher self-reported adherence was believing that the therapy was helpful. This highlights the fact that patient beliefs influence the way self-management behaviors are performed and may be further evidence of the importance of standard patient education, with ultrasound being one method [39].

Perhaps the most salient aspect of this study design is the delivery of the intervention by a rheumatologist compared to other healthcare providers. The majority of JIA-focused adherence interventions were prior to biologic therapies and/or utilized psychologists, nurses or peer-mentors to perform the interventions [6, 40–42]. Since the advent of biologics, families of children with JIA have navigated more complex treatment regimens. Our prior work studying adherence barriers in JIA indicated that worry about JIA treatments was common for caregivers and patients [10], which suggests a need for more communication regarding specific concerns. Further, in a study assessing perceptions of adolescents prescribed biologic therapy, most adolescents preferred an active and involved role with dedicated education during their clinic visits [43]. Real-time, objective ultrasound interventions performed by rheumatologists, informs the patients of up-to-date disease status and presents the opportunity for additional questions or concerns regarding care. In some cases, it also justifies the need for therapy in the absence of perceived symptoms as well as the reverse. Our intervention not only included a review of normal joint anatomy and how ultrasounds can be useful in JIA, but patients were encouraged to actively participate in the ultrasound examination by seeing exactly what fluid or synovitis looks like in their own joints. This prompted many patients to have further discussions with their rheumatologists following the examination with a new sense of knowledge that they would have lacked prior. Previous work has established that both patients and providers value the information provided by ultrasounds [44]; however, more research is needed to measure the potentially compound effects that the receipt of an ultrasound can provide.

One unanticipated finding from this study was the benefit of adjunctive MSKUS for clinical care of patients with JIA. Despite the study being short-term, MSKUS aided in the detection of subclinical disease and informed therapeutic change. In our sample, the rate of abnormalities on ultrasound examination was 87.5% with two-thirds of those being discrepant to the rheumatologist's physical examinations. Our rate of subclinical disease discovery was higher than prior study in pediatrics [15]. There was no recruitment screening done for patients presumed to be in active disease; thus, many of the rheumatology providers were surprised by the ultrasound findings. Outcomes in our sample revealed improvement overall, likely related to attainment of disease control based on optimized medication therapy. This is further supported by the fact that in the subset of patients that were started on a biologic during the intervention visit, the interval improvement in cJADAS score was more clinically meaningful as compared to patients that did not incur a therapeutic change. While unable to be correlated during this study, uncovering subclinical disease is one clear factor that could help to engage patients to adhere more closely to therapies and activate providers to screen for nonadherence more vigorously. This was mentioned by several rheumatologists upon hearing the results of their patient's ultrasounds in our study.

As this was a proof-of-concept study, there are several important opportunities for improvement. Our small sample size was composed of a heterogeneous collection of participants including differences in therapy regimens, duration of disease and disease severity. Standardizing these parameters, increasing the sample, and testing the intervention via a randomized-controlled trial would increase our ability to detect the impact of our intervention on outcomes. An attention control arm including a verbal-education only group would aid in assessing the true effect of ultrasound imaging as an educational intervention. Also, the inclusion of two participants that received their intervention despite having a baseline adherence rate of 100% may have altered results due to ceiling effects. Any subsequent work in this area should exclude patients who demonstrate high adherence and thus do not need adherence interventions. Adherence interventions in other disease populations have successfully used this approach [32, 45]. Additionally, our short study duration of 12 weeks may have not provided sufficient time to examine behavioral changes over time. A longer study duration would also better demonstrate changes in our secondary outcomes (i.e. HRQOL and cJADAS) as these typically require longer monitoring to display changes over time. Furthermore, the medication regimen changes made during the study in several patients, may have altered the treatment routines of patients, thus potentially adding or subtracting barriers to adherence. However, the ethical need to respond to new information provided by the ultrasound, precludes avoidance of these therapeutic changes. Additional specific improvements that could be made to the ultrasound intervention itself include multi-provider blinded testing as to decrease biases imparted by the study team.

This study emphasizes the continuing importance of the development of adherence interventions for use in JIA. Following more rigorous testing, a multimodal adherence intervention including visual demonstration of disease using ultrasound could become common practice as either primary or secondary adherence promotion. There is still much work to be done in order to understand and encourage our patients to better navigate self-care and participate in their health. As providers of children with chronic illnesses in the midst of advancing technologies, we must continue to seek solutions to better bridge the patient-provider gap and deliver education to improve outcomes.

Conclusions

Our study highlights an additional beneficial and novel use of MSKUS as a patient education tool. In this proof-of-concept trial, patients and families saw the purpose and helpfulness of real-time disease demonstration via ultrasound. We document that quantitative, electronically -measured adherence to methotrexate is, not only less than self-reported measures, but also below acceptable thresholds for therapy. We have also contributed to growing literature that establishes the utility of MSKUS as a useful clinical tool, with the potential to be harnessed for use in patient activation.

Abbreviations

BAT: Barriers assessment tool; CARQ: Child adherence report questionnaire; cJADAS: Clinical juvenile arthritis disease activity score; DMARD: Disease modifying anti-rheumatic drug; JIA: Juvenile idiopathic arthritis; MEMS: Medication event monitoring system; MSKUS: Musculoskeletal ultrasound; PARQ: Parent adherence report questionnaire; PD: Power Doppler; PedsQL: Pediatric quality of life inventory; RA: Rheumatoid arthritis; SH: Synovial hypertrophy; VAS: Visual analog scale

Acknowledgments

The team would like to acknowledge Dr. Daniel Lovell for his guidance in study conceptualization and design.

Funding

This work was funded by a training grant through the Center for Adherence and Self-Management at Cincinnati Children's Hospital Medical Center. The National Institutes of Health. Grant Award/Number: T32HD068223.

Author's contributions

LF, AM and TT all contributed to study design. LF coordinated enrollment and data collection. LF and TT preformed all ultrasound interventions and interpreted imaging findings. LF and AM analyzed and interpreted the data. All authors were contributors to the writing of the manuscript and formation of tables and figures. All authors read and approved the final manuscript.

Consent for publication

All 11 adolescents who were enrolled completed a written assent and their respective caregivers completed a written consent to participate and have this work published.

Competing interests

The authors declare that they have no competing interests.

References

1. Oen KG, Cheang M. Epidemiology of chronic arthritis in childhood. Semin Arthritis Rheum. 1996;26(3):575–91.
2. Wallace CA, Giannini EH, Spalding SJ, Hashkes PJ, O'Neil KM, Zeft AS, et al. Clinically inactive disease in a cohort of children with new-onset polyarticular juvenile idiopathic arthritis treated with early aggressive therapy: time to achievement, total duration, and predictors. J Rheumatol. 2014;41(6):1163–70.
3. Ringold S, Seidel KD, Koepsell TD, Wallace CA. Inactive disease in polyarticular juvenile idiopathic arthritis: current patterns and associations. Rheumatology. 2009;48(8):972–7.
4. Guzman J, Oen K, Huber AM, Watanabe Duffy K, Boire G, Shiff N, et al. The risk and nature of flares in juvenile idiopathic arthritis: results from the ReACCh-out cohort. Ann Rheum Dis. 2016;75:1092–8.

5. Modi AC, Pai AL, Hommel KA, Hood KK, Cortina S, Hilliard ME, et al. Pediatric self-management: a framework for research, practice, and policy. Pediatrics. 2012;129(2):e473–85.
6. Rapoff MA, Lindsley CB. Improving adherence to medical regimens for juvenile rheumatoid arthritis. Pediatr Rheumatol Online J. 2007;5:10.
7. Toupin April K, Feldman DE, Zunzunegui MV, Duffy CM. Association between perceived treatment adherence and health-related quality of life in children with juvenile idiopathic arthritis: perspectives of both parents and children. Patient Prefer Adherence. 2008;2:121–8.
8. Feldman DE, De Civita M, Dobkin PL, Malleson PN, Meshefedjian G, Duffy CM. Effects of adherence to treatment on short-term outcomes in children with juvenile idiopathic arthritis. Arthritis Rheum. 2007;57(6):905–12.
9. Ringold S, Grant S, Girdish C, Wallace CA, Sullivan SD. Methotrexate and injectable tumor necrosis factor-alpha inhibitor adherence and persistence in children with rheumatic diseases. J Rheumatol. 2013;40(1):80–6.
10. Favier LA, Taylor J, Rich KL, Jones KB, Vora SS, Harris JG, Gottlieb BS, Robbins L, Lai JT, Lee T, Kohlheim M, Ferraro K, Gil J, Bouslaugh L, Young A, Griffin N, Modi AC. Barriers to adherence in juvenile idiopathic arthritis: a multicenter collaborative experience and preliminary results. J Rheumatol. 2018;45(5):690–6.
11. Wu YP, Pai ALH. Health care provider-delivered adherence promotion interventions: a meta-analysis. Pediatrics. 2014;133(6):e1698–707.
12. Colebatch-Bourn AN, Edwards CJ, Collado P, D'Agostino MA, Hemke R, Jousse-Joulin S, et al. EULAR-PReS points to consider for the use of imaging in the diagnosis and management of juvenile idiopathic arthritis in clinical practice. Ann Rheum Dis. 2015;74(11):1946–57.
13. Collado P, Jousse-Joulin S, Alcalde M, Naredo E, D'Agostino MA. Is ultrasound a validated imaging tool for the diagnosis and management of synovitis in juvenile idiopathic arthritis? A systematic literature review. Arthritis Care Res (Hoboken). 2012;64(7):1011–9.
14. Magni-Manzoni S, Scirè CA, Ravelli A, Klersy C, Rossi S, Muratore V, et al. Ultrasound-detected synovial abnormalities are frequent in clinically inactive juvenile idiopathic arthritis, but do not predict a flare of synovitis. Ann Rheum Dis. 2013;72(2):223–8.
15. Magni-Manzoni S, Epis O, Ravelli A, Klersy C, Visconti C, Lanni S, et al. Comparison of clinical versus ultrasound-determined synovitis in juvenile idiopathic arthritis. Arthritis Care Res (Hoboken). 2009;61(11):1497–504.
16. Rebollo-Polo M, Koujok K, Weisser C, Jurencak R, Bruns A, Roth J. Ultrasound findings on patients with juvenile idiopathic arthritis in clinical remission. Arthritis Care Res (Hoboken). 2011;63(7):1013–9.
17. Joplin S, van der Zwan R, Joshua F, Wong PKK. Medication adherence in patients with rheumatoid arthritis: the effect of patient education, health literacy, and musculoskeletal ultrasound. Biomed Res Int. 2015;2015:1–10.
18. Joplin SK, van der Zwan R, Bagga H, Joshua F, Wong PKK. Pilot study assessing the novel use of musculoskeletal ultrasound in patients with rheumatoid arthritis to improve patient attitudes and adherence to medication. Int J Rheum Dis. 2014. https://doi.org/10.1111/1756-185X.12402.
19. Kumar K, Raza K, Gill P, Greenfield S. The impact of using musculoskeletal ultrasound imaging and other influencing factors on medication adherence in patients with rheumatoid arthritis: a qualitative study. Patient Prefer Adherence. 2016;10:1091–100.
20. Modi AC, Guilfoyle SM, Rausch J. Preliminary feasibility, acceptability, and efficacy of an innovative adherence intervention for children with newly diagnosed epilepsy. J Pediatr Psychol. 2013;38(6):605–16.
21. Ingerski LM, Hente EA, Modi AC, Hommel KA. Electronic measurement of medication adherence in pediatric chronic illness: a review of measures. J Pediatr. 2011;159(4):528–34.
22. McGrady ME, Holbein CE, Smith AW, Morrison CF, Hommel KA, Modi AC, Pai AL, Ramsey RR. An independent evaluation of the accuracy and usability of electronic adherence monitoring devices. Ann Intern Med. 2018.
23. Rapoff MA. Adherence to pediatric medical regimens. Second Edition J Dev Behav Pediatr. 2010;31:476.
24. De Civita M, Dobkin PL, Ehrmann-Feldman D, Karp I, Duffy CM. Development and preliminary reproducibility and validity of the parent adherence report questionnaire: a measure of adherence in juvenile idiopathic arthritis. J Clin Psychol Med Settings. 2005;12(1):1–12.
25. Toupin April K, Higgins J, Ehrmann FD. Application of Rasch analysis to the parent adherence report questionnaire in juvenile idiopathic arthritis. Pediatr Rheumatol. 2016;14(1):45.
26. Simons LE, McCormick ML, Devine K, Blount RL. Medication barriers predict adolescent transplant recipients' adherence and clinical outcomes at 18-month follow-up. J Pediatr Psychol. 2010;35(9):1038–48.
27. Modi AC, Monahan S, Daniels D, Glauser TA. Development and validation of the pediatric epilepsy medication self-management questionnaire. Epilepsy Behav. 2010;18(1–2):94–9.
28. Modi AC, Crosby LE, Guilfoyle SM, Lemanek KL, Witherspoon D, Mitchell MJ. Barriers to treatment adherence for pediatric patients with sickle cell disease and their families. Child Heal Care. 2009;38(2):107–22.
29. Consolaro A, Ruperto N, Bazso A, Pistorio A, Magni-Manzoni S, Filocamo G, et al. Development and validation of a composite disease activity score for juvenile idiopathic arthritis. Arthritis Rheum. 2009;61(5):658–66.
30. Varni JW, Seid M, Knight TS, Burwinkle T, Brown J, Szer IS. The PedsQL in pediatric rheumatology: reliability, validity, and responsiveness of the pediatric quality of life inventory generic Core scales and rheumatology module. Arthritis Rheum. 2002;46(3):714–25.
31. Ting TV, Vega-Fernandez P, Oberle EJ, De Ranieri D, Bukulmez H, Lin C, et al. A Novel Ultrasound Image Acquisition Protocol and Scoring System for the Pediatric Knee. Arthritis Care Res. 2018; Epub ahead of print.
32. Collado P, Vojinovic J, Nieto JC, Windschall D, Magni-Manzoni S, Bruyn GA, et al. And Omeract ultrasound pediatric group. Toward standardized musculoskeletal ultrasound in pediatric rheumatology: Normal age-related ultrasound findings. Arthritis Care Res. 2016;68(3):348–56.
33. Roth J, Ravagnani V, Backhaus M, Balint P, Bruns A, Bruyn GA, et al. Preliminary definitions for the sonographic features of synovitis in children. Arthritis Care Res. 2017;69(8):1217–23.
34. Maddux M, Ricks S, Delurgio S, Hommel K. A pilot study evaluating the impact of an adherence-promoting intervention among nonadherent youth with inflammatory bowel disease. J Pediatr Nurs. 2017;35:72–7.
35. Drotar D. Promoting adherence to medical treatment in chronic childhood illness: concepts, methods, and interventions: Psychology Press; 2000.
36. Modi AC, Rausch JR, Glauser TA. Patterns of nonadherence to antiepileptic drug therapy in children with newly diagnosed epilepsy. JAMA. 2011;305(16):1669.
37. Mulligan K, Wedderburn LR, Newman S. The experience of taking methotrexate for juvenile idiopathic arthritis: results of a cross-sectional survey with children and young people. Pediatr Rheumatol. 2015;13:58.
38. Feldman DE, De Civita M, Dobkin PL, Malleson P, Meshefedjian G, Duffy CM. Perceived adherence to prescribed treatment in juvenile idiopathic arthritis over a one-year period. Arthritis Care Res (Hoboken). 2007;57(2):226–33.
39. Janz NK, Becker MH. The health belief model: a decade later. Health Educ Q. 1984;11(1):1–47.
40. Rapoff MA, Belmont JM, Lindsley CB, Olson NY, Morris J, Padur J. Prevention of nonadherence to nonsteroidal anti-inflammatory medications for newly diagnosed patients with juvenile rheumatoid arthritis. Health Psychol. 2002; 21(6):620.
41. Rapoff MA, Belmont JM, Lindsley CB, Olson NY. Electronically monitored adherence to medications by newly diagnosed patients with juvenile rheumatoid arthritis. Arthritis Care Res (Hoboken). 2005;53(6):905–10.
42. Stinson J, McGrath P, Hodnett E, Feldman B, Duffy C, Huber A, et al. Usability testing of an online self-management program for Adolescents with Juvenile Idiopathic Arthritis. J Med Internet Res. 2010;12(3).
43. Lipstein EA, Muething KA, Dodds CM, Britto MT. "I'm the one taking it": adolescent participation in chronic disease treatment decisions. J Adolesc Health. 2013;53(2):253–9.
44. Harry O, Huggins JL, Taylor J, Holland MJ, Ting TV. Assessing the utility and impact of musculoskeletal ultrasound in a large pediatric rheumatology clinic. Arthritis Rheumatol. 2017;69.
45. Modi AC, Guilfoyle SM, Mann KA, Rausch JR. A pilot randomized controlled clinical trial to improve antiepileptic drug adherence in young children with epilepsy. Epilepsia. 2016;57(3):e69–75.

18

Protective parents and permissive children: what qualitative interviews with parents and children can tell us about the feasibility of juvenile idiopathic arthritis trials

Frances C. Sherratt[1*], Louise Roper[1], Simon R. Stones[2], Flora McErlane[3,4], Matthew Peak[5], Michael W. Beresford[6,7], Helen Foster[3,4], Athimalaipet V. Ramanan[8], Madeleine Rooney[9], Eileen Baildam[6] and Bridget Young[1]

Abstract

Background: Patient recruitment can be very challenging in paediatric studies, especially in relatively uncommon conditions, such as juvenile idiopathic arthritis (JIA). However, involving children and young people (CYP) in the design of such trials could promise a more rapid trajectory towards making evidence-based treatments available. Studies involving CYP are advocated in the literature but we are not aware of any early stage feasibility studies that have qualitatively accessed the perspectives of parents and CYP with a long term condition to inform design and conduct of a trial. In the context of a feasibility study to inform the design of a proposed randomised controlled trial of corticosteroid induction regimen in JIA, we explored families' perspectives on the proposed trial and on JIA trials generally.

Methods: We analysed interviews with 27 participants (8 CYP aged 8–16 years and 19 parents) from four UK paediatric rheumatology centres. CYP had recently received corticosteroids to treat JIA. Audio-recorded interviews were transcribed and analysed thematically, drawing on the Framework Method.

Results: Both parents and CYP were capable of engaging with the logic of the proposed trial but pointed to challenges with its design. Treatment preferences influenced willingness to participate in the proposed trial. The preferences of older children and their parents often differed, with CYP being more willing to participate in the proposed trial than parents. Families' current treatment preferences were largely informed by past positive and negative treatment experiences. Some participants also indicated that their treatment preferences were influenced by those of their clinicians.

Conclusion: Previous research has typically focused on deficits in patients' understandings of trials. We found that both parents and CYP understood trial concepts and were able to identify potential flaws in the proposed trial. We propose recommendations to optimise the design of a planned corticosteroid induction regimen trial in JIA. Accessing both parents' and CYP's perspectives helps to identify and address recruitment challenges, which will ultimately optimise informed consent and future recruitment.

Keywords: Juvenile idiopathic arthritis, JIA, Randomised controlled trial, Recruitment, Corticosteroids, Qualitative, Children, Feasibility, Parents, Patients

* Correspondence: sherratt@liverpool.ac.uk
[1]Department of Psychological Sciences, University of Liverpool, Whelan Building, Brownlow Hill, Liverpool L69 3GB, UK
Full list of author information is available at the end of the article

Introduction

Juvenile idiopathic arthritis (JIA) refers to a collection of inflammatory arthritides (commonly divided into several subtypes) with symptom onset at, or before the age of 16 years [1]. There has been a recent increase in the number of JIA randomised controlled trials [2]. Recruitment is crucial to the success of such trials, and poor recruitment can inflate costs [3], result in underpowered trials, and lead to potentially effective interventions being abandoned or delayed [4]. Approximately 45% of UK multi-centre trials do not achieve their original recruitment target, often resulting in costly recruitment extensions [5].

Patient recruitment can be especially challenging in paediatric studies, and in relatively uncommon conditions, such as JIA [6, 7]. Compared with trials in adult rheumatology, consent seeking can be more complex due to the need to involve both child and parents in enrolment decisions [8], and some drug treatments may be poorly tolerated by younger children [9]. Innovative trial methodology and involving parents and children and young people (CYP) in the design of JIA trials promises a more rapid trajectory towards making evidence-based treatments available to young patients [10, 11].

Increasingly, researchers are using qualitative methods to explore patients' views of trial feasibility, and to proactively identify and address problems that may otherwise undermine a trial [12, 13]. Early stage feasibility studies, without a randomised component, are a distinct subtype of feasibility study. These are often used to resolve fundamental questions, such as which treatments to compare, or uncertainties about the 'in principle' acceptability of a trial to patients and recruiters before committing resources to a pilot or full randomised trial.

Although studies involving CYP are advocated in the literature [14, 15], we are aware of only one early stage feasibility study that has qualitatively investigated perspectives of both parents and CYP to inform the design and conduct of a trial [14]. This recent study focused on the experiences of CYP with acute osteomyelitis or septic arthritis, whereas the current study explored the perspectives of CYP with JIA. JIA is a long term condition, CYP with JIA may find the prospect of trial participation especially challenging due to preferences arising from their ongoing experiences of the condition and different treatments [15]. Research is needed to shed light on such issues. This article explores what an early phase qualitative feasibility study, involving interviews with both parents and CYP, can tell us about the viability of a proposed JIA trial of corticosteroid induction regimens. We also report on the wider barriers and opportunities for recruitment in JIA trials.

Methods

We adopted a qualitative approach involving semi-structured interviews. Qualitative research provides in-depth insights on participants' experiences and perspectives. Such studies are typically characterised by smaller sample sizes but rich, voluminous data [16]. Qualitative research has been used to identify and address key uncertainties in planning and designing proposed trials for adult patients [12]. Semi-structured interviews are a qualitative research method well suited to exploring the perceptions of patients regarding complex and sensitive issues [17], as these enable families to raise matters of importance to them, and for interviewers to inform families about trials and clarify any misunderstandings.

A Research Ethics Committee in the North East of England (The North East – Newcastle and North Tyneside 2) approved this study (16/NE/0047).

Participant selection

Within four UK paediatric and adolescent rheumatology centres, clinicians approached families of children and young people who met the eligibility criteria (Table 1), briefly described the study and requested verbal permission for a researcher to contact families. Children and young people had a confirmed diagnosis of JIA in line with current guidance [1, 18]. FS and LR, both experienced in qualitative research in health settings, conducted the interviews after seeking informed consent from parents and assent or consent from CYPs. Interviews took place from August 2016 to March 2017 and were audio recorded and transcribed. The research team monitored sampling characteristics to ensure these were inclusive of patients of varying ages, and of families from a range of treatment centres and socioeconomic backgrounds. Sampling for interviews ceased when data saturation was reached, that is, when further interviews were no longer contributing new information [19].

Interview protocol

Semi-structured, topic-guided interviews (Additional file 1: Appendix A) were conversational to allow participants to raise and reflect on matters of concern to them. While we interviewed all parents regardless of their child's age, only children aged eight years and over were interviewed. We developed separate topic guides for

Table 1 Inclusion criteria for qualitative interviews with families

Inclusion criteria
• CYP ≤ 16 years.
• CYP has received a clinical diagnosis of JIA.
• CYP has recent experience (≤ 12 months) of at least one of four corticosteroid delivery routes: (a) oral prednisolone (tablets); (b) intravenous methylprednisolone (IV); (c) intra-articular injection(s) (IACI), or; (d) intra-muscular injection (IM).

parents, children (8–12 years), and young people (13–16 years), and adapted these throughout the study, guided by the ongoing analysis. We also developed stimulus materials to facilitate the interviews, including a video, a flow chart illustrating the proposed trial, and prompt cards detailing potential benefits and side effects of the four corticosteroid delivery routes (Additional file 2: Appendix B). Consultant paediatric rheumatologists advised on the development of the prompt cards. These cards listed key points about the delivery routes that the rheumatologists perceived relevant to patients and families. The cards were intended to facilitate discussion in the interviews, rather than to provide an exhaustive list of benefits and side effects of the delivery routes.

In brief, the proposed trial was described to participants as comparing four corticosteroid delivery routes (hereon referred to as treatments): (a) oral prednisolone (referred to herein as tablets); (b) intravenous methylprednisolone (IV); (c) intra-articular injection(s) (IACI), and; (d) intra-muscular injection (IM). These four treatments are widely used in clinical practice for JIA, although the only informative evidence-base of effectiveness and efficacy is for IACI [20, 21]. Referring to the prompt cards the interviewer described the four delivery routes to families, including the process of delivery (e.g. duration) and potential pros and cons. While a trial could help to establish which of the treatments is most effective in treating JIA, the feasibility of such a trial is uncertain.

Qualitative analysis

We drew on The Framework Method [16], an approach to the thematic analysis of qualitative of data [22], and used NVivo 10 to assist with data indexing and coding [23]. FS, LR and BY initially read a selection of transcripts and discussed the developing analysis. FS and LR double-coded approximately 10% of transcripts, discussing divergences and their resolution, leading to the development of a preliminary coding framework. Remaining transcripts were coded by either FS or LR and further analysis meetings were organised involving the research team (BY, LR, and FS) throughout the course of analysis to discuss convergences and divergences, identify quotes for report writing, and review data saturation.

In quantitative research, numbers contribute to the persuasive "power" of the findings, whereas, in qualitative research, the words of participants enable the reader to judge whether the research team's interpretations of the data are grounded in the experience of the participants [24]. The research team selected participant quotes for this report to illuminate and explicate the researchers' synopsis of the themes identified through systematic data analysis [25, 26]. A draft report of the analysis containing extensive data extracts was circulated to the wider study team. This enabled investigator triangulation helping to 'test' and refine the analysis. Participants were sent a summary of the study findings.

Results

Participants

All 26 eligible families identified by clinicians agreed to researcher contact. Of these, nine could not be contacted and two declined. Twenty-eight participants from 15 families completed or attempted an interview (58% response rate), comprising nine patients and 19 parents (Table 2). In one of the 28 interviews, we were unable to sufficiently engage the patient (C8) in discussing the concepts that we wished to explore. As no meaningful data were obtained this patient's interview was not transcribed or analysed, although his parents' interview was. Another patient's interview (C11) was unusually short (six minutes) as the family had limited time but her parent was interviewed and child and parent interviews were analysed. Excluding the outlier interview (C11), interviews lasted from 23 to 76 min (Median = 43 [IQR = 35–54] minutes).

Participants were interviewed in their homes ($n = 9$), in a private setting in the paediatric rheumatology clinic ($n = 4$), in a parent's workplace ($n = 1$) or by telephone ($n = 1$). Of the nine CYP, two were interviewed jointly with their parents, while seven were interviewed separately. Of 19 parents, 14 were interviewed separately while five were interviewed with their child present, including the two noted above, and three parents whose children were ≤ 7 years and ineligible for interview.

As Table 2 shows, CYP's ages ranged from 1 to 16 years, and most were female ($n = 9/16$, 56%). One family had two CYP with JIA. All but two families ($n = 13/15$) had experienced at least two treatments, and most CYP had established JIA with a recent disease flare ($n = 10/16$). IACI was the most common treatment experienced ($n = 14/16$). While the inclusion criteria stated that patients needed to have had corticosteroids within the past 12 months (see Table 1), all families reported that patients were treated within the past 6 months and almost a third ($n = 4/15$) were actively receiving at least one corticosteroid treatment at the time of interview. We obtained families' postcodes wherever possible and used the Indices of Multiple Deprivation (IMD), a measure of socio-economic status, to inform sampling and ensure representation from all socio-economic groups: 6/13 (46%) families lived in areas of high deprivation (IMD decile 1–3), 5/13 (38%) in areas of moderate deprivation (IMD decile 4–6), and 2/13 (15%) in the least deprived (IMD decile 7–10) areas of England [27].

Table 2 Characteristics of participants in the study

Family number	Parent interviewed	Child/young person's age	Child/young person's JIA status (reported by clinician)	Treatments experienced by the child/young person[b]			
				Tablets	IV	IM	IACI
1 [a]	Mo, Fa	11–13	Flare	✓	✓	✓	✓
2	Mo	5–7	Flare	✓			✓
3 [a]	Mo	14–16	Flare	✓	✓		✓
4[c]	Mo, Fa	1–4, 5–7	Diagnosis, Flare	✓			✓
5	Mo	1–4	Diagnosis				✓
6	Mo	5–7	Diagnosis	✓			✓
7	Mo, Fa	1–4	Diagnosis				✓
8 [a]	Mo, Fa	8–10	Flare	✓			✓
9 [a]	Mo	11–13	Diagnosis		✓		✓
10 [a]	Mo	14–16	Flare	✓	✓	✓	✓
11 [a]	Mo	8–10	Flare	✓			✓
12 [a]	Mo	11–13	Diagnosis	✓	✓		
13 [a]	Mo	14–16	Flare		✓		✓
14 [a]	Mo	14–16	Flare			✓	✓
15	Fa	14–16	Flare	✓	✓		

Mo = Mother, *Fa* = Father, Tablets = Oral prednisolone, *IV* = Intravenous methylprednisolone, *IM* = Intra-muscular injection, *IACI* = Intra-articular injection(s). JIA status as reported by clinician
[a]Families where the child/young person was also interviewed, [b]Reported by parents, [c]Family with two children with JIA

Willingness to participate: Protective parents and permissive children

Participant is indicated (Mo = mother, Fa = father, or C = child) with family number (see Table 2 for family number reference). Patients' age categories are provided (e.g. 14-16y). Ellipsis (...) indicate omitted text and square brackets indicate explanatory text.

Families recognised the need for JIA trials and some expressed enthusiasm for the proposed trial: *"I would [participate] 'cause I've always been up for like helping with research* (Mo2_5-7y)"; *"It is a very good topic to actually do a research on [...] it's one that's needed because there are many ways of [delivering] steroids"* (C3_14-16y). CYP often suggested that participation in the proposed trial could be of benefit to either themselves or others: *"I'd try it [the trial], yeah... It seems fine... If it's going to help, it's going to help"* (C14_14-16y).

How CYP and parents perceived randomisation influenced their views of the trial. For the most part, both parties appeared to grasp the rationale for randomisation as a means to avoid bias: *"I do think it will be best if it's chosen by a computer because some patients might be biased."* (C3_14-16y). However, at times some parents struggled to reconcile randomisation with a need to trust in clinicians' expertise: *"I'd go with just whatever's the best one and that's why, that's why I'm trusting [the doctors] to get her better... I wouldn't be comfortable with the computer randomly selecting what would be the best course of treatment for her."* (Fa15_14-16y).

Others struggled to reconcile randomisation with their need as parents to have confidence in the care being provided for their child: *"We were told the steroid injections would help her, so that sort of put confidence in us. But for someone to say we're not quite sure which one the best one is, so we're going to do it randomly, I think that would put a lot of sort of discomfort in us."* (Mo7_1-4y). In contrast, only one young person was opposed to participating in the proposed trial, rejecting randomisation in favour of a clinician-informed treatment: *"I would have said no because... the doctor needs to tell you what's best for you and not a computer because a computer doesn't know that."* (C12_11-13y).

The comments of other CYP indicated they were open to participating and some expressed a degree of nonchalance to their treatment being randomised as part of research participation: *"I'd be like 'It's been happening for this long, I don't care anymore, you can do whatever, do anything with my body, it's alright!'"* (C13_14-16y). In some of the joint interviews, CYP were more permissive about research than their parents and suggested that they would be more willing to participate in such a trial:

> C13: *[At diagnosis] I haven't experienced any of them [treatments] so far so it wouldn't hurt to try any of them...*

Mo13: *I think I might have been a little bit more concerned 'cause I think I would want, at the beginning when we didn't know a lot about it, I think I would have been thinking, oh no, I need to have the consultant say what's best for him.* (14-16y)

This permissive attitude among CYP may have been founded in part on feeling confident that clinicians would always prioritise their care over the trial: "*I'd probably take part in it just to like help the research and, 'cause I think if something didn't work on me I know that... they'd just put me on something else like in the end.*" (C9_11-13y).

Barriers and facilitators to participation

Our analysis identified several potential recruitment barriers and facilitators to the proposed trial, some of which were voiced by parents but not CYP and vice versa. For example, some parents questioned or remarked on the number of visits to clinic that the proposed trial would entail, noting that it was already challenging to attend clinic appointments due to work or school commitments. Parents thereby implied that their willingness to participate would hinge on the convenience or otherwise of the trial: "*Would that entail, mean more hospital visits though, to do this trial? 'Cause obviously with work we'd be struggling, it depends how often that would be.*" (Mo2_5-7y). Some CYP acknowledged these factors but did not suggest that this would be a barrier to participation: "*Mam doesn't really mind going to the hospital and that, because obviously she does it because it helps me.*" (C14_14-16y).

Past treatment experiences

Families spoke of their experience of different treatments over numerous disease flares since diagnosis. This experience heavily influenced their views on the proposed trial and their willingness to participate. Reflecting on a treatment that "*had worked*", one mother indicated that she would like her child to receive the same treatment if they experienced a future flare-up: "*When you're first diagnosed you will try any of the medication, but now we know what works for [my child] I would want to stick with that.*" (Mo14_14-16y). Conversely, on realising that joining the trial could mean her child receiving a treatment that had previously "*not worked*", another mother questioned the logic of offering the same treatment in the context of a trial: "*If it's not worked this time, what makes them think it's going to work the second time?*" (Mo6_5-7y). That is, parents struggled to see the logic behind randomising a child to a treatment that they had previously experienced as ineffective, and this was an important issue they would want clinicians to address should such a trial be offered to them.

Older children and their parents frequently differed in their treatment preferences, with both parties often noting drawbacks of treatments that the other had not identified:

C12: *I'd rather [have IV].*
Mo12: *You'd rather have [IV] than just have a needle in your bum? I think I'd rather have the needle in my bum than be sat here.*
C12: *Wouldn't [IM] hurt? That would hurt more surely?*
Mo12: *... well you've had to come here for three days [for IV].*
C12: *It doesn't bother me. It's like an hour on this and then it's done.* (11-13y)
Mo13: *... to me, [IM] would be a lot less painful going in your butt 'cause you've got that little meatiness, do you know, something to put it in.*
C13: *Any muscle anywhere else I probably would have been fine. Like you could just stick it in my thigh or something that's okay but I don't want to have to get the moon out for you.* (14-16y)

Some CYP were receiving corticosteroids at the time they were interviewed. Despite being unable to assess the effect of the current treatment in reducing symptoms at that point in time, one young person explained that he preferred his current treatment over other treatments, even ones he had not been prescribed: "*I'd say [I prefer] this one... because my experience right now... I feel quite, quite fine on this. Probably [would then have] tablets since I haven't experienced those [tablets]*" (C13_14-16y), implying that treatment side effects also weighed heavily in his treatment preferences.

CYP with multiple affected joints often received corticosteroids via several delivery routes, either simultaneously or consecutively, which made it difficult for them and their parents to differentiate the effect of an individual treatment: "*I don't know [which is best] because like I feel like the intravenous and the tablets go along with each other in a way because I'm on both at the minute.*" (C12_11-13y). Most families also had experience of non-corticosteroid treatments for JIA, such as other immunosuppressive medication, hydrotherapy, or physiotherapy, and some were concerned about the possibility that interactions between corticosteroid and non-corticosteroid treatments could jeopardise the validity of the proposed trial's findings if non-corticosteroid treatment effects were not controlled for: "*The challenge is that they don't have this treatment independently of other things, do they? It's always combined with something else or it has been in our experience. So, it'll be steroids plus something else.*" (Mo10 14-16y). Some parents also queried whether they could continue with existing treatments if their child was to participate in a trial of corticosteroids: *"I don't know, would they stop the methotrexate or would they just carry it on?"* (Mo4 1-4y, 5-7y). These illustrate further issues that clinicians would need to address when inviting families to take part in JIA trials.

Perceived treatment suitability

While families did not view any one of the four delivery routes as unsuitable overall to be evaluated in the proposed trial, they did perceive certain treatments as more or less acceptable for certain CYP. Families held these views even when they did not have direct experience of the treatment concerned. Parents believed that treatment suitability depended on a child's age. For example, a mother anticipated that her eight-year-old would not tolerate IV: *"He's not going to want to stand there for hours... I would imagine if he got lots and lots of flare-ups, and he is older and he understands it, I can see the logic behind that."* (Mo11 8-10y). While a child's age seemed important to parents in making decisions about treatments, and therefore in designing the trial, CYP did not comment on this.

Both parents and CYP believed that treatments varied in their suitability for different patient groups or JIA subtypes. For example, one child suggested that IV is more suitable when a child has more than one joint affected: *"If you have a flare and it doesn't just affect one joint, then [IV], it'd kind of help you more."* (C9_ 11-13y). Similarly, a mother of a child with localised JIA echoed the view that treatments varied in their suitability for different JIA subtypes and implied that IV could also be potentially harmful for her child due to its systemic nature: *"The intravenous one would affect the whole body, so I don't know whether that would be a good thing or not. I've never experienced that, we've only ever had the joint injections."* (Mo2 5-7y). Parents and some children therefore struggled to see the logic of a trial in which they might receive a treatment, that, based on their knowledge of JIA and how treatments worked, was ill suited to their subtype of JIA.

Being approached about research at diagnosis

Given the powerful influence of past treatment experiences on current treatment preferences, it was unsurprising that most participants were more comfortable with the idea of participating in the trial if invited at diagnosis when treatments would be new to families: *"[We would participate] at the beginning when he had it, probably it will be different but now, no way... we had such a big, big problems with his injection..."* (Mo8_ 8-10y). Nevertheless, there were some exceptions. Several parents recalled the emotional upheaval of learning that their child had a life changing condition and their strong desire for certainty at that time. One mother explained that if she was asked to enter her child into a trial in the aftermath of diagnosis: *"I'd probably say 'Not yet'"* (Mo9_ 11-13y).

CYP did not view trial recruitment at diagnosis to be problematic, again pointing to divergence in the views of the two parties. Overall, parents often described their children as resilient and CYP themselves rarely described the emotional upheaval of receiving a diagnosis but they did reflect on how the diagnosis had affected their parents:

> I: *What was it like being told about having arthritis?*
> C9: *I don't know, I think I took it a bit better than my mum, 'cause mums are mums, so they get a bit worried.* (11-13y)

Families' accounts of clinicians' treatment preferences

Both parents and CYP referred to the relationships they had with their clinician and how they trusted them to accurately inform them about treatments and provide them with optimal care: *"The doctors have been so good... I've got to trust what they are telling me and what they think is best"* (Fa15_ 14-16y).

> I: *Who do you think would be the best person to give you more information about the research study?*
> C1: *Probably doctors and that so you know it's true, in case like random people just say this works.* (11-13y)

Families spoke about treatment preferences that their clinician had voiced when making recommendations about treatment during routine consultations and that clinicians' preferences too depended on a child's age, medical history and JIA subtype: *"And age thing as well, and how long they've had [JIA]. Because [the doctor] tends to do it with their age doesn't she?"* (Mo1_ 11-13y). Participants indicated that clinician treatment preferences influenced their perception of treatment efficacy and suitability: *"Probably the joint injections [would be best] 'cause [the doctor] said they work better 'cause it's straight into the joint."* (C9_ 11-13y).

Discussion

This is the first, pre-trial qualitative feasibility study that has involved both parents and CYP with a long term condition. Although studies involving CYP are advocated in the literature [14, 15], we are aware of only one other early stage feasibility study that qualitatively investigated both parents' and CYP's input in trial design and conduct [14]. This explored families' views on the feasibility of a trial to determine optimum duration of intravenous antibiotic therapy for children with acute osteomyelitis or septic arthritis The current study recruited CYP with a long term condition, for whom trial participation can be especially challenging [15]. While much research has focused on deficits in patients' understanding of trials [4], we found that parents and CYP were able to engage with the logic of the proposed trial and identify potential flaws in its design, despite the scenario being hypothetical [28, 29]. This suggests that pre-trial, qualitative feasibility studies with families can inform and optimise trial design, thereby aiming to avoid common recruitment pitfalls [3, 4], by drawing on the in-depth knowledge and insight families acquire in coping with a long term condition.

Contrary to previous research [30], we found that parents and CYP frequently differed in their willingness to participate in the proposed trial and in their treatment preferences. While CYP were more permissive towards the trial than parents, they sometimes identified concerns that parents did not raise. This also echoes a previous pre-trial feasibility study which found that patients with acute osteomyelitis or septic arthritis often downplayed the impact of the illness or focused on different issues to their parents [14]. Previous research has found that parents often adopt an executive or managerial role in their child's treatment and care [31], working to identify, anticipate and meet their child's needs [32]. Based on this previous work and findings from the current study, we propose that CYP's permissiveness reflects their reliance upon their parents to protect them from harm and coordinate their care. CYP also trusted clinicians with their care and, unlike parents, they did not identify trial inconveniences (e.g. travel), which may have also contributed to their permissive orientation. Current guidance encourages recruiters to support families in sharing decisions regarding research [14]. Given that our study and others show that CYP can offer valuable input to trial design [14], the viewpoints of both parents and CYP are likely to be valuable in informing and improving future paediatric clinical trials and clinical practice. The findings have helped us in developing recommendations for a proposed corticosteroid induction regimen trial (Table 3). Several of these recommendations will be useful in developing future trials in JIA more broadly and in avoiding common recruitment pitfalls.

Table 3 Summary of the recommendations for the design of a future corticosteroid induction regimen trial in JIA

1. The views of parents and children and young people are important in informing trial design and conduct.
2. Although families may not deem one treatment as unsuitable overall, trialists need to establish whether *all* treatments are suitable for *all* patients with JIA. If this is not possible, amendments to the eligibility criteria or fewer treatments will be needed.
3. Further qualitative work should explore clinicians' views on a future corticosteroid induction regimen trial in JIA, to establish clinical equipoise and support for the trial.
4. Trialists should consider methods of making a future trial more accessible to parents and children and young people, such as combining trial follow-up assessments with clinic appointments.

While families did not deem any single treatment as unsuitable to evaluate in the proposed trial, they believed that treatments needed to be tailored to CYP depending on factors such as age and JIA subtype. Previous experience of treatments also influenced such beliefs. Our findings indicate that where families have treatment preferences that are experience-based (e.g. trials evaluating established treatments), rather than anticipated (e.g. trials of treatments that are new to families), recruitment and randomisation is likely to be especially challenging [33–36]. This is pertinent as CYP with JIA receive treatments on repeated occasions [21]. Clinicians recruiting to such trials will need to be prepared to respond to questions from families who have previously experienced a particular treatment to be ineffective. Trialists should consider which treatment options can be evaluated in a trial and will be tolerated by CYP with JIA. Some trials may need to adapt the eligibility criteria or the treatments included to make the trial more acceptable to families. It is also currently unclear how decision-making about trial participation is managed within families when treatment preferences conflict; further research would be beneficial.

Families described how clinicians had shaped their treatment preferences via previous discussions about the suitability of different treatments, based on factors, such as a child's age and the number of joints affected. Such discussions are part of good care in routine clinical practice, but equally, when invited to consider participation in a trial, families cannot be expected to put aside knowledge they have previously gleaned from clinicians. While clinician and patient treatment preferences are often regarded as separate entities, our findings indicate that the two can be intertwined and that the influence of previous clinician-family discussions about treatments needs to be considered when communicating with families about trials. For example, clinicians will need to respond to families' concerns about using a treatment that clinicians may have previously told them was unsuitable. Indeed, clinicians and their treatment preferences can often be a considerable barrier to patient participation in paediatric trials [37, 38]. Further qualitative work exploring clinicians' views of future JIA trials would help to address such potential difficulties.

Similar to previous research [39], we found that trial inconvenience, such as additional appointments, will also likely be a recruitment barrier for parents. Trialists will need to explore options to reduce burden, such as completing follow-up appointments by telephone or Skype, and arranging appointments at participants' convenience (e.g. out of school hours).

We interviewed socio-economically diverse families from across England with children of different ages and varied treatment experiences. While we had interview data from only one patient aged under 10 years, our sample did include parents of children aged 1–16 years. Additionally, we interviewed families of patients who had different sub-types of JIA and numbers of affected joints, although we did not actively sample for these clinical characteristics. In accessing the perspectives of CYP our approach is consistent with current guidance on including the voices of children in research [14]. Furthermore, the competence of chronically ill children in communicating about health related matters can often exceed their chronological age [40]. We did not interview families with a JIA diagnosis who had not yet been treated with corticosteroids, and we acknowledge that the views of such families may differ markedly from our findings. However, interviewing families at diagnosis, but before corticosteroid treatment, would likely have been challenging, particularly given the difficulties families experience at this time [41], which we also reported here. This study's sample size is typical and appropriate for a qualitative study given that the inferences drawn are not about prevalence or statistical distribution [16]. Rather, our inferences concern the nature of families' perspectives and the value of these in informing the design of JIA trials. Similar to deliberative engagement methods [42], we used stimulus materials (see Additional file 2: Appendix B) and discursive interviews to enable families to raise matters of importance to them, and for us to inform families about trials and clarify any key misunderstandings.

Conclusion

This pre-trial qualitative feasibility study demonstrated that families could engage in the logic of a proposed trial in JIA and provide valuable input into trial design before further investment of resources. We identified potential barriers to recruitment for a corticosteroid induction regimen trial in JIA, divergent views between parents and CYP and areas for further exploration, including clinician treatment preferences. This study highlights the importance of including families in pre-trial feasibility work to illuminate barriers to recruitment and to inform strategies to improve informed consent and recruitment.

Abbreviations

C: Child; CYP: Children and young people; Fa: Father; HTA: Health Technology Assessment; IACI: Intra-articular injection(s); IM: Intra-muscular injection; IMD: Indices of Multiple Deprivation; IV: Intravenous methylprednisolone; JIA: Juvenile Idiopathic Arthritis; Mo: Mother; NIHR: National Institute for Health Research; SIRJIA: Steroid Induction Regimen for Juvenile Idiopathic Arthritis

Acknowledgements

We would like to thank children and parents who took part in an interview and health professionals who helped to identify eligible families for the study. We would like to thank Katie Littler for her drawings and helping to design the interview stimulus materials, Alexandra Fewtrell for her input in designing the summary of results leaflet for families, and Gloria Nkoma and Ashley Jones for their input into the study set-up and progress.

Funding

This study is part of the Steroid Induction Regimen for Juvenile Idiopathic Arthritis (SIRJIA) project and is funded by the National Institute for Health Research (NIHR) Health Technology Assessment (HTA) Programme (Ref: 14/167/01).

Authors' contributions

EB and BY conceived the idea for the study and all authors contributed to the design of the study. FM, HF, and AR identified eligible potential participants for the study. FS and LR conducted the interviews. FS, LR and BY analysed the data. All authors contributed to the drafting of the paper, approved the final version, and agreed to be accountable for all aspects of the work.

Consent for publication

Informed consent was obtained for all participants. As part of this, participants were informed that their data would be used in a study report but that it would not be identifiable to others.

Competing interests

The authors declare that they have no competing interest.

Author details

[1]Department of Psychological Sciences, University of Liverpool, Whelan Building, Brownlow Hill, Liverpool L69 3GB, UK. [2]School of Healthcare, University of Leeds, Leeds, UK. [3]Great North Children's Hospital, Newcastle upon Tyne, UK. [4]Institute Cellular Medicine, Newcastle University, Newcastle upon Tyne, UK. [5]Clinical Research Division, Alder Hey Children's NHS Foundation Trust, Liverpool, UK. [6]Department of Paediatric Rheumatology, Alder Hey Children's NHS Foundation Trust, Liverpool, UK. [7]Department of Women's and Children's Health, Institute of Translational Medicine, University of Liverpool, Liverpool, UK. [8]University Hospitals Bristol NHS Foundation Trust & Bristol Medical School, University of Bristol, Bristol, UK. [9]School of Medicine, Dentistry and Biomedical Sciences, Queens University of Belfast, Belfast, UK.

References

1. Petty RE, Southwood TR, Manners P, Baum J, Glass DN, Goldenberg J, et al. International league of associations for rheumatology classification of juvenile idiopathic arthritis: second revision, Edmonton, 2001. J Rheumatol. 2004;31(2):390–2.
2. Ruperto N, Giannini EH, Pistorio A, Brunner HI, Martini A, Lovell DJ. Is it time to move to active comparator trials in juvenile idiopathic arthritis?: a review of current study designs. Arthritis & Rheumatism. 2010;62(11):3131–9.
3. Salman RA-S, Beller E, Kagan J, Hemminki E, Phillips RS, Savulescu J, et al. Increasing value and reducing waste in biomedical research regulation and management. Lancet. 2014;383(9912):176–85.
4. Fletcher B, Gheorghe A, Moore D, Wilson S, Damery S. Improving the recruitment activity of clinicians in randomised controlled trials: a systematic review. BMJ Open. 2012;2(e000496):1–14.

5. Sully BGO, Julious SA, Nicholl J. A reinvestigation of recruitment to randomised, controlled, multicenter trials: a review of trials funded by two UK funding agencies. Trials. 2013;14(1):166.
6. Tishler CL, Reiss NS. Pediatric drug-trial recruitment: enticement without coercion. Pediatrics. 2011;127(5):949–54.
7. Berard RA, Laxer RM. Learning the hard way: clinical trials in juvenile idiopathic arthritis. Ann Rheum Dis. 2017;77:1–2.
8. Caldwell PHY, Murphy SB, Butow PN, Craig JC. Clinical trials in children. Lancet. 2004;364(9436):803–11.
9. Smyth RL, Weindling AM. Research in children: ethical and scientific aspects. Lancet 1999;354 Suppl 2:Sii21–Sii24.
10. Balevic SJ, Becker ML, Cohen-Wolkowiez M, Schanberg LE. Clinical trial Design in Juvenile Idiopathic Arthritis. Paediatric drugs. 2017;19(5):379–89.
11. Douglas SLA. Consumer perspective on embedding research in paediatric rheumatology. Rheumatology (Oxford). 2014;53(11):1915–6.
12. O'Cathain A, Hoddinott P, Lewin S, Thomas KJ, Young B, Adamson J, et al. Maximising the impact of qualitative research in feasibility studies for randomised controlled trials: guidance for researchers. Pilot and feasibility studies. 2015;1:32.
13. O'Cathain A, Thomas KJ, Drabble SJ, Rudolph A, Goode J, Hewison J. Maximising the value of combining qualitative research and randomised controlled trials in health research: the QUAlitative research in trials (QUART) study--a mixed methods study. Health Technol Assess. 2014;18(38):1–197 v-vi.
14. Nuffield Council on Bioethics. Children and clinical research: ethical issues 2015 23rd February 2018. Available from: http://nuffieldbioethics.org/wp-content/uploads/Children-and-clinical-research-full-report.pdf.
15. Shaw C, Brady, L-M., Davey, C. Guidelines for Research with Children and Young People 2011 23rd February 2018. Available from: https://www.ncb.org.uk/sites/default/files/field/attachment/NCB%20guidelines%20CYP.pdf.
16. Ritchie J, Lewis J. Qualitative research practice: a guide for social science students and researchers. London: Sage; 2003.
17. Barriball KL, While A. Collecting data using a semi-structured interview: a discussion paper. J Adv Nurs. 1994;19(2):328–35.
18. Petty RE, Southwood TR, Baum J, Bhettay E, Glass DN, Manners P, et al. Revision of the proposed classification criteria for juvenile idiopathic arthritis: Durban, 1997. J Rheumatol. 1998;25(10):1991–4.
19. Fusch PI, Ness LR. Are we there yet? Data saturation in qualitative research. Qual Rep. 2015;20(9):1408–16.
20. Cleary AG, Murphy HD, Davidson JE. Intra-articular corticosteroid injections in juvenile idiopathic arthritis. Arch Dis Child. 2003;88(3):192.
21. Marti P, Molinari L, Bolt IB, Seger R, Saurenmann RK. Factors influencing the efficacy of intra-articular steroid injections in patients with juvenile idiopathic arthritis. Eur J Pediatr. 2008;167(4):425–30.
22. Gale NK, Heath G, Cameron E, Rashid S, Redwood S. Using the framework method for the analysis of qualitative data in multi-disciplinary health research. BMC Med Res Methodol. 2013;13(1):117.
23. QSR International Pty Ltd. NVivo qualitative data analysis software. 10th ed; 2012.
24. Morrow SL. Quality and trustworthiness in qualitative research in counseling psychology. J Couns Psychol. 2005;52(2):250–60.
25. O'Brien BC, Harris IB, Beckman TJ, Reed DA, Cook DA. Standards for reporting qualitative research: a synthesis of recommendations. Acad Med. 2014;89(9):1245–51.
26. Tong A, Sainsbury P, Craig J. Consolidated criteria for reporting qualitative research (COREQ): a 32-item checklist for interviews and focus groups. Int J Qual Health Care. 2007;19(6):349–57.
27. Department for Communities and Local Government. English indices of deprivation 2015 2015 [Available from: http://imd-by-postcode.opendatacommunities.org/.
28. Boland L, McIsaac DI, Lawson ML. Barriers to and facilitators of implementing shared decision making and decision support in a paediatric hospital: a descriptive study. Paediatr Child Health. 2016;21(3):e17–21.
29. Zwaanswijk M, Tates K, van Dulmen S, Hoogerbrugge PM, Kamps WA, Beishuizen A, et al. Communicating with child patients in pediatric oncology consultations: a vignette study on child patients', parents', and survivors' communication preferences. Psycho-Oncol. 2011;20(3):269–77.
30. Madden L, Shilling V, Woolfall K, Sowden E, Smyth RL, Williamson PR, et al. Questioning assent: how are children's views included as families make decisions about clinical trials? Child Care Health Dev. 2016;42(6):900–8.
31. Young B, Dixon-Woods M, Windridge KC, Heney D. Managing communication with young people who have a potentially life threatening chronic illness: qualitative study of patients and parents. BMJ. 2003;326(7384):305.
32. Williams C. Alert assistants in managing chronic illness: the case of mothers and teenage sons. Sociology of Health & Illness. 2000;22(2):254–72.
33. Ross S, Grant A, Counsell C, Gillespie W, Russell I, Prescott R. Barriers to participation in randomised controlled trials: a systematic review. J Clin Epidemiol. 1999;52(12):1143–56.
34. Mills EJ, Seely D, Rachlis B, Griffith L, Wu P, Wilson K, et al. Barriers to participation in clinical trials of cancer: a meta-analysis and systematic review of patient-reported factors. Lancet Oncol. 2006;7(2):141–8.
35. King M, Nazareth I, Lampe F, Bower P, Chandler M, Morou M, et al. Impact of participant and physician intervention preferences on randomized trials: a systematic review. JAMA. 2005;293(9):1089–99.
36. Elliott D, Husbands S, Hamdy FC, Holmberg L, Donovan JL. Understanding and improving recruitment to randomised controlled trials: qualitative research approaches. Eur Urol. 2017;72(5):789–98.
37. Shilling V, Williamson PR, Hickey H, Sowden E, Beresford MW, Smyth RL, et al. Communication about children's clinical trials as observed and experienced: qualitative study of parents and practitioners. PLoS One. 2011;6(7):e21604.
38. Caldwell PHY, Butow PN, Craig JC. Pediatricians' attitudes toward randomized controlled trials involving children. J Pediatr. 2002;141(6):798–803.
39. Prescott RJ, Counsell CE, Gillespie WJ, Grant AM, Russell IT, Kiauka S, et al. Factors that limit the quality, number and progress of randomised controlled trials. Health Technol Assess. 1999:3.
40. Alderson P. Competent children? Minors' consent to health care treatment and research. Soc Sci Med. 2007;65(11):2272–83.
41. Gómez-Ramírez O, Gibbon M, Berard R, Jurencak R, Green J, Tucker L, et al. A recurring rollercoaster ride: a qualitative study of the emotional experiences of parents of children with juvenile idiopathic arthritis. Pediatr Rheumatol Online J. 2016;14:13.
42. Morain SR, Whicher DM, Kass NE, Faden RR. Deliberative engagement methods for patient-centered outcomes research. The patient. 2017;10(5):545–52.

Body composition and phase angle as an indicator of nutritional status in children with juvenile idiopathic arthritis

Paweł Więch[1*], Izabela Sałacińska[1], Dariusz Bazaliński[1] and Mariusz Dąbrowski[1,2]

Abstract

Background: Juvenile idiopathic arthritis (JIA) is the most common chronic, systemic autoimmune connective tissue disease diagnosed in children and adolescents. An important aspect of monitoring of children with JIA is a precise assessment of the nutritional status to identify children and adolescents at risk of malnutrition. The aim of the study was to assess the body composition and phase angle in children diagnosed with JIA in comparison to age and sex matched healthy children since there are scarce reports in paediatric patients.

Methods: A total of 46 children and adolescents aged 4–18 years, with JIA were included in the cross-sectional study. Controls were selected from the group of healthy children and adolescents. Children with diagnosed JIA and healthy children were strictly matched for age and gender. In both groups BIA with phase angle calculation was performed.

Results: Phase angle score was significantly lower in the study group compared to control group (5.45 ± 0.64 vs. 5.85 ± 0.80, $p = 0.010$). Also lower percentage of body cell mass (50.63 ± 3.46 vs. 52.70 ± 4.06, p = 0.010) and muscle mass (46.02 ± 6.32 vs. 49.53 ± 6.67, $p = 0.005$) were revealed. In the analysis of subtypes of JIA we found significant differences between children and adolescents with polyarthritis compared to control group, while no significant differences were found between patients with oligoarthritis and control group.

Conclusions: The obtained results indicate a higher risk of malnutrition in children and adolescents with JIA compared to healthy peers, predominantly in patients with polyarthritis.

Keywords: Bioelectrical impedance, Juvenile idiopathic arthritis, Phase angle, Children, Malnutrition

Background

Juvenile idiopathic arthritis (JIA) is the most common chronic, systemic autoimmune connective tissue disease diagnosed in children and adolescents [1]. An important aspect of monitoring of children with JIA is a precise assessment of the nutritional status to identify children and adolescents at risk of undernourishment. However, the available data in medical databases also indicate the risk of development of overweight and obesity in this group of children. Discrepancy in research in this area probably depends on the subtype of the disease and the pharmacological treatment used [2, 3]. Bioelectrical impedance analysis (BIA) is currently frequently used as a method of body composition assessment, due to ease of use, safety and low cost of this procedure [4, 5]. BIA is the measure of resistance and reactance of the body. The body is made up of both conductive and non-conductive tissues. The conducting tissues are lean tissues with large amount of water and conducting electrolytes. In nonconductive tissues like bone and fat, the fluid content and conducting electrolytes are low. BIA is used indirectly to measure the body fat composition. The total impedance is the total sum of impedance of different tissues. Body fat, total body water and extra cellular water offer electric resistance to electrical current. Cell membranes and tissues interfaces offer capacitive reactance. [6].

To assess the nutritional status of children, regardless of their clinical condition, both fat mass (FM) and fat

* Correspondence: p.k.wiech@gmail.com
[1]Institute of Nursing and Health Sciences, Faculty of Medicine, University of Rzeszów, Al. mjr. W. Kopisto 2 a, 35-310 Rzeszów, Poland

free mass (FFM) should be measured. The phase angle (PhA) reflects nutritional and functional status of the studied subject and is calculated from the equation:

$$\mathrm{PhA} = \left(\frac{Xc}{R}\right) x \left(\frac{180^{\circ}}{\Pi}\right)$$

where Xc is reactance and R is resistance obtained in BIA [4]. PhAis a linear method of measuring the relationship between electric resistance (R) and reactance (Rc) in series or parallel circuits [6]. Low phase angle score is considered as an indicator of impaired cellular membrane integrity and also indicates the shift of body water from intracellular to extracellular compartments [7]. PhA is an important prognostic factor in numerous disease entities [8, 9]. The European Society for Clinical Nutrition and Metabolism (ESPEN) recommends the assessment of PhA as a prognostic measure of nutrition and a reliable prognostic marker. PhA can be treated as a screening tool to identify patients at risk of deterioration of nutritional status and functionality [10, 11].

The primary aim of the study was to assess the body composition and phase angle in children diagnosed with JIA in comparison to age and sex matched healthy children since there are scarce reports in paediatric patients. We did not find any study assessing both body composition and phase angle in pediatric patients with diagnosed JIA with analysis of subtypes of JIA according to ILAR criteria.

Methods

Ethics

The study was approved by the institutional Bioethics Committee at the University of Rzeszów (Resolution No. 5/02/2012) and by all appropriate administrative bodies. The study was conducted in accordance with ethical standards laid down in an appropriate version of the Declaration of Helsinki (as revised in Brazil in 2013) and in Polish national regulations. The study was conducted according to the STROBE criteria.

Subject

The study group consisted of 46 children diagnosed with JIA, in the Provincial Clinical Hospital No. 2 in Rzeszów at the Pediatric and the Pediatric Neurology Departments. For the purpose of the study, newly diagnosed children and children at various stages of treatment were included. According to the criteria by Ringold and Wallace, an inactive disease phase was indicated in 38 children [12]. Children took only medicines associated with JIA in monotherapy or combination treatment: azathioprine, methotrexate, sulfasalazine, TNF inhibitors, glucocorticosteroids. Due to the combination of more than one drug in many children and hence the inability to allocate to a specific group of drugs, these parameters were not analyzed quantitatively and qualitatively.

Inclusion criteria for the study group were: diagnosed JIA, age of the examined children from 4 to 18 years, lack of other autoimmune or chronic disease that may affect the growth, weight or nutritional status. In addition, legal guardians had to express written consent for children to participate in the study, and adolescents aged 16 and over also had to give their own written consent to participate in the study.

Controls were selected from the group of healthy children and adolescents from primary, middle and high schools from the neighboring urban and rural areas. Children with diagnosed JIA and healthy children were strictly matched for age and gender i.e. every participant with JIA had his/her comparator with the same gender and possibly the nearest date of birth. Detailed characteristics of both groups are presented in the Table 1.

Table 1 Demographic and anthropometric parameters of the study participants

Parameter	Juvenile Idiopathic Arthritis (JIA) ($n = 46$) (mean ± SD)	Control for JIA ($n = 46$) (mean ± SD)	*P value*
Age (years)	12.74 ± 3.85	12.70 ± 3.80	0.956
Girls	12.85 ± 3.96	12.79 ± 3.90	0.951
Boys	12.42 ± 3.66	12.42 ± 3.66	1.000
Body weight (kg)	45.39 ± 18.12	46.90 ± 15.26	0.665
Girls	44.84 ± 18.58	45.12 ± 13.08	0.811
Boys	46.93 ± 17.45	51.97 ± 20.05	0.519
Height (cm)	149.33 ± 21.61	153.82 ± 19.07	0.341
Girls	148.03 ± 21.80	153.06 ± 19.02	0.425
Boys	153.00 ± 21.54	155.96 ± 19.91	0.931
BMI (kg/m^2)	19.42 ± 4.06	19.24 ± 3.06	0.827
Girls	19.40 ± 4.23	18.77 ± 2.65	0.463
Boys	19.47 ± 3.69	20.60 ± 3.80	0.466
Classification systems (ILAR JIA):			
Systemic arthritis	1	n/a	n/a
Oligoarthritis	18	n/a	n/a
Polyarthritis	22	n/a	n/a
Psoriatic arthritis	2	n/a	n/a
Enthesitis-related arthritis	3	n/a	n/a
Undifferentiated arthritis	0	n/a	n/a
Duration of the disease:			
New diagnosis	6	n/a	n/a
More than 6 months	40	n/a	n/a

SD Standard deviation, *BMI* Body mass index, *z-score* Standard score, *ILAR JIA* The International League of Associations for Rheumatology classification of juvenile idiopathic arthritis [1]; *n/a* Not applicable

Assessments

In every study participant, body weight, height were measured and BMI (Body Mass Index) was calculated. Subsequently, bioelectrical impedance analysis with phase angle calculation was performed using the AKERN BIA - 101 analyzer (Akern SRL, Pontassieve, Florence, Italy) to assess nutritional status and body composition. The results were analyzed using dedicated software (Bodygram1_31 from AKERN, Pontassieve, Florence, Italy). Detailed description of methodology was described elsewhere [13].

The parameters of body composition analyzed in BIA included: fat mass (FM), fat free mass (FFM), muscle mass (MM) (kg and %), total body water (TBW), intra- and extra-cellular water (ICW and ECW) (liters and %), body cell mass (BCM) (kg and %) and body cell mass index (BCMI). Upon resistance and reactance results, the phase angle score was calculated. In addition, we also calculated two other indices: fat mass index (FMI) and fat free mass index (FFMI).

Statistical analysis

Statistical analysis of the data was performed using SigmaPlot for Windows, version 12.5 (Systat Software Inc., San Jose, CA, USA). We performed comparative analysis between two groups as a whole, separate analysis according to gender. Since the most numerous subtypes of JIA were poly- and oligoarthritis, we performed additional comparative analysis between children with these subtypes of JIA and their comparators. The continuous data are presented as mean and SD (standard deviation). Differences between two groups were analyzed using an unpaired two-tailed Student's t-test after checking normality of distribution by Shapiro-Wilk test and after performing constant variance test. In case of normality and/or constant variance test failure, the Mann-Whitney rank sum test was performed. A *P* value of < 0.05 was considered statistically significant.

Results

No significant differences in demographic and anthropometric parameters between study and control groups were found (Table 1).

The value of the phase angle in the children with JIA was significantly lower than in the control group of healthy children ($p = 0.010$). The individual parameters of the body composition did not differ statistically between the study group and the control group. Among the children with JIA muscle mass and body cell mass were significantly different in comparison to children from the control group (BCM: $p = 0.005$; MM: p = 0.010) (Table 2).

In the analysis according to gender, the phase angle, muscle mass and body cell mass were significantly lower in the girls with JIA compared to control group. In boys, although the differences in these parameters were similar, statistical significance was not reached (Table 3).

An important finding was observation that in the analysis with regards to the most two prevalent JIA subtypes, significant differences between case and control groups were found only for polyarthritis (lower MM, BCM, BCMI an phase angle) and not oligoarthritis. Despite significantly older age of children with polyarthritis, they had significantly lower percentage of muscle mass compared to children with oligoarthritis ($p = 0.027$). No other significant differences between these groups (also with regards to weight and height) were revealed. We also found a trend towards lower percentage of body cell mass (BCM%), higher FMI and lower PA in children with polyarthritis, compared to group with oligoarthritis, but the level of statistical significance was not attained (Table 4).

Table 2 Bioelectrical Impedance Analysis results in study participants

Parameter	Juvenile Idiopathic Arthritis (JIA) (*n* = 46) (mean ± SD)	Control (*n* = 46) (mean ± SD)	*P value*
FM (kg)	12.38 ± 6.96	11.08 ± 4.64	0.617
FM (%)	26.62 ± 8.46	23.89 ± 7.58	0.107
FMI	5.34 ± 2.56	4.66 ± 1.89	0.339
FFM (kg)	33.01 ± 13.24	35.82 ± 12.67	0.300
FFM (%)	73.38 ± 8.46	76.11 ± 7.58	0.107
FFMI	14.04 ± 2.48	14.56 ± 2.38	0.310
MM (kg)	20.89 ± 8.96	23.64 ± 9.56	0.175
MM (%)	**46.02 ± 6.32**	**49.53 ± 6.67**	**0.005**
TBW (liters)	25.12 ± 9.34	27.10 ± 9.08	0.304
TBW (%)	56.55 ± 7.80	58.00 ± 6.07	0.322
ECW (liters)	11.22 ± 4.48	12.01 ± 3.97	0.295
ECW (%)	44.60 ± 4.21	44.49 ± 2.77	0.585
ICW (liters)	13.89 ± 5.40	15.09 ± 5.25	0.271
ICW (%)	55.40 ± 4.21	55.52 ± 2.77	0.585
BCM (kg)	16.90 ± 7.30	19.21 ± 7.91	0.166
BCM (%)	**50.63 ± 3.46**	**52.70 ± 4.06**	**0.010**
BCMI	7.16 ± 1.53	7.76 ± 1.78	0.098
R – resistance (Ohm)	699.57 ± 117.99	656.15 ± 94.83	0.055
X – reactance (Ohm)	66.30 ± 12.19	66.28 ± 7.49	0.784
PhA	**5.45 ± 0.64**	**5.85 ± 0.80**	**0.010**

SD Standard deviation, *FM* Fat mass, *FMI* Fat mass index, *FFM* Fat free mass, *FFMI* Fat free mass index, *MM* Muscle mass, *TBW* Total body water, *ECW* Extracellular water, *ICW* Intracellular water, *BCM* Body cell mass, *BCMI* Body cell mass index, *PhA* Phase angle. Bold characters indicate significant values ($p<0.05$)

Discussion

JIA is the most common systemic disease of autoimmune connective tissue in children and adolescents.

Table 3 BIA results in JIA participants according to gender

Parameter	Girls		*P value*	Boys		*P value*
	Juvenile Idiopathic Arthritis (JIA), n = 34	Control, *n* = 34		Juvenile Idiopathic Arthritis (JIA), n = 12	Control, *n* = 12	
	Mean ± SD	Mean ± SD		Mean ± SD	Mean ± SD	
FM (kg)	12.81 ± 7.27	11.05 ± 4.16	0.512	11.16 ± 6.12	11.16 ± 6.02	1.000
FM (%)	27.12 ± 6.89	24.34 ± 6.30	0.109	25.20 ± 12.13	22.64 ± 10.67	0.589
FMI	5.45 ± 2.41	4.64 ± 1.60	0.329	5.01 ± 3.04	4.71 ± 2.65	0.840
FFM (kg)	32.03 ± 12.13	34.07 ± 10.06	0.394	35.78 ± 16.25	40.81 ± 17.79	0.386
FFM (%)	72.88 ± 6.89	75.67 ± 6.30	0.109	74.81 ± 12.14	77.36 ± 10.67	0.590
FFMI	13.91 ± 2.30	14.11 ± 1.81	0.702	14.40 ± 3.02	15.84 ± 3.30	0.278
MM (kg)	20.00 ± 8.10	22.05 ± 7.15	0.209	23.43 ± 11.06	28.13 ± 13.81	0.436
MM (%)	**44.99 ± 4.39**	**48.54 ± 5.04**	**0.003**	48.95 ± 9.65	52.33 ± 9.70	0.402
TBW (liters)	24.13 ± 8.25	25.68 ± 7.01	0.387	27.91 ± 11.88	31.14 ± 12.87	0.583
TBW (%)	55.73 ± 7.21	57.48 ± 5.32	0.258	58.88 ± 9.22	59.47 ± 7.92	0.868
ECW (liters)	10.82 ± 3.87	11.44 ± 3.20	0.462	12.38 ± 5.94	13.62 ± 5.48	0.453
ECW (%)	44.91 ± 3.97	44.66 ± 2.68	0.762	43.74 ± 4.91	44.00 ± 3.09	0.507
ICW (liters)	13.14 ± 4.68	14.23 ± 3.93	0.270	16.03 ± 6.84	17.53 ± 7.59	0.616
ICW (%)	55.09 ± 3.97	55.34 ± 2.68	0.762	56.26 ± 4.91	56.00 ± 3.09	0.507
BCM (kg)	16.17 ± 6.62	17.89 ± 5.88	0.191	18.98 ± 8.95	22.96 ± 11.46	0.354
BCM (%)	**49.87 ± 3.03**	**51.97 ± 3.79**	**0.014**	52.80 ± 3.79	54.77 ± 4.23	0.243
BCMI	6.99 ± 1.42	7.39 ± 1.32	0.235	7.64 ± 1.76	8.81 ± 2.45	0.194
Resistance (ohm)	714.27 ± 104.30	679.82 ± 74.54	0.122	657.92 ± 147.48	589.08 ± 116.11	0.217
Reactance (ohm)	65.85 ± 9.25	67.35 ± 7.71	0.470	67.58 ± 18.67	63.25 ± 6.12	0.840
PhA	**5.30 ± 0.53**	**5.70 ± 0.73**	**0.011**	5.87 ± 0.78	6.27 ± 0.88	0.249

SD Standard deviation, *FM* Fat mass, *FMI* Fat mass index, *FFM* Fat free mass, *FFMI* Fat free mass index, *MM* Muscle mass, *TBW* Total body water, *ECW* Extracellular water, *ICW* Intracellular water, *BCM* Body cell mass, *BCMI* Body cell mass index, *PhA* Phase angle. Bold characters indicate significant values ($p < 0.05$)

Not only joints are affected by the disease but is also characterized by non-articular changes and systemic complications [14, 15].

We did not find significant difference in BMI between study and control groups. Some authors found that patients with JIA have worse nutritional status and lower BMI values compared to healthy children. They explained it as a result of the disease itself and factors such as the inflammatory process, medications and their effects, limited physical activity or increased energy expenditure [14, 16, 17]. Inversely, some other studies indicate higher prevalence of overweight and obesity in affected children [18–20]. Studies in the US demonstrated presence of obesity in 18% of patients with JIA [19]. In Germany as many as 15% of children with JIA were overweight and 7% were obese [20]. Differences between our research and those cited above most often result from the difference in the average age of the examined children or the different activity of the disease.

Analysis of the results with respect to gender showed that the phase angle, muscle mass and body cell mass were significantly lower in girls with JIA. In the group of boys, the size of differences in these parameters was similar, but the statistical significance was not achieved, probably due to the small number of affected boys. Our results confirm the facts, that men have higher phase angles than women due to the higher amount of body muscle mass. Moreover, phase angle increases with increasing BMI due to the increased number of muscle and fat cells. PhA decreases with increasing age, due to a reduction in reactance which parallels the loss of muscle mass and an increase in resistance due to the declining proportion of body water at the expense of increasing fat mass in higher age [4].

Also our patients differences in nutritional status were associated with the JIA subtype, specifically polyarthritis. We found significantly lower percentage of muscle mass in children with polyarthritis compared to patients with oligoarthritis. Furthermore a trend towards lower body cell mass (BCM%), higher FMI and lower PhA in these children was observed. It is in line with other observations. Guzman et al. observed an increase in body mass in various subtypes of JIA in the studied group of children in addition to systemic arthritis [3]. Also Lofthouse et al. in their research pointed out that 18.1% of children with JIA had body mass below the third percentile and

Table 4 BIA results in JIA participants according to predominant classification systems

Parameter	Oligoarthritis, *n* = 18		Control		*P value*	Polyarthritis, *n* = 22		Control, n = 22		*P value*	*P value poly vs. oligo*
	Mean	SD	Mean	SD		Mean	SD	Mean	SD		
Age	10.89	4.50	10.89	4.50	1.000	14.00	3.02	13.91	2.93	0.925	**0.037**
Gender (girls/boys)	13/5		13/5		N/A	18/4		18/4		N/A	0.705
BMI	17.86	3.68	19.08	4.15	0.357	19.68	3.59	19.27	2.29	0.655	0.123
FM (kg)	9.57	6.06	10.48	5.78	0.580	13.03	6.96	11.48	3.35	0.673	0.105
FM (%)	24.32	8.65	24.69	8.85	0.950	27.08	7.94	23.46	5.63	0.089	0.299
FMI	4.43	2.23	4.86	2.48	0.537	5.47	2.29	4.53	1.22	0.149	0.077
FFM (kg)	30.31	16.49	31.65	16.03	0.681	33.35	10.29	38.13	8.87	0.113	0.328
FFM (%)	75.69	8.65	75.31	8.85	0.950	72.92	7.94	76.54	5.63	0.089	0.298
FFMI	13.38	2.80	14.21	2.96	0.367	14.18	2.09	14.72	1.91	0.371	0.312
MM (kg)	19.67	11.32	20.86	12.22	0.692	**20.69**	**7.09**	**25.17**	**6.51**	**0.035**	0.730
MM (%)	48.42	6.98	48.25	6.82	0.943	**44.78**	**5.47**	**50.32**	**5.48**	**0.002**	**0.027**
TBW (liters)	23.00	11.99	24.32	11.52	0.728	25.39	6.70	28.46	6.29	0.110	0.308
TBW (%)	58.12	8.23	58.49	7.27	0.887	56.37	7.59	57.37	4.46	0.445	0.491
ECW (liters)	10.48	5.74	10.48	4.61	0.704	11.28	3.33	12.80	2.88	0.113	0.328
ECW (%)	45.23	3.48	43.84	3.43	0.164	44.45	4.91	44.96	1.98	0.869	0.572
ICW (liters)	12.85	6.93	13.84	7.02	0.635	13.84	3.98	15.66	3.52	0.098	0.399
ICW (%)	54.77	3.48	56.16	3.43	0.164	55.55	4.91	55.04	1.98	0.869	0.572
BCM (kg)	15.91	9.20	16.97	10.16	0.716	**16.73**	**5.80**	**20.46**	**5.38**	**0.032**	0.734
BCM (%)	51.61	3.64	51.88	4.42	0.841	**49.58**	**3.38**	**53.31**	**3.72**	**0.001**	0.077
BCMI	6.97	1.75	7.48	2.20	0.537	**7.07**	**1.35**	**7.91**	**1.38**	**0.049**	0.605
Resistance (ohm)	716.00	134.65	673.56	115.23	0.317	703.14	106.60	648.50	76.66	0.058	0.738
Reactance (ohm)	69.89	13.25	65.94	8.15	0.267	64.36	11.00	67.14	7.41	0.269	0.108
PhA	5.63	0.73	5.69	0.89	0.899	**5.26**	**0.58**	**5.96**	**0.72**	**< 0.001**	0.074

SD Standard deviation, *FM* Fat mass, *FMI* Fat mass index, *FFM* Fat free mass, *FFMI* Fat free mass index, *MM* Muscle mass, *TBW* Total body water, *ECW* Extracellular water, *ICW* Intracellular water, *BCM* Body cell mass, *BCMI* Body cell mass index, *PhA* Phase angle. Bold characters indicate significant values ($p < 0.05$)

patients with polyarticular disease showed significantly more signs of malnutrition than patients with pauciarticular disease. In the polyarticular subtype, in comparison with the control group, they revealed significantly lower body weight, percentage of adipose tissue and total body water [21]. In children with JIA reduced muscle mass and increased fat mass and higher caloric requirements can be noticed. Some researchers recommend bone examination with the assessment of lean mass in this group of children [15, 22, 23].

The prognostic value of our findings should be determined in subsequent studies carried out in this population. ESPEN strongly recommended PhA as a prognostic nutritional measure [24, 25]. The possibility of predicting the occurrence or exacerbation of a given disease is emphasized by many researchers around the world [8, 9, 26, 27]. Hui et al. in their research phase angle retained its prognostic significance in the context of many known prognostic factors. Thus, to being a marker of cellular function, muscle mass and nutritional status, PhA may be a predictive factor of the risk of different complications. Moreover, PhA was weakly but significantly associated with other prognostic variables, suggesting that it captures some additional information compared to existing prognostic factors [26]. There is a promising prognostic tool to use in treatment planning, but further studies (also in JIA) are needed.

One of the most important limitations of the study is the small number of the children with diagnosed JIA included to the study. It did not allow us to demonstrate other significant differences between the study and control groups. In addition, the studied group of children was not analyzed a nutritional status with regards to the pharmacological treatment and disease activity. Nevertheless, our research has shown significant differences in the nutritional status between the study and control groups. Moreover, these differences depended mainly on the subtype of the disease. Also, due to the fact that assessment of important markers of nutritional status (lipids profile, glucose, TSH etc.) was not done in all the children, we were not able to analyze association of these variables with BIA and PhA results. Searching for such relationships would be an intriguing implication for further research.

In the summary, significant differences in body composition and nutritional status between children with JIA and control group indicate the need for implementation of BIA with a phase angle assessment to the routine clinical practice. It can be useful in identifying children at risk of malnutrition in this group of patients, especially among children with polyarthritis.

Conclusions

The results of this study showed that selected body composition parameters and nutritional indicators, including the phase angle, are lower in children and adolescents with JIA compared to healthy peers. Differences in the nutritional status in the study group depend on the subtype of the disease and children with polyarthritis are at the highest risk of malnutrition. Further prospective studies should be conducted in this group of children to indicate the prognostic value of the results obtained.

Abbreviations

BCM: Body cell mass; BCMI: Body cell mass index; BIA: Bioelectrical impedance analysis; BMI: Body mass index; ECW: Extra-cellular water; ESPEN: European Society for Clinical Nutrition and Metabolism; FFM: Fat free mass; FFMI: Fat free mass index; FM: Fat mass; FMI: Fat mass index; ICW: Intra-cellular water; ILAR: International League of Associations for Rheumatology; JIA: Juvenile idiopathic arthritis; MM: Muscle mass; PhA: Phase angle; PsA: Psoriatic arthritis; RF: Rheumatoid factor; TBW: Total body water

Acknowledgments

We thank Lonc Monika, MD and Dąbrowska Małgorzata, MD from Pediatric Department, Clinical Provincial Hospital No. 2 in Rzeszów, for prepering a data of this manuscript. Also the study was co-financed under the grant for statutory activity (Research Potential) of the Institute of Nursing and Health Sciences, Faculty of Medicine, University of Rzeszów for 2018 and 2019 years (Resolution No. WM/21/2018/P-M).

Funding

The study was conducted as the project of the Natural and Medical Center for Innovative Research in the University of Rzeszów, and it was co-financed by the Regional Operational Program for the Podkarpackie Province for the years 2007–2013, contract number UDA-RPPK.01.03.00–18-004/12–00.

Authors' contributions

PW, IS, and DB made substantial contributions to conception and design, acquisition of data, analysis and interpretation of data, and drafting the manuscript. MD made substantial contributions to conception and design and critical revision of the manuscript. All authors read and approved the final manuscript.

Competing interests

The authors declare that they have no competing interests.

Author details

[1]Institute of Nursing and Health Sciences, Faculty of Medicine, University of Rzeszów, Al. mjr. W. Kopisto 2 a, 35-310 Rzeszów, Poland. [2]Diabetic Outpatient Clinic, Medical Center "Beta-Med", Pl. Wolności 17, 35-073 Rzeszów, Poland.

References

1. Petty RE, Southwood TR, Manners P, Baum J, Glass DN, Goldenberg J, et al. International league of associations for rheumatology classification of juvenile idiopathic arthritis: second revision, Edmonton, 2001. J Rheumatol. 2004;31(2):390–2.
2. Caetano MC, Ortiz TT, Terreri MTSRLA, Sarni ROS, Silva SGL, Souza FIS, et al. Inadequate dietary intake of children and adolescents with juvenile idiopathic arthritis and systemic lupus erythematosus. J Pediatr. 2009;85(6): 509–15.
3. Guzman J, Kerr T, Ward LM, Ma J, Oen K, Rosenberg AM, et al. Growth and weight gain in children with juvenile idiopathic arthritis: Results from the ReACCh-Out cohort. Pediatr Rheumatol. 2017;15(1):68.
4. Norman K, Stobäus N, Pirlich M, Bosy-Westphal A. Bioelectrical phase angle and impedance vector analysis - clinical relevance and applicability of impedance parameters. Clin Nutr. 2012;31(6):854–61.
5. Rodríguez-Rodríguez F, Cristi-Montero C, González-Ruíz K, Correa-Bautista JE, Ramírez-Vélez R. Bioelectrical impedance vector analysis and muscular fitness in healthy men. Nutrients. 2016;8(7):407.
6. Kumar S, Dutt A, Hemraj S, Bhat S, Manipadybhima B. Phase angle measurement in healthy human subjects through bio-impedance analysis. Iran J Basic Med Sci. 2012;15(6):1180–4.
7. Khalil SF, Mohktar MS, Ibrahim F. The theory and fundamentals of bioimpedance analysis in clinical status monitoring and diagnosis of diseases. Sensors (Basel). 2014;14(6):10895–928.
8. Schulz K-H, Patra S, Spielmann H, Klapdor S, Schlüter K, van Eckert S. Physical condition, nutritional status, fatigue, and quality of life in oncological out-patients. SAGE Open Med. 2017;5:2050312117743674.
9. Dittmar M, Reber H, Kahaly GJ. Bioimpedance phase angle indicates catabolism in type 2 diabetes. Diabet Med. 2015;32(9):1177–85.
10. Lee SY, Lee YJ, Yang J-H, Kim C-M, Choi W-S. The association between phase angle of bioelectrical impedance analysis and survival time in advanced Cancer patients: preliminary study. Korean J Fam Med. 2014;35(5):251–6.
11. Caccialanza R, Cereda E, Klersy C, Bonardi C, Cappello S, Quarleri L, et al. Phase angle and handgrip strength are sensitive early markers of energy intake in hypophagic, non-surgical patients at nutritional risk, with contraindications to enteral nutrition. Nutrients. 2015;7(3):1828–40.
12. Ringold BS, Wallace CA. Measuring clinical response and remission in juvenile idiopathic arthritis. Curr Opin Rheumatol. 2007;19(5):471–6.
13. Więch P, Dabrowski M, Bazaliński D, Sałacińska I, Korczowski B, Binkowska-Bury M. Bioelectrical impedance phase angle as an indicator of malnutrition in hospitalized children with diagnosed inflammatory bowel diseases—a case control study. Nutrients. 2018;10(4):499.
14. Jednacz E, Rutkowska-Sak L. Assessment of the body composition and parameters of the cardiovascular risk in juvenile idiopathic arthritis. Biomed Res Int. 2015;2015:619023.
15. Bechtold S, Simon D. Growth abnormalities in children and adolescents with juvenile idiopathic arthritis. Rheumatol Int. 2014;34(11):1483–8.
16. Cleary AG, Lancaster GA, Annan F, Sills JA, Davidson JE. Nutritional impairment in juvenile idiopathic arthritis. Rheumatology. 2004;43(12):1569–73.
17. Knops N, Wulffraat N, Lodder S, Houwen R, de Meer K. Resting energy expenditure and nutritional status in children with juvenile rheumatoid arthritis. J Rheumatol. 1999;26(9):2039–43.
18. Sherman G, Nemet D, Moshe V, et al. Disease activity, overweight, physical activity and screen time in a cohort of patients with juvenile idiopathic arthritis. Clin Exp Rheumatol. 2018; [Epub ahead of print].

19. Pelajo CF, Lopez-Benitez JM, Miller LC. Obesity and disease activity in juvenile idiopathic arthritis. Pediatr Rheumatol Online J. 2012;10(1):3.
20. Niewerth M, Minden K, Foeldvari I, et al. Prevalence of being overweight among children and adolescents with juvenile idiopathic arthritis. Ann Rheum Dis. 2006;65:449.
21. Lofthouse CM, Azad F, Baildam EM, Akobeng AK. Measuring the nutritional status of children with juvenile idiopathic arthritis using the bioelectrical impedance method. Rheumatology (Oxford). 2002;41(10):1172–7.
22. Roth J, Bechtold S, Borte G, Dressler F, Girschick HJ, Borte M. Osteoporosis in juvenile idiopathic arthritis--a practical approach to diagnosis and therapy. Eur J Pediatr. 2007;166(8):775–84.
23. Frost HM, Schönau E. The "muscle-bone unit" in children and adolescents: a 2000 overview. J Pediatr Endocrinol Metab. 2000;13(6):571–90.
24. Rinninella E, Ruggiero A, Maurizi P, Triarico S, Cintoni M, Mele MC. Clinicaltoolstoassessnutritional risk and malnutrition in hospitalized children and adolescents. Eur Rev Med Pharmacol Sci. 2017;21:2690–701.
25. Cederholm T, Barazzoni R, Austin P, Ballmer P, Biolo G, Bischoff SC, Compher C, Correia I, Higashiguchi T, Holst M, et al. ESPEN guidelines on definitions and terminology of clinical nutrition. Clin Nutr. 2017;36:49–64.
26. Hui D, Bansal S, Morgado M, Dev R, Chisholm G, Bruera E. Phase angle for prognostication of survival in patients with advanced Cancer: preliminary findings. Cancer. 2014;120(14):2207–14.
27. Axelsson L, Silander E, Bosaeus I, Hammerlid E. Bioelectrical phase angle at diagnosis as a prognostic factor for survival in advanced head and neck cancer. Eur Arch Otorhinolaryngol. 2018;275(9):2379–86.

20

Arterial properties in adults with long-lasting active juvenile idiopathic arthritis compared to healthy controls

Hanne Aaserud Aulie[1,2*], Mette-Elise Estensen[3], Anne Marit Selvaag[1], Vibke Lilleby[1], Berit Flatø[1,4] and Svend Aakhus[5,6]

Abstract

Background: The data on cardiovascular risk and systemic arterial properties in patients with long-lasting juvenile idiopathic arthritis (JIA) is limited. The objective of this study was to describe systemic arterial properties including characteristic impedance (Z_0), total arterial compliance (C), and peripheral vascular resistance (R) in patients with long-lasting active JIA compared with matched controls, and to assess the relation to JIA disease variables and traditional cardiovascular risk factors.

Findings: *Methods:* Eighty-one JIA patients (median age 38.6) with at least 15 years of active disease were reexamined after median 29 years of disease duration and compared to 41 healthy controls. With use of echocardiography and calibrated right common carotid artery tonometric pulse traces, noninvasive estimates of pressure and blood flow from the aortic root were obtained and used to estimate the systemic arterial parameters Z_0, C and R.
Results: The patients had higher Z_0 as assessed by Windkessel model (mean ± SD 65.0 ± 30.1 versus 53.4 ± 18.8 10^{-3} mmHg/ml/s, $p = 0.027$), lower C as assessed by either Windkessel model or ratio of stroke volume and pulse pressure (1. 57 ± 0.46 versus 1.80 ± 0.65 ml/mmHg, $p = 0.030$, 1.29 ± 0.37 versus 1.43 ± 0.34 ml/mmHg, $p = 0.038$), and similar R compared to the controls. Years on daily prednisolone and insulin resistance were the most important correlates of $Z_{0.}$ Metotrexat use, polyarticular disease course and erythrocyte sedimentation rate were also associated with a higher $Z_{0.}$

Conclusion: Our results indicate that JIA patients had altered arterial properties as compared to controls. Years on daily prednisolone and insulin resistance were the most important correlates of altered arterial properties.

Keywords: Juvenile idiopathic arthritis, Inflammation, Cardiovascular disease, Arterial stiffness

Introduction

Juvenile idiopathic arthritis (JIA) is a chronic inflammatory rheumatic disease with symptom onset in childhood and persists into adulthood in about 50% of the patients [1, 2].

Arterial stiffness is an established independent predictor of cardiovascular disease (CVD) [3]. Whereas adult onset inflammatory arthritis is known to be related to increased arterial stiffness [4], little is known of systemic arterial properties and cardiovascular risk in those with long-lasting JIA.

Pulse wave velocity (PWV) is the most frequently used method for the measurement of arterial stiffness reflecting large arterial stiffness [5]. However, the properties of the arterial system can be described in more detail by use of system level parameters, as characteristic impedance (Z_0), arterial compliance (C) and vascular resistance (R) [6].

We have previously reported an increased prevalence of hypertension and arterial stiffness as measured by PWV in adults with long-lasting active JIA [7]. However, Z_0, C and R have hitherto not been described in this patient group. The present study was therefore designed to characterize systemic arterial properties in detail in JIA patients as compared to matched controls. We also wanted to assess the associations between JIA disease variables, cardiovascular risk factors and arterial properties.

* Correspondence: hanneaulie@hotmail.com
[1]Department of Rheumatology, Oslo University Hospital, Rikshospitalet, Oslo, Norway
[2]Department of Internal Medicine, Diakonhjemmet Hospital, Oslo, Norway

Methods

Patients and controls

Totally 134 JIA patients with clinically active disease for at least 15 years of disease duration were invited to a combined rheumatologic and cardiologic follow-up study after median 29 years. The patients were initially referred to the Oslo University hospital between 1980 and 85, and re-examined after median 15 and 23 years before the present study [2]. Between May 2011 and March 2012, 90 patients were included in the study. Nine were excluded after inclusion due to pregnancy ($n = 3$), recordings of suboptimal quality ($n = 5$), or severe heart disease without presumed relation to JIA ($n = 1$). The 81 participants were not different from the 53 eligible but not participating patients regarding gender, disease duration and age (data not shown).

Forty-six healthy, age- and gender-matched controls were selected randomly from the Norwegian population register. Responders with a history of diabetes mellitus, hypertension, or inflammatory arthritis were not included. Five were excluded after inclusion due to suboptimal recordings.

Clinical examination and cardiovascular risk assessments

The 81 patients underwent a clinical examination performed by a specialist in rheumatology, the controls were clinically examined by a physician.

JIA was classified according to the International League of Associations for Rheumatology criteria [8]. Active disease was defined as the lack of remission off anti-rheumatic medication [9].

Family history of CVD was defined as a first degree having CVD before the age of 65 (women) and 55 (men). Information about smoking habits and physical activity was obtained through a questionnaire. Insulin resistance was derived from the assessments of insulin and glucose [10].

Three measurements of systolic blood pressure (SBP) and diastolic blood pressure (DBP) with a difference of < 5 mmHg were averaged and taken in all participants after 5 min rest in a supine position. Arterial hypertension was defined as SBP > 140 mmHg and/or DBP > 90 mmHg, and/or use of antihypertensive medication.

Blood samples were drawn after an overnight fast and analysed for high sensitive C-reactive protein (CRP), erythrocyte sedimentation rate (ESR), insulin, glucose and cholesterol.

Non-invasive assessment of arterial properties

Tonometry

We recorded the arterial pulse waveform from the right common carotid artery with the patient in a supine position, using a high-fidelity external applanation tonometric device (Millar SPT-301, Millar Instruments Inc., Houston, USA). Recordings were obtained semi-simultaneously with echocardiographic doppler recordings (Vivid 7 ultrasound scanner, GE Vingmed ultrasound, Norway) of blood flow from the left ventricular outflow tract and the parasternal short axis midventricular cineloops. The tonometric signal was amplified and transferred to a personal computer for processing in Matlab 7 application [11]. We selected at least three cardiac cycles for analysis. The carotid pulse trace peak and nadir were then calibrated with the systolic and diastolic brachial arterial pressures, respectively.

Systemic arterial properties

A 3-element electrical analogue Windkessel model of the systemic circulation was used to assess Z_0, R and C [11]. In order to obtain estimates of systemic parameters independent of any assumed model, we also assessed Z_0 in the frequency domain as the average of the high frequency harmonics of the input impedance modulus [6]. C was also estimated as stroke volume (mL) over arterial pulse pressure (mmHg).

Statistics

The JIA patients and controls, and the patient subgroups were compared using a 2-sided independent sample *t*-test for the continuous normally distributed variables, the Mann-Whitney *U*-test for the continuous not normally distributed values, and the χ^2 test for the categorical variables. For the continuous normally distributed variables, central tendencies were given as the mean ± SD and for the continuous not normally distributed values, median inter-quartile range. A p value < 0.05 (2 tailed) were regarded as statistically significant for all the analyses. Pearson's Correlation coefficients and multivariate linear regression analysis were used to investigate associations between disease variables, cardiovascular risk factors and arterial properties. SPSS Version 20 (SPSS, Chicago, USA) was used for the statistical analyses.

Results

Demographics and cardiovascular risk factors

The characteristics of patients and controls are summarized in Table 1. Hypertension was present in 11% of the patients, and in none of the controls ($p = 0.028$).

Systemic arterial properties

Z_0 estimated by Windkessel model was significantly higher (21.7%, $p = 0.027$, Table 2) in the patients, and Z_0 by frequency domain analyses although numerically higher in the patients, the difference was not statistically different between the groups. C by either of Windkessel model or ratio of stroke volume and pulse pressure was significantly lower in the patients compared to controls

Table 1 JIA disease characteristics and traditional cardiovascular risk factors

Variables	JIA patients ($n = 81$)	Controls ($n = 41$)
Demographics		
Male gender; n (%)	20 (25)	9 (22)
Age (years); median (IQR)	38.6 (34.9–40.7)	37.7 (34.8–40.5)
Disease duration (years); median (IQR)	29.3 (28.3–30.6)	
Onset age (years); median (IQR)	8.9 (4.9–11.8)	
JIA subtype distribution		
Systemic arthritis; n (%)	4 (5)	
RF negative polyarthritis; n (%)	11 (14)	
RF positive polyarthritis; n (%)	5 (6)	
Persistent oligoarthritis; n (%)	14 (17)	
Extended oligoarthritis; n (%)	13 (16)	
Entesitis related arthritis; n (%)	18 (22)	
Psoriatic arthritis; n (%)	14 (17)	
Unclassified arthritis; n (%)	2 (3)	
Current medication at 29-year follow-up		
Anti-TNF; n (%)	25 (31)	
Metotrexat; n (%)	19 (24)	
NSAIDs daily; n (%)	23 (28)	
Prednisolone; n (%)	5 (6.2)	
Cardiovascular risk factors		
BMI (kg/m^2); mean (SD)	25.7 (5.0)	25.3 (3.9)
Waist circumference (cm); mean (SD)	92.7 (12.7)	92.7 (9.0)
Daily smokers; n (%)	18 (22)	5 (12)
CVD in first degree relative; n (%)	46 (57)	19 (46)
Hypertension; n (%)	9 (11)	0 (0)*
Myocardial infarction; n (%)	1 (1)	0 (0)
Total cholesterol (mmol/L); mean (SD)	4.9 (1.1)	4.9 (0.8)
LDL cholesterol (mmol/L); mean (SD)	3.0 (1.0)	3.0 (0.8)
hs-CRP (mg/L); median (IQR)	1.8 (0.7–5.0)	0.7 (0.0–1.9)*
Insulin resistance	1.1 (1.1)	0.9 (0.6)

JIA Juvenile idiopathic arthritis, *IQR* inter-quartile range, *RF* rheumatoid factor, anti-*TNF* anti-tumor necrosis factor, *NSAIDs* nonsteroidal anti-inflammatory drugs, *BMI* body mass index, *LDL* low density lipoprotein, *CVD* cardiovascular disease, *hs-CRP* high sensitivity C-reactive protein

* $p < 0.05$ compared with values in previous column

(12.8 and 9.8%, $p = 0.030$ and $p = 0.038$, respectively). Heart rate was slightly higher in the patients ($p = 0.026$), however R was similar in patients and controls.

The association between JIA disease variables, cardiovascular risk factors and systemic arterial properties

Z_0 by Windkessel model was significantly higher in the patients with present or previous use of metotrexat, using prednisolone, and/or had polyarticular disease course as compared to the other patients (Fig. 1), and was correlated to higher ESR area under the curve (AUC), years on daily prednisolone and insulin resistance (Table 3). When including these variables in a multiple linear regression analysis, years on daily prednisolone and insulin resistance were determinants of Z_0 (ß = 0.003,$p = 0.021$, ß = 0.006,$p = 0.042$).

Findings

The present long-term follow-up study indicates that JIA patients with long-term active disease have altered systemic arterial properties as demonstrated by a higher Z_0 by Windkessel and a lower C when compared to controls. Years on daily prednisolone and insulin resistance were the most important correlates of Z_0. Furthermore, the use of metotrexat, polyarticular disease course and ESR AUC correlated with higher Z_0.

Table 2 Arterial haemodynamics and arterial properties

Variables	JIA Patients ($n = 81$)	Controls ($n = 41$)	Difference (%)	*P*-value
Height, cm	170.5 (8.4)	170.3 (8.3)	0	0.881
Weight, kg	74.9 (16.7)	73.3 (12.1)	2.2	0.603
Heart rate, beats/minute	65 (11)	61 (9)	6.6	0.026
Systolic blood pressure, mmHg	119 (18)	113 (11)	5.3	0.054
Diastolic blood pressure, mmHg	70 (10)	67 (9)	4.5	0.091
Mean arterial pressure; mmHg	90 (13)	85 (9)	5.9	0.026
R, mm Hg/ml/s	1.02 (0.27)	1.00 (0.22)	0.02	0.636
C WK, ml/ mm Hg	1.57 (0.46)	1.80 (0.65)	12.8	0.030
C SV/PP, ml/ mmHg	1.29 (0.37)	1.43 (0.34)	9.8	0.038
Z_0 WK, 10^{-3} mmHg/ml/s	65.0 (30.1)	53.4 (18.8)	21.7	0.027
Z_0 FD	96.1 (37.2)	91.5 (31.4)	5.0	0.497

Values are the mean (SD)

R total peripheral resistance, *C WK* compliance estimated by Windkessel model, *C SV/PP* compliance estimated as ratio of stroke volume and pulse pressure, *Z_0 WK* characteristic impedance estimated by Windkessel model, *Z_0 FD* characteristic impedance estimated by frequency domain analyses

Whereas Z_0 reflects the combined effect of size and stiffness (a high Z_0 implies a stiffer and/or small sized aorta) of predominantly the ascending aorta, C reflects the volume compliance of the entire systemic arterial tree. R is mainly determined by the small muscular arterioles [6]. Considering both C and the Z_0 by Windkessel, our findings suggest that the central conduit arteries are altered more than peripheral arteries in adult JIA patients. Previous reports have emphasized the importance of large arterial stiffness rather than alterations of microvascular resistance in the prediction of cardiovascular risk in patients with hypertension [12, 13]. Importantly, lower C and higher Z_0 are associated with increased cardiovascular risk in the adult general population [14, 15].

Our data support a previous study from the same patient cohort, showing higher PWV in adult JIA patients compared to controls [7]. Thus, increased arterial stiffness has been demonstrated to be present by different noninvasive techniques in JIA patients.

In the patient group, 8 had hypertension while controls with hypertension were excluded in order to maintain a healthy control group. However, when compared to controls, the differences in SBP and DBP were only marginal numerically, and not of statistical significance. Thus, we

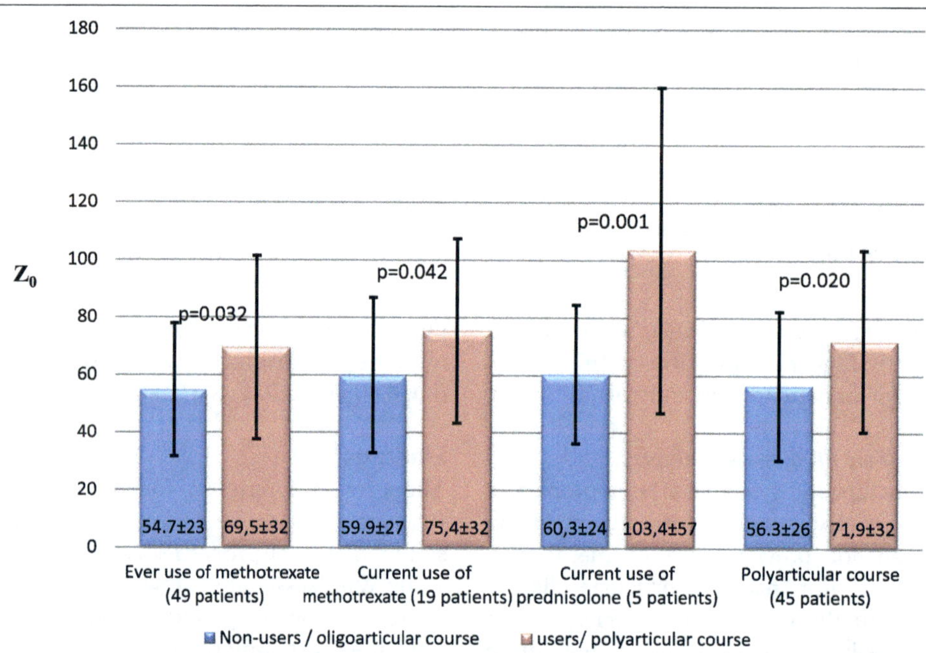

Fig. 1 The influence of JIA anti-rheumatic medication and JIA disease burden on systemic arterial properties; legends: JIA = Juvenile idiopathic arthritis, Z_0 Windkessel model = characteristic impedance estimated by Windkessel model

Table 3 Correlations of JIA disease variables, traditional cardiovascular risk factors and arterial properties assessed by Z_0 Windkessel model

	R	*P*-value
JIA disease variables		
CRP area under the curve[a]	0.095	0.402
ESR area under the curve[a]	0.238	0.037
Years on daily prednisolone	0.346	0.002
Years on daily NSAIDs	0.152	0.177
Years on daily metotrexat	0.094	0.403
Disease duration	−0.193	0.085
JADAS	−0.084	0.465
Number of active joints	0.035	0.758
Traditional cardiovascular risk factors		
Age	−0.117	0.296
BMI	0.180	0.108
Waist circumference	0.213	0.060
Insulin resistance	0.273	0.015
Daily smoking	0.072	0.526
Vigorous physical activity (hours/ week)	−0.111	0.347
Moderate physical activity (hours/ week)	−0.189	0.118

Variables assessed at 29-year follow-up unless otherwise stated
[a]Calculated from parameters assessed at 15-year and 29-year follow-up (CRP), disease onset, 15-year and 29-year follow-up (ESR)
JIA juvenile idiopathic arthritis, *CRP* C-reactive protein, *ESR* erythrocyte sedimentation rate, *NSAIDs* nonsteroidal anti-inflammatory drugs, *JADAS* Juvenile Arthritis Disease Activity Score, *BMI* body mass index

do not think that the difference in arterial properties between the JIA patients and controls can be fully explained by blood pressure variations. On the other hand, increased vascular stiffness predicts incident hypertension [16] underscoring the bidirectional relationship between arterial properties and blood pressures. In our previous study not excluding hypertensive controls we found an increased prevalence of hypertension in the JIA patients as compared to the controls [7].

We found an association between use of antirheumatic medication, polyarticular disease course and higher ESR AUC and insulin resistance and altered arterial properties. Larger prospective controlled studies are needed to identify determinants of altered arterial properties in JIA patients. Our findings add to the previously reported association between prednisolone use and increased arterial stiffness in JIA patients from our cohort [7].

The strengths of this study are the inclusion of a well-defined cohort of JIA patients followed for 29 years and the fact that detailed information of arterial properties has not been presented in JIA patients before. However, the number of included participants was relatively small, and because of a cross sectional study design the prognostic value of our findings is unknown.

In conclusion, our results suggest that adult patients with long-lasting active JIA had stiffer proximal aorta, and lower total arterial compliance but similar systemic resistance compared to matched controls from the general population. Years on daily prednisolone and insulin resistance were the most important correlates of altered arterial properties. Whether our findings indicate that JIA patients should enter a regular BP monitoring program needs to be determined in future longitudinal follow-up studies.

Abbreviations
AUC: Area under the curve; C: Total arterial compliance; CRP: C-reactive protein; CVD: Cardiovascular disease; DBP: Diastolic blood pressure; ESR: Erythrocyte sedimentation rate; JIA: Juvenile idiopathic arthritis; PVW: Pulse wave velocity; R: Peripheral vascular resistance; SBP: Systolic blood pressure; Z_0: Characteristic impedance

Acknowledgements
We are indebted to prof. Patrick Segers, IBIT IBiTech-bioMMeda, Ghent University, Belgium for his valuable comments on this manuscript. We would also like to thank Pia Elisabeth Bryde, Richard Massey and Lene Annette Rustad for valuable assistance with echocardiographic and tonometric recordings. Further we thank Torhild Garen for help with preparation of questionnaires, Lars Mørkrid for valuable help obtaining laboratory assessments, and Inge-Margrethe Gilboe and Øyvind Molberg for administrative support.

Funding
The study was founded by the Norwegian Rheumatism Association science foundation, Consultant Jan A Pahles and Storstuens legat, and the Norwegian ExtraFoundation for Health and Rehabilitation.

Authors' contributions
HAA organised the study, examined the patients/controls, performed the statistics, wrote the manuscript and developed the tables and figure, MEE, AMS and VL examined the patients and contributed in writing the manuscript, BF conceived and planned the project, examined the patients and supervised the project and contributed to the manuscript, SA contributed to the design of study and the manuscript preparation. All authors read and approved the final manuscript.

Competing interests
The authors declare that they have no competing interests.

Author details
[1]Department of Rheumatology, Oslo University Hospital, Rikshospitalet, Oslo, Norway. [2]Department of Internal Medicine, Diakonhjemmet Hospital, Oslo, Norway. [3]Department of Cardiology, Oslo University Hospital, Rikshospitalet, Oslo, Norway. [4]Institute for Clinical Medicine, Medical Faculty, University of Oslo, Oslo, Norway. [5]Department of Circulation and Imaging, Faculty of Medicine and Health Science, Norwegian University of Science and Technology, NTNU, Trondheim, Norway. [6]Clinic of Cardiology, St. Olavs Hospital, Trondheim, Norway.

References

1. Bertilsson L, Andersson-Gare B, Fasth A, Petersson IF, Forsblad-D'elia H. Disease course, outcome, and predictors of outcome in a population-based juvenile chronic arthritis cohort followed for 17 years. J Rheumatol. 2013;40:715–24.
2. Selvaag AM, Aulie HA, Lilleby V, Flato B. Disease progression into adulthood and predictors of long-term active disease in juvenile idiopathic arthritis. Ann Rheum Dis. 2016;75:190–5.
3. Mitchell GF, Hwang SJ, Vasan RS, Larson MG, Pencina MJ, Hamburg NM, et al. Arterial stiffness and cardiovascular events: the Framingham heart study. Circulation. 2010;121:505–11.
4. Ambrosino P, Tasso M, Lupoli R, Di MA, Baldassarre D, Tremoli E, et al. Non-invasive assessment of arterial stiffness in patients with rheumatoid arthritis: a systematic review and meta-analysis of literature studies. Ann Med. 2015; 47:457–67.
5. Laurent S, Cockroft J, Bortel L, Boutouyrie P, Giannattasio C, Hayoz D, et al. Expert consensus document on arterial stiffness: methodological issues and clinical applications. Eur Heart J. 2006;26:2588–605.
6. Segers P, Rietzschel ER, De Buyzere ML, Vermeersch SJ, De BD, Van Bortel LM, et al. Noninvasive (input) impedance, pulse wave velocity, and wave reflection in healthy middle-aged men and women. Hypertension. 2007;49:1248–55.
7. Aulie HA, Selvaag AM, Gunther A, Lilleby V, Molberg O, Hartmann A, et al. Arterial haemodynamics and coronary artery calcification in adult patients with juvenile idiopathic arthritis. Ann Rheum Dis. 2015;74:1515–21.
8. Petty RE, Southwood TR, Manners P, Baum J, Glass DN, Goldenberg J, et al. International league of associations for rheumatology classification of juvenile idiopathic arthritis: second revision, Edmonton, 2001. J Rheumatol. 2004;31:390–2.
9. Wallace CA, Ruperto N, Giannini E. Preliminary criteria for clinical remission for select categories of juvenile idiopathic arthritis. J Rheumatol. 2004;31:2290–4.
10. Matthews DR, Hosker JP, Rudenski AS, Naylor BA, Treacher DF, Turner RC. Homeostasis model assessment: insulin resistance and beta-cell function from fasting, plasma glucose and insulin concentrations in man. Diabetologia. 1985;28:412–9.
11. Rietzschel ER, De Buyzere ML, Bekaert S, Segers P, De Bacquer D, Cooman L, et al. Rationale, design, methods and baseline characteristics of the Asklepios study. Eur J Cardiovasc Prev Rehabil. 2007;14:179–91.
12. Millar JA, Lever AF, Burke V. Pulse pressure as a risk factor for cardiovascular events in the MRC mild hypertension trial. J Hypertens. 1999;17:1065–72.
13. Blacher J, Staessen JA, Girerd X, Gasowski J, Thijs L, Liu L, et al. Pulse pressure not mean pressure determines cardiovascular risk in older hypertensive patients. Arch Intern Med. 2000;160:1085–9.
14. Lilly SM, Jacobs D, Bluemke DA, Duprez D, Zamani P, Chirinos J. Resistive and pulsatile arterial hemodynamics and cardiovascular events: the multiethnic study of atherosclerosis. In: J am heart Assoc published online: 11 des; 2014. https://doi.org/10.1161/JAHA.114.001223.
15. Cooper LL, Rong J, Benjamin EJ, Larson MG, Levy D, Vita JA, et al. Components of hemodynamic load and cardiovascular events: the Framingham heart study. Circulation. 2015;131:354–61.
16. Dernellis J, Panaretou M. Aortic stiffness is an independent predictor of progression to hypertension in nonhypertensive subjects. Hypertension. 2005;45:426–31.

21

Clinical and MRI outcome of cervical spine lesions in children with juvenile idiopathic arthritis treated with anti-TNFα drugs early in disease course

Damjana Ključevšek[1*], Nina Emeršič[2], Nataša Toplak[2,3] and Tadej Avčin[2,3]

Abstract

Backgrounds: The purpose of the study was to evaluate the clinical and magnetic resonance imaging (MRI) outcome of cervical spine arthritis in children with juvenile idiopathic arthritis (JIA), who received anti-TNFα early in the course of cervical spine arthritis.

Methods: Medical charts and imaging of JIA patients with cervical spine involvement were reviewed in this retrospective study. Data, including age at disease onset, JIA type, disease activity, treatment and clinical outcome were collected. Initial and followup MRI examinations of cervical spine were performed according to the hospital protocol to evaluate the presence of inflammation and potential chronic/late changes.

Results: Fifteen JIA patients with MRI proved cervical spine inflammation (11 girls, 4 boys, median age 6.3y) were included in the study: 9 had polyarthritis, 3 extended oligoarthritis, 2 persistent oligoarthritis and 1 juvenile psoriatic arthritis. All children were initially treated with high-dose steroids and methotrexate. In addition, 11 patients were treated with anti-TNFα drug within 3 months, and 3 patients within 7 months of cervical spine involvement confirmed by MRI. Mean observation time was 2.9y, mean duration of anti-TNFα treatment was 2.2y. Last MRI showed no active inflammation in 12/15 children, allowing to stop biological treatment in 3 patients, and in 3/15 significant reduction of inflammation. Mild chronic changes were found on MRI in 3 children.

Conclusions: Early treatment with anti-TNFα drugs resulted in significantly reduced inflammation or complete remission of cervical spine arthritis proved by MRI, and prevented the development of serious chronic/late changes. Repeated MRI examinations are suggested in the follow-up of JIA patients with cervical spine arthritis.

Keywords: Juvenile idiopathic arthritis, Cervical spine arthritis, Magnetic resonance, Anti-TNFα, Outcome

Background

Cervical spine arthritis is a well-recognized complication of juvenile idiopathic arthritis (JIA), usually presenting in patients with systemic or polyarticular forms of the disease [1]. More commonly, the upper cervical spine is affected because the atlanto-occipital and the atlanto-axial joints are synovial and are thus primary targets for rheumatic inflammation [2]. Early detection of cervical involvement is essential for identification of children that require more aggressive treatment including early introduction of biologic therapy. Untreated chronic inflammation of the cervical joints can lead to morphological changes and functional impairment, which can be even life-threatening due to instability and potential risk of spinal cord injury.

Clinical signs and symptoms of cervical spine arthritis may include neck pain, stiffness, torticollis, limited range of motion (LROM), headache, facial and ear pain, and signs of cervical myelopathy. Absence of clinical symptoms does

* Correspondence: damjana.kljucevsek@gmail.com
[1]Radiology Unit, University Children's Hospital Ljubljana, Ljubljana, Slovenia

not exclude subclinical inflammation and imaging abnormalities of cervical spine [3].

Imaging modalities used in assessment of cervical spine arthritis include radiography, computer tomography and magnetic resonance imaging (MRI) [4–6]. Radiography has been most evaluated imaging modality for assessment of cervical spine lesions and is particularly useful for evaluation of malalignment, functional impairment, morphological changes of bones, and vertebral body growth disturbances [3, 7–9]. In general, MRI is the method of choice in evaluation of cervical spine arthritis and is most useful in detecting synovitis with hypertrophic, enhanced synovia and pannus formation, joint effusion, erosions, bone marrow edema and possible neural structure compressions [10, 11]. The diagnostic accuracy and predictive value of conventional MRI in JIA patients with axial joint involvement have been poorly investigated [12]. The role of MRI in detecting early changes in cervical spine in JIA was first evaluated in a Turkish study showing higher sensitivity of MRI compared to radiography for detection of erosions in children [13]. More recently, a German study evaluating MR changes of cervical spine arthritis at diagnosis and response to treatment in 13 patients with JIA was published [14]. It was concluded that close MRI monitoring of these patients appears to be sensitive tool for early diagnosis and may help to detect further disease progression and complications.

In the last two decades, highly effective biologic therapies became available. The efficacy of treatment with anti-TNFα should be assessed and validated by standardized imaging protocols for data acquisition and interpretation. MRI scoring for patients with rheumatoid arthritis is a good alternative, but it was not adapted and validated for joint involvement in children with JIA [15]. The main problem in assessment of arthritis in children and adolescents are difficulties to differentiate between physiologic and pathologic joint findings [16–18]. Therefore, there is a clear need for development of tools for more accurate monitoring of therapeutic responses for both disease activity and structural damage to the joint [15].

According to ACR 2011 Recommendations, cervical spine arthritis was considered a poor prognostic factor that may require escalation of therapy [19]. We decided to introduce anti-TNFα treatment in all children with proven cervical spine arthritis on MRI [20]. Therefore, the objective of our study was to evaluate the clinical and MRI outcome of cervical spine arthritis in a group of consecutive patients with JIA who received anti-TNFα treatment early in disease course. Our preposition was that treatment with anti-TNFα early in the course of cervical spine arthritis could provide a good response to active inflammation with potential less chronic changes.

Methods

The study was designed as a retrospective cohort study with longitudinal follow-up of clinical and MRI data in children with JIA. The charts of 407 children with JIA treated at the University Children's Hospital between September 2010 and July 2016 were reviewed and all children with cervical spine involvement confirmed by MRI examination were included in the study.

In all children clinical signs of neck involvement (LROM, neck pain, stiffness and torticollis) and involvement of other axial and peripheral joints were assessed at the time of initial presentation of cervical arthritis and at their last follow-up visit. MRI of cervical spine was performed in all children within 3 weeks of clinical notion of cervical spine involvement and evaluated according to the hospital protocol. All MRI examinations of cervical spine included at least one short Tau inversion recovery (STIR) (usually in coronal or sagittal plane), T2 TSE and T1 TSE in sagittal and axial plane, T1 TSE FS axial, and postcontrast sequences T1 TSE FS in 2 or 3 planes (Magnetom Aera or Avanto 1.5 T MR Siemens Healthcare). MRI evaluation of cervical spine consisted on determination of synovitis, bone changes and the presence of malalignment. Synovitis was evaluated as presence of synovial thickening in cervical spine (predental and paradental space of atlanto-axial joint, atlanto-occipital joints and facet joints), presence of fluid in these joints, and evaluation of ligaments in this region (transversus, alar and apical ligaments). Enhancement of synovia and joints after i.v. administration of paramagnetic contrast medium was determined. Bone evaluation consisted of presence or absence of bone edema and morphologic changes of bone (dens deformation, thinned corticalis of bone in involved region, erosions, ankyloses). Malalignment was evaluated as abnormal position of articular surfaces of atlanto-occipital (basilar invagination), atlanto-axial (anterior atlanto-axial subluxation - aAAS), facet joints (subaxial subluxation), and narrowing of craniocervical spinal canal. In children with suspected malalignment radiography of cervical spine in antero-posterior and lateral position was performed.

Data about therapy including the type of medication and time from disease onset and treatment introduction was collected for all patients.

Follow-up examinations included clinical evaluation and serial follow-up MRI examinations of cervical spine. The timeframe of follow-up MRI examinations depended on the severity of cervical spine inflammation found on the initial MRI and treatment efficacy. Persistent clinical signs (more than 3 months) were indication for earlier MRI follow-up. If at least three compartments of AA and AO joints were involved, or additional facet joints inflammation, in case of abounded pannus resulting in malalignement, and presence of bone edema even in the case of good clinical response, follow-up MRI was performed 5 to 6 months after the initial one to make an objective evaluation of treatment response. In other children the first follow-up MRI was performed 9 to 12 months later. On average, patients had 2.4 (range 1–8) follow-up MRI examinations with mean time interval between the initial and the first follow-up examination 6.5 months (range 2 to 14 months) and between initial and the last MRI examination 27.9 months (range 6 to 71 months). Initial and follow-up MRI findings were compared and the response to therapy was determined as no response (same), partial improvement (reduced inflammation compared to previous MRI), and no inflammation (no MRI signs of active inflammation or minimal residual patchy enhancement). Serial MRI examinations enabled not only evaluation of treatment response, but also evaluation of the development of chronic bone changes during the observation period.

In addition, suspected malalignment was assessed on cervical radiography in antero-posterior and lateral projections in 3 children. Cervical radiography in antero and retroflexion positions was performed at the time when the patient had no signs of active inflammation.

Descriptive statistics was used to summarize the study.

Results

Initial presentation of cervical spine arthritis

Cervical spine involvement was identified in fifteen out of 407 (3.7%) children with JIA (4 boys and 11 girls) ranging in age from 2.5 to 15.1 years (mean 6.3 years). Eight children were diagnosed with rheumatoid factor (RF) negative polyarthritis (pJIA), 1 with RF positive polyarthritis, 3 with extended oligoarthritis (oJIA), 2 with persistent oJIA, and 1 with juvenile psoriatic arthritis (jPsA).

Cervical spine involvement occurred in 9/15 (60%) children within the first 6 months from the disease onset including 3 patients with cervical arthritis as the initial manifestation of JIA. Six out of 15 patients (40%) developed cervical spine arthritis more than 1 year after the disease onset. Mean disease duration at the time of diagnosis of cervical spine arthritis including 14 patients in our cohort was 5.2 months (range 1 month to 13 months), excluding the patient #11, who presented with cervical arthritis 13.5 years after the disease onset. All children clinically presented with LROM, two of them had stiff neck and one torticollis. Twelve children complained about the pain in the neck. None of our patients developed cervical spine involvement as the isolated manifestation of JIA. Mean number of active peripheral joints at the time of diagnosis of cervical spine arthritis was 18.1 (range 2 to 40 active peripheral joints). Three out of 15 patients (20%) had signs of temporomandibular joint (TMJ) arthritis together with cervical spine arthritis. One patient had associated uveitis.

Laboratory examinations at the time of presentation revealed normal erythrocyte sedimentation rate (ESR) in 2 and elevated ESR in 13 patients with the mean value of 36 mm/h (range 9 to 77), mean white blood cell (WBC) count 8.9 × 10^9/L (range 5.7–19.3), mean hemoglobin109 g/L (range 92–133) and mean platelet count 457 × 10^9/L (range 109–782). Ten out of fifteen (67%) patients had positive antinuclear antibody (ANA) titres. Only one out of 11 patients had positive human leukocyte antigen (HLA) B27. Fourteen patients had negative RF and one patient (#12) was RF positive.

Initial MRI examination demonstrated in all children atlanto-axial synovitis with enhanced synovia during i.v. application of paramagnetic contrast medium, 9 had also fluid in predental space. Co-existed atlanto-occipital synovitis was found in 6 children, and additional fluid in joint space was found in 3. Involvement of facet joints was seen in 8 children including one child with 6 affected facet joints. Bone edema of masse lateralis and thickened ligaments were found in 2 children. Anterior atlanto-axial subluxation at presentation was seen in one girl (patient # 8). No morphological changes of bone (cortical thinning or dens deformation) or erosions were seen in the initial MRI examinations.

All children were initially treated with high-dose intravenous pulse methylprednisolone therapy followed by oral corticosteroid and methotrexate (MTX, 10-15 mg/m2/once per week per os). Eleven out of 15 (73.3%) patients were additionally treated with anti-TNFα drug within 3 months of clinical signs of cervical spine involvement confirmed by MRI (6 with infliximab, 3 with etanercept, and 2 with adalimumab). There was a delay in introduction of biological treatment in 3/15 children. The delay of 4 months between the initial sign of cervical spine involvement and treatment with biologics in one patient (#14) was due to parents concerns regarding the safety of biological treatment. Two patients in our cohort (#12 and # 13) were initially treated only with corticosteroids and MTX according to the decision of the treating physician and received treatment with infliximab 6 months after the beginning of cervical spine involvement due to unsatisfactory results with initial treatment seen in the follow-up MRI. Both patients were later treated with infliximab and achieved a sustained remission. One patient (#15) from our cohort was treated only with MTX and pulse methylprednisolone therapy and did not receive biologics due to parent refusal. This patient also achieved inactive disease state.

Follow-up

The mean observation time from diagnosis of cervical spine arthritis to July 2016 was 2.9 year (from 0.5 to 6.8 years).

At the last follow-up examination 4 children had still some cervical LROM, but all children were without pain, torticollis or neck stiffness. Peripheral joint arthritis persisted only in 4 patients with 1 to 5 active peripheral joints. ESR significantly decreased to mean value of 11 mm/h (range 4–25 mm/h). Decreases were also noted in the mean value of WBC (7.3 × 10^9/L (range 2.9–11.7)) and mean platelet count (308 × 10^9/L (range 128–411)), while hemoglobin level increased to the mean value of 123 g/L (range 107–141)).

Mean duration of treatment with biologics in our cohort was 2.2 years (range 0.5 to 4.5 years). In three patients treatment with biologics was stopped after a mean period of remission on treatment for 3.4 years (range 2.1 to 4.5 years). After stopping treatment with anti-TNFα two patients remained in sustained remission without any treatment for more than 2 years, and one patient continued treatment with MTX. A girl with jPsA (patient # 7) who stopped treatment with biologics after 2.1 years remained in remission without treatment for 2.3 years, and then presented with reactivation of cervical spine arthritis with MRI signs of synovitis of atlanto-axial, atlanto-occipital and right C2-C3 facet joints. She was retreated with infliximab and again achieved a stable remission for 1.5 years.

The last follow-up MRI revealed no signs of inflammation in 12 patients (6 with no signs of arthritis and 6 with minimal residuals in a form of minor patchy enhancement of cervical synovia, which could be considered as normal), in 2 patients improvement of arthritis, but with MRI signs of persistent active inflammation (remnants of synovial thickening with moderate contrast enhancement in patients # 5 and # 6, both received anti-TNFα for 6 months)(Fig. 1), and in one significant improvement of arthritis, but with mild to moderate MRI signs of active inflammation (patient#8) (Fig. 2).

Chronic changes (late sequels) in cervical spine due to inflammation were seen in 3 patients at the last follow-up MRI examination. Two of them (patients #12 and #15) had minor chronic changes in a form of irregular bone contour of dens and thinned corticalis. In addition, the girl with RF positive polyarthritis (patient #12) had thickened transverse ligament not compromising the spinal canal, and the boy (patient #15) had borderline aAAS (5 mm) without additional increase of the distance during functional radiography of cervical spine. More severe chronic changes were found in a girl (patient #8) who initially presented with severe inflammation in upper cervical spine and significant a AAS (13 mm), narrowing of spinal canal at this level with compression of the spinal cord at the initial MRI (Fig. 2a). At the last follow-up MRI the aAAS reduced to 6 mm with remnants of thickened ligament in anterior atlanto-axial space and morphologically deformed enlarged dens with bulging dorsal contour (Fig. 2b). There were no signs of chronic changes in other children.

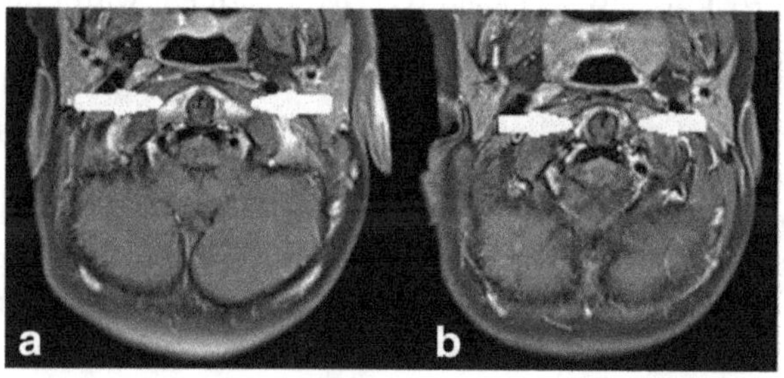

Fig. 1 MRI of cervical spine (patient #5) (T1 TSE FS axial with a contrast medium): **a** inital MRI showed an intense contrast enhancement of the thickened synovia in pre- and paradental space (white arrows), **b** follow-up MRI 6 months later showed a reduction of synovial thickening and a significantly less intense enhancement (white arrows)

Discussion

Cervical spine involvement in children with JIA is considered a poor prognostic factor and could be life threatening [19]. Therefore, obtaining a good insight into its frequency, clinical and imaging presentation is of vital importance.

According to published data, symptoms and signs correlate poorly with the degree of cervical spine inflammation and possible subluxations. In adult population, cervical spine involvement is seen in 35–65% of patients with JIA [3]. This wide range of reported cervical spine involvement in adult patients with juvenile-onset idiopathic arthritis could, to some extent, reflects recruitment bias since some studies were focused on clinical manifestations and others on radiographs or MRI changes [3, 9, 21, 22]. In our study, all children had LROM, 80% had neck pain, two neck stiffness and only one torticollis. These findings are in line with the German study suggesting that the LROM in cervical spine and not pain is a leading clinical sign of cervical spine arthritis [14]. The frequency of cervical spine involvement in our cohort of patients with JIA is estimated to be 4%. It is difficult to compare epidemiological data with other prevalence studies, because the duration of observation of patients in different studies varied or the studies were conducted only in selected JIA subtypes such as polyarticular and systemic forms of the disease. It is also important to note that different treatment modalities and protocols were used in the era before biologics, and more aggressive treatment, which is being used recently, may prevent some symptoms to develop. In addition, our study was conducted only in patients with cervical spine symptoms and some asymptomatic patients may have been missed.

A significant clinical observation in our study was that all children had peripheral joints involvement and in

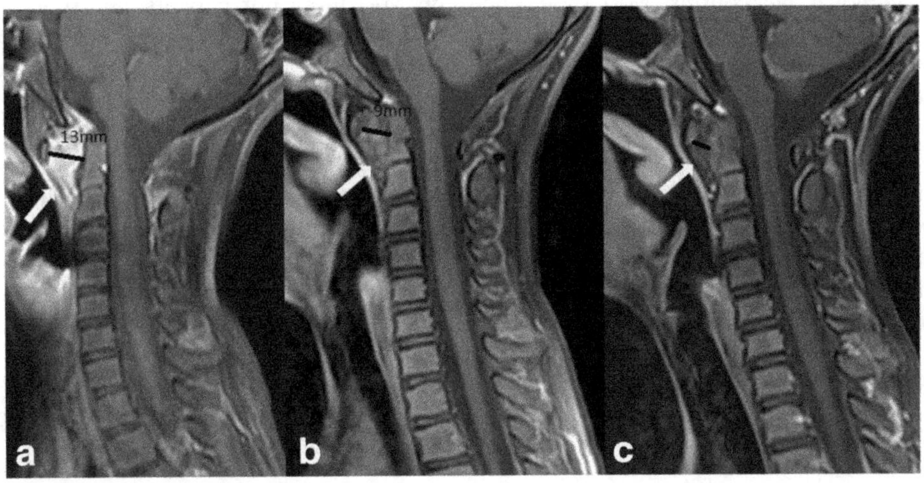

Fig. 2 MRI of cervical spine (patient #8)(T1 TSE FS sagittal with a contrast medium): **a** initial MRI (January, 2013) showed an intense contrast enhancement of a huge synovial thickening (white arrow) in predental space with a huge anterior atlanto-axial subluxation (aAAS)(black line, 13 mm) and a compression of the anterior liquor space, normal shape of the dens, **b** follow-up MR (January, 2014): the evaluation of the treatment with anti-TNFα showed a reduction of synovial thickening and a less intense contrast-enhancement and less significant aAAS, normal width of the anterior liquor space, but with initial morphological changes of the dens, **c** follow-up MRI (March, 2016): the evaluation of the treatment with anti-TNFα showed a significant reduction of synovial thickening in the predental space and aAAS, only patchy contrast enhancement, but with morphological changes of the dens and a thinned corticalis

addition, 20% of them had co-existing unilateral or bilateral TMJ arthritis. The TMJ MRI examinations from our patients with TMJ involvement showed severe TMJ inflammation in all cases with intensive synovitis, joint fluid and significant morphological changes of mandibular condyles. In only few TMJ MRI examinations atlanto-axial joint was seen on T2 coronal sequence and we found in one patient signs of inflammation in atlanto-axial joint without clinical complains of pain and LROM. To identify patients with TMJ arthritis and possible clinically covert cervical spine involvement we suggest to include the atlanto-axial joints in coronal plane also on standard TMJ MRI examinations.

Imaging in patients with JIA is particularly important for joints that are difficult to assess clinically such as hip, sacroiliac joint and spine. In adults radiography of the cervical spine is accepted as mandatory in rheumatoid arthritis patients with neck pain and it is well standardized. On the other hand, studies reported low sensitivity of radiography in children because it provides morphological and structural information more typical for late phase of inflammation (dens deformation, erosive changes) and various forms of malalignment and ankylosis, which are rare in children as a first manifestation of cervical spine arthritis [13, 23]. At least in the initial stage cervical spine radiography is not a routine imaging in children, but it can be useful in children with malalignment and persistent changes seen on MR to obtain functional information of cervical spine. The most frequently noted abnormalities seen on cervical radiography are apophyseal joint ankyloses or fusion at C2-C3, followed by aAAS, subaxial subluxation at levels between second and seventh cervical vertebrae, and erosions of the dens resulting in an “apple core” deformity [9]. Atlantoaxial impaction (AAI) is another serious complication of longstanding rheumatoid arthritis, rarely seen in childhood. In our cohort radiography of cervical spine was performed in 20% of children to evaluate the malalignment and morphological changes of bones due to persistent LROM or signs of aAAS presented on MRI. Contrast-enhanced MRI of cervical spine has become the method of choice in evaluation of inflammation in this region [11, 14]. Standardization of MRI protocol enables more reliable follow-up examinations and comparison of initial MRI with controls [15, 24]. The main advantage of MRI is its ability to detect early, often subclinical disease by directly visualizing not only soft tissues changes in a form of synovial thickening/enhancement, joint effusion, facet joints inflammation, and ligament evaluation, but also bone changes in a form of edema, cortical thinning, morphological changes (especially dens deformation, evaluation of bone erosions), and malalignment. The presence of bone marrow edema was recognized as a strong predictor of future erosions and it is considered as pre-erosive abnormality in adults and indication for treatment initiation to prevent permanent joint damage [25]. Early detection of joint pathology is of outmost importance with regards to the prompt therapeutic intervention. It is important to note that normal synovia in childhood can provide some degree of enhancement, and that there are no imaging criteria to clearly distinguish normal findings from early signs of arthritis. Moreover, postcontrast MRI should be performed during first 5–10 min of injection, because beyond this time diffusion of contrast material into the joints limits differentiation between enhancing synovia and adjunct joint fluid [26]. Rheumatoid arthritis MR imaging score (RAMRIS) has been shown to have acceptable applicability to children in evaluation of the inflammation and response to treatment despite differences in the pediatric and adult skeletons, but was primarily designed for peripheral joint and not for assessment of cervical spine [27, 28]. Synovitis of atlanto-axial joints was present on MRI in all our patients, and more than half of them had synovitis in other cervical joints compartments and facet joints. The degree of inflammation presented on MRI varied from mild (unilateral atlanto-axial inflammation) to moderate (bilateral inflammation) (Fig. 1) and severe (extensive pannus in atlanto-axial region)(Fig. 2). The early introduction of anti-TNFα in treatment of JIA patients with severe form of the disease provides an opportunity to delay or even prevent severe joint inflammation and subsequent destruction [20, 29]. MRI as objective imaging method has important role in evaluation

Table 1 Clinical and MRI examination data in patients with cervical spine involvement

	G	JIA	iMRI age (y)	Biologics	Treatment duration with biologics(y)	last MRI results		Clinical outcome
						Inflam	Chronic changes	
1	M	pJIA ANA+	4.1	ETA ADA	0.7 1.3	no	no	no inflam.
2	F	pJIA	7.6	IFX	1.8	no	no	no inflam.
3	F	pJIA ANA+	6.9	ETA	1	no	no	no inflam.
4	F	oJIA	3.2	ETA	2.8	no	no	no inflam.
5	M	pJIA ANA+ HLAB27+	2.4	IFX	0.5	peristent	no	Inflam. in 2 perif.joints
6	M	pJIA	14.8	IFX	0.5	persistent	no	LROM Inflam. in 5 perifer. joints
7	F	jPsA	3.6	IFX	2.1	no	no	no treatment for 2.3y
			8.2	IFX	1.5	no	no	LROM no inflam.
8	F	pJIA ANA+	8.7	IFX	3.5	peristent	yes	LROM Inflam. in 2 perif. joint
9	F	oJIA ANA+	15.1	IFX	1.2	no	no	no inflam.
10	F	pJIA	2.7	ADA TOC ETA	0.3 1.3 1.7	no	no	LROM no inflam.
11	F	oJIA	14.6	ADATOC	0.4 0.8	no	no	Inflam. in 1perif.joint
12	F	poJIA ANA+ RF+	3.1	IT IFX	0.5 4.5	no	yes	no inflam. uveitis noanti-TNFα for 2y MTX
13	F	poJIA ANA+	4.8	IT IFX	0.6 3.6	no	no	no inflam. no treatment for 2.2y
14	F	pJIA	2.5	IT ETA ADA	0.3 0.5 0.4 2.4	no	no	no inflam.
15	M	pJIA ANA+	4.2	IT MTX only	1.5 2.5	no	yes	no treatment for 1.4y

G gender, *F* female, *M* male, *pJIA* polyarticular juvenile idiopatic arthritis, *oJIA* extended oligoarthritis JIA, *poJIA* persistent oligoarthritis JIA, *jPsA* juvenile psoriatic arthritis, *iMRI* age of child when initial magnetic resonance imaging of cervical spine confirmed cervical spine arthritisBiologics, *IFX* infliximab, *ETA* etanercept, *ADA* adalimumab, and Anti IL-6, *TOC* tocilizumab, *IT* initial treatment with corticosteroids and methotrexate (MTX) received all children, duration of IT was written only in children with delay introduction of biologics Last MR: Inflam – no inflammation, persistent inflammation of cervical spine seen on last MRI, chronic changes - no chronic changes, yes- chronic changes seen on last MRI Clinical outcome: no inflammation – no inflammation in other peripheral joints, X periph.joints- number of peripheral joints presented with inflammation

of treatment response. The evaluation of early treatment with biologics is usually done by comparing initial and follow-up MRI examinations in each child. No official scoring system for MRI evaluation of cervical spine arthritis in children is available [15]. The only MRI based follow up study of cervical spine arthritis in children treated with anti-TNFα was done by Hospach et al. [14]. The cohort of patients in this study was comparable to our patients and included 13 children, 12 of whom were treated with biologics, but with longer median disease duration of 1.7 years after the diagnosis of JIA (in our cohort 5.2 months) and shorter observation time. A variable duration of treatment with MTX and biologics has not been specified. Our study was in concordance with the abovementioned study in evaluation of inflammation, and showing a significant reduction of MRI signs of inflammation in cervical spine. The most significant difference between the study of Hospach et al. and our study was the evaluation of "chronic/late" changes. The follow-up MRI examinations in the study of Hospach et al. described more chronic changes in a form of malalignment in 3 patients after treatment, ankyloses in 3, erosion in 2, and narrowing of spinal canal in 3. In our study, half of the children with delayed biologic treatment had minor chronic changes compared to children with early introduction of biologics, where only one girl (#8) with severe and persistent inflammation developed more severe chronic changes, including dens deformation with bulging into spinal canal, thickened transverse ligament and persistent aAAS (Fig. 2). The low rate of long term consequences in our study could be due to earlier recognition with shorter disease duration and early aggressive treatment with biologics.

In 3 children we were able to withdraw the anti-TNFα after 2.1, 3.6 and 4.5 years, respectively. The duration of treatment depended on clinical signs of arthritis not only in cervical spine, but also in peripheral joints. In one patient (#7) disease relapse occurred after 2.3 years of inactive disease with a good response to reintroduction of anti-TNFα treatment. In 4 children the anti-TNFα was changed due to disease relapse in peripheral joints or unsatisfactory treatment result of cervical inflammation; two of our refractory JIA patients received also anti-IL-6 therapy as specified in the Table 1.

Limitations of our study include the retrospective design and small cohort of patients. Additional limitation is also the lack of a real gold standard in determination of the severity of neck arthritis. In spite of the limited number of patients, our results demonstrated that early and aggressive treatment of cervical spine arthritis with anti-TNFα could provide good results with elimination of inflammation (early response) and has a potential to reduce/deminish the chronic changes. According to our experience, in all children with persistent LROM MRI should be performed and if inflammation is confirmed, anti-TNFα treatment should be considered [20]. The follow-up MRI examinations are individually addressed. However, according to our and others experiences [14], we suggest the first follow-up MRI after 9 months, and if the clinical and laboratory responses are satisfactory, the second follow-up MRI should be performed 1 year later to evaluate possible development of chronic/late sequels. If the clinical signs of cervical arthritis persist, MRI should be performed earlier (after 6 months). Due to high incidence of co-existing TMJ inflammation (20% in our cohort), we suggest that the transversal plane during MR examination of cervical spine include TMJ (at least one of the fluid sensitive sequences). On the contrary, in children with MRI examination of TMJ atlanto-axial joint should be included in one of the fluid sensitive coronal sequences.

Conclusions

In conclusion, in children with JIA and cervical spine involvement the early treatment with anti-TNFα drugs showed good results evaluated with follow-up MR examinations. Prompt treatment led to significantly reduced inflammation or complete remission, and prevented the development of chronic/late changes. To determine the prevalence and severity of chronic changes in patients with early cervical arthritis treated with "biologics" further long term studies should be performed in larger population of JIA patients.

Abbreviations

aAAS: Anterior atlanto-axial subluxation; ANA: Antinuclear antibody; ESR: Erythrocyte sedimentation rate; HLA: Human leukocyte antigen; JIA: Juvenile idiopathic arthritis; jPsA: Juvenile psoriatic arthritis; LROM: Limited range of motion; MRI: Magnetic resonance imaging; MTX: Methotrexate; oJIA: Juvenile oligoarthritis; pJIA: Juvenile polyarthritis; RAMRIS: Rheumatoid arthritis MR imaging score; RF: Rheumatoid factor; STIR: Short Tau inversion recovery; TMJ: Temporomandibular joint; WBC: White blood cell

Acknowledgements

Not applicable.

Funding

There were no extra funding related to this study.

Author's contributions

TA and DK accompanied in designing the study. NT and NE analysed and interpreted the patient data regarding the clinical and laboratory data. DK analysed and interpreted the MRI examinations. All authors collaborated in writing the manuscript, read and approved the final manuscript.

Competing interests
TA declares speakers bureau (AbbVie, Pfizer, Octapharma) and advisory board (Bristol-Myers Squibb, Octapharma, Boehringer-Ingelheim). DK, NE and NT declare that they have no competing interest.

Consent for publication
Not applicable.

Author details
[1]Radiology Unit, University Children's Hospital Ljubljana, Ljubljana, Slovenia. [2]Department of Allergology, Rheumatology and Clinical Immunology, University Children's Hospital Ljubljana, Ljubljana, Slovenia. [3]Department of Pediatrics, Medical Faculty, University of Ljubljana, Ljubljana, Slovenia.

References

1. Wolfs JF, Arts MP, Peul WC. Juvenile chronic arthritis and the craniovertebral junction in the paediatric patient: review of the literature and management considerations. Adv Tech Stand Neurosurg. 2014;41:143–56.
2. Reiter MF, Boden SD. Inflammatory disorders of the cervical spine. Spine (Phila Pa 1976). 1998;23(24):2755–66.
3. Elhai M, Wipff J, Bazeli R, et al. Radiological cervical spine involvement in young adults with polyarticular juvenile idiopathic arthritis. Rheumatology (Oxford). 2013;52:267–75.
4. Jurik AG. Imaging the spine in arthritis – a pictorial review. Insight Imaging. 2011;2:177–91.
5. Sheybani EF, Khanna G, White AJ, Demertzis JL. Imaging of juvenile idiopathic arthritis: a multimodality approach. Radiographics. 2013;33:1253–73.
6. Tins BJ, Bulter R. Imaging in rheumatology: reconciling radiology and rheumatology. Insight Imaging. 2013;4:799–810.
7. Joaquim AF, Ghizoni E, Tedeschi H, Appenzeller S, Riew KD. Radiological evaluation of cervical spine involvement in rheumatoid arthritis. Neurosurg Focus. 2015;38(4):E4.
8. Bouchaud-Chabot A, Lioté F. Cervical spine involvement in rheumatoid arthritis. A review. Joint Bone Spine. 2002;69:141–54.
9. Kjellberg H, Pavlou I. Changes in the cervical spine of children with juvenile idiopathic arthritis evaluated with lateral cephalometric radiographs: a case control study. Angle Orthod. 2011;81:447–52.
10. Damasio MB, Malattia C, Martini A, Tomà P. Synovial and inflammatory diseases in childhood: role of new imaging modalities in the assessment of patients with juvenile idiopathic arthritis. Pediatr Radiol. 2010;40:985–98.
11. Damasio MB, de Horatio LT, Boavida P, et al. Imaging in juvenile idiopathic arthritis (JIA): an update with particular emphasis on MRI. Acta Radiol. 2013;54:1015–23.
12. Munir S, Patil K, Miller E, et al. Juvenile idiopathic arthritis of the axial joints: a systematic review of the diagnostic accuracy and predictive value of conventional MRI. AJR. 2014;202:199–210.
13. Oren B, Oren H, Osma E, Cevik N. Juvenile rheumatoid arthritis: cervical spine and MRI in early diagnosis. Turk J Pediatr. 1996;38:189–94.
14. Hospach T, Maier J, Műller-Abt P, Patel A, Horneff G, von Kalle T. Cervical spine involvement in patients with juvenile idiopathic arthritis - MRI follow-up study. Pediatr Rheumatol Online J. 2014 Mar 4;12:9.
15. Nusman C, Ording Müller LS, Hemke R, et al. Current status of efforts on standardizing magnetic resonance imaging of juvenile idiopathic arthritis: report from the OMERACT MRI in JIA working group and health-e-child. J Rheumatol. 2016;43:239–44.
16. Müller LS, Avenarius D, Damasio B, et al. The paediatric wrist revisited: redefining MR findings in healthy children. Ann Rheum Dis. 2011;70:605–10.
17. Ording Müller LS, Boavida P, Avenarius D, et al. MRI of the wrist in juvenile idiopathic arthritis: erosions or normal variants. A prospective case-control study. Pediatr Radiol. 2013;43:785–95.
18. Boavida P, Lambot-Juhan K, Müller LS, et al. Carpal erosions in children with juvenile idiopathic arthritis: repeatability of a newly devised MR-scoring system. Pediatr Radiol. 2015;45:1972–80.
19. Beukelman T, Patkar NM, Saag KG, Tolleson-Rinehart S, Cron RQ, DeWitt EM, et all. American College of Rheumatology recommendations for the treatment of juvenile idiopathic arthritis: initiation and safety monitoring of therapeutic agents for the treatment of arthritis and systemic features. Arthritis Care Res. 2011; 63(4):465-482.
20. Blazina S, Markelj G, Avramovič ZM, Toplak N, Avčin T. Management of Juvenile Idiopathic Arthritis: a clinical guide. Paediatr Drugs. 2016;18(6):397–412.
21. Laiho K, Savolainen A, Kautiainen H, Kekki P, Kauppi M. The cervical spine in juvenile chronic arthritis. Spine J. 2002;2(2):89–94.
22. Hofer MF, Cimaz R. Is cervical spine involvement in juvenile polyarthritis under-recognized? Rheumatology (Oxford). 2013;52(2):221–2.
23. Fried JA, Arhtreya B, Gregg JR, Das M, Doughty R. The cervical spine in juvenile rheumatoid arthritis. Clinical Orthopedics Relat Res. 1983;179:102–6.
24. Colebatch-Bourn AN, Edwards CJ, Collado P, et al. EULAR-PReS points to consider for the use of imaging in the diagnosis and management of juvenile idiopathic arthritis in clinical practice. Ann Rheum Dis. 2015;74(11):1946–57.
25. Narváez JA, Narváez J, de Albert M. De Lamae, Serrallonga M, Nolla JM. Bone marrow edema in the cervical spine of symptomatic rheumatoid arthritis patients. Semin Arthritis Rheum. 2009;38(4):281–8.
26. Østergaard M, Klarlund M. Importance of timing of post-contrast MRI in rheumatoid arthritis: what happens during the first 60 minutes after IV gadolinium-DTPA? Ann Rheum Dis. 2001;60(11):1050–4.
27. Hemke R, Doria AS, Tzaribachev N, Maas M, van der Heijde DM, van Rossum MA. Selecting magnetic resonance imaging (MRI) outcome measures for juvenile idiopathic arthritis (JIA) clinical trials: first report of the MRI in JIA special interest group. J Rheumatol. 2014;41(2):354–8.
28. Malata C, Damasio BM, Pistorio A. Development and preliminary validation of a paediatric-targeted MRI scoring system for the assessment of disease activity and damage in juvenile idiopathic arthritis. Ann Rheum Dis. 2011;70:440–6.
29. Ilowite NT. Update on biologics in juvenile idiopathic arthritis. Curr Opin Rheumatol. 2008;20:613–8.

Early feeding and risk of Juvenile idiopathic arthritis: a case control study in a prospective birth cohort

Erik Kindgren[1,2*], Mats Fredrikson[3,4] and Johnny Ludvigsson[2]

Abstract

Background: Juvenile idiopathic arthritis (JIA) is considered to be an autoimmune disease, but the etiology is unknown. We decided to study the influence of early nutrition on later development of JIA.

Methods: All parents with children born between October 1, 1997 and October 1, 1999 in Southeast Sweden were asked to participate in the ABIS prospective cohort study (All Babies in Southeast Sweden), At 1 year, questionnaires with information on breastfeeding and introduction of foods were completed by 10,565 families. We identified 32 children with JIA and 111 children with non-chronic arthritis with completed questionnaires after delivery and after 1 year. A multivariable logistic regression model, adjusted for relevant factors, was performed to calculate the association between JIA and feeding during the first year of life.

Results: An increased risk for JIA was found in children who had breast fed for less than 4 months, as opposed to those who were continued on breast milk beyond 4 months of age (aOR 3.5, 95% CI 1.4-8,5; $p = 0.006$). A short duration of exclusive as well as total breastfeeding was associated with an increased risk of JIA (aOR 1.3, 95% CI 1.1-1.6; $p = 0.008$ and aOR 1.2, 95% CI 1.1-1.3; $p < 0.001$). All associations between breastfeeding and JIA persisted after adjustment. There was no relationship between early nutrition and non-chronic arthritis.

Conclusions: Our results indicate that there are different disease mechanisms for different types of arthritis in childhood. Longer duration of breastfeeding (both total and exclusive) may protect against development of JIA. Mothers should be encouraged to breast-feed their babies exclusively, if at all possible, for 4 months and continue partial breastfeeding for an extended time when foreign proteins are introduced.

Keywords: Juvenile idiopathic arthritis (JIA), Arthritis, Epidemiology, Autoimmunity, Nutrition, Reactive arthritis, Breastfeeding, Rheumatic disease

Background

Juvenile idiopathic arthritis (JIA), the most common chronic rheumatic disease of childhood, is a collection of chronic pediatric arthritis characterized by onset before 16 years of age and the presence of arthritis (inflammation of the synovium with thickening of the synovial lining and accumulation of synovial fluid) for at least 6 weeks [1].

JIA is considered to be an autoimmune disease, which is a result of an immune reaction caused or triggered by environmental factors in a genetically susceptible individual. The starting point of autoimmunity leading to this disease is still unknown.

The mother's immunological memory is transferred to her infant via breast milk, and breast milk contains a variety of immune-modulating compounds, both immune cells and their products such as cytokines. Breastfeeding leads to immunological imprinting and programming of the infant [2], and thereby contributes to the maturity of the infant's immune system [3–5]. It has been proposed that breastfeeding might protect against the development of JIA [6]. Another study noted a tendency of shorter breastfeeding among children who later developed oligoarticular JIA [7]. However, breastfeeding did not show

* Correspondence: erik@kindgren.org
[1]Department of Pediatrics, Västervik Hospital, Västervik, Sweden
[2]Division of Pediatrics, Department of Clinical and Experimental Medicine, Linköping University, Linköping, Sweden

any protective effect against JIA in subsequent studies [8–10]. A cohort study from UK recently showed that breastfeeding is associated with milder onset of JIA [11]. Previous studies have been retrospective case-control studies. To get more reliable unbiased results, we have analyzed data on early feeding of children in a prospective cohort study of the general population, the ABIS study (All Babies in Southeast Sweden). The primary aim of this study was to explore feeding factors, such as breastfeeding, in relation to risk of later development of JIA. Increased knowledge of the role of early nutrition of the child and its association with autoimmunity is of great importance for public health, as dietary recommendations may help to prevent these chronic diseases.

Methods

In Sweden, all children aged 0-18 years with diagnosed JIA or Rheumatoid Arthritis (RA) are treated at pediatric clinics in hospitals or pediatric rheumatology clinics. The Swedish National Patient Register is maintained by the Swedish National Board of Health and Welfare (http://www.socialstyrelsen.se/english). This population-based register, was launched in 1964, but complete coverage of all in-patient care in Sweden did not begin until 1987 [12]. Currently, more than 99% of all somatic and psychiatric hospital discharges are registered. Since 2001 the register also covers outpatient visits from both private and public caregivers. Diseases are coded using International Classification of Diseases (ICD) codes and for each healthcare contact several items are recorded, including personal identity number (PIN - a unique 10-digit number assigned to all Swedish residents) [13], date of admission and discharge, hospital and primary and secondary diagnoses.

The Swedish JIA-registry started in 2009 with the primary goal to follow all children on cytokine modulators, but later expanded to all children with JIA. In 2014 there were 1700 patients included and coverage was almost complete. Through the unique PIN, information on each individual patient can be linked to other registries.

Participants and design

All parents with children born between October 1,1997 and October 1,1999 in Southeast Sweden (n = 21,700) were asked to participate in the ABIS study, a prospective cohort study. 17,055 (78.6%) out of the 21,700 families who were asked gave their informed consent to participate. Questionnaires were completed at birth and then at the ages 1, 2.5, 5, 8 and 11-13. Different biological samples were collected. A diary was used for daily registration of certain facts related to nutrition, infections etc. during the first year of life. In the questionnaires, parents were asked for the duration of breastfeeding. Exclusive breastfeeding is defined as the infant receiving only breast-milk. Partial breastfeeding is defined as breastfeeding in addition to formula or other food (corresponding to WHO's definition of complementary feeding) [14]. Total duration of breastfeeding is defined as the length of any kind of breastfeeding.

We also have considered a possible influence by the introduction of infant formula or gruel, cow's milk and gluten, heredity, mode of delivery, and various socioeconomic variables such as civil status, parental age, education, smoking habits, and whether or not the parents were born outside Sweden. Questions pertaining to the duration of exclusive breastfeeding and total duration of breastfeeding, as well as the time for introduction of formulas and other semi-solid (infant formula, follow-on formula) and solid foods (porridge, first solid food) had response alternatives of months (after birth), usually from 1 to ≥9. The 1 year questionnaires were completed by 10,883 families, and in addition a detailed diary during the first year of life, including the exact time (date) of weaning and introduction of different food items, was collected for 9849 children. All subjects with missing values were excluded from the statistical model.

Using the Swedish personal identification number [13], we linked data between the ABIS-cohort and The Swedish National Patient Register [12]. Diagnoses are classified according to the ICD, versions 8 to 10. We identified 59 children, born between October 1, 1997 and October 1, 1999 in the ABIS region, with inpatient hospital discharges or outpatient visits who had a diagnostic code of JIA (M08-09 on ICD 8-10) and had accepted to participate in ABIS. After communication with all pediatric rheumatologists at local hospitals who reviewed the medical records of all 59 patients, 17 patients were excluded due to misdiagnosis (mostly arthritis that later proved to be reactive arthritis). Three of the 59 children had moved out of the ABIS region, but could be found with the PIN. Of the remaining 42 children, 41 guardians had completed the screening questionnaire after delivery, and 32 of them had completed both the screening questionnaire after delivery and the 1 year follow up questionnaire. 29 of 32 had also completed the diary during the first year. All cases of JIA were controlled via The Swedish pediatric JIA-registry.

We identified 111 patients in the same cohort with an episode of a transient non-chronic arthritis, with only one joint involved with a maximum duration of 6 weeks. 12% (13/111) of them were diagnosed with reactive arthritis and 88% (95/111) with unspecified arthritis (M02 respective M13 on ICD 8-10). The risk of rheumatic disease is considered to be minimal in this group, with only one period of monoarthritis with a short duration throughout the 17-19 year-long follow up period.

Data were analyzed as a case-control study with two groups of cases (JIA and non-chronic arthritis) and remaining children as controls.

Statistics

The normality for independent variables was revised both graphically and by the Shapiro–Wilk test and, subsequently, homogeneity of variance was tested using Levene's test.

Univariate logistic regression was used to calculate odds ratio (OR) and 95% confidence intervals (95% CIs). We used JIA as the dependent variable. Duration of breastfeeding (continuous as months from the 1-year questionnaire and as days from the diary), age of introduction of food (continuous as months) and possible confounding factors (listed below) associated with incidence of JIA were analyzed. In the second statistical model we used the same covariates but changed the dependent variable to non-chronic arthritis. Duration of breastfeeding was also dichotomized to shorter or longer than 4 and 6 months respectively, according to the recommendation to introduce solid food during 4 to 6 months. Adjusted odds ratio (aOR) was calculated in the final multivariable logistic regression model. Variables with $p < 0.1$ in the univariate analyses were included in the adjusted model as possible confounding factors associated breastfeeding. Attributable risk percent was calculated using the formula two in Rockhill et al. [15].

All *P*-values are two-tailed. A *P*-value below 0.05 and a 95% CI not overlapping the null value 1.00 for the OR were regarded as statistically significant.

Possible confounding factors were: heredity for rheumatism (JIA or RA in first- and second-degree relatives), parity, mode of delivery, preterm birth, introduction of formula,

parent-reported infections during child's first year of life (cold, fever, throat infection/tonsillitis, influenza, otitis media, pneumonia, measles, rubella, mumps, pertussis, varicella, urinary tract infection, gastroenteritis and other infection), mother's civil status, parental age, education, smoking habits, and whether or not the parents were born outside Sweden.

Statistics were calculated using the Statistical Package for Social Science (SPSS 20.0 software; SPSS Inc., Chicago, IL, USA).

Results

Cases

32 cases of JIA with complete questionnaires after delivery and at the 1 year follow up were identified. The most common JIA category was oligoarticular disease (Table 1). The unclassified based on the ILAR-criteria [1], either not fulfill criteria for any category or they meet categorization for 2 subtypes. Family history of RA/JIA in first-degree family member was present in only one patient in both the JIA-group (3%) and the group with non-chronic arthritis (1%) compared with 130 controls (1%) (Table 1). A family history of RA/JIA in a second-degree family member was more common; three patients in the JIA-group (9%), 16 in the group with non-chronic arthritis (14%), and 940 of the controls (9%).

Exclusive breastfeeding

One-year post-birth questionnaire data from the whole ABIS cohort 1 year after birth showed that the mean duration of exclusive breastfeeding was four and a half months, the same for boys and girls. The corresponding mean in the JIA-group was three and a half months. At the age of 3 months 78.4% of the unaffected children were exclusively breastfed compared to 61.3% in the affected (JIA) group (Fig. 1). A short duration of exclusive breastfeeding was significantly associated with an increased risk of JIA in logistic regression with continuous variables, both by months (from the one-year post-birth questionnaire) and by days (from the diary).

Dichotomized, exclusive breastfeeding less than 4 months, had highest statistical significance, associated with increased risk of developing JIA (aOR 2.50, 95% CI 1.20-5.56, $p = 0.029$), and attributable risk percent at 60.02%. Stratified data for end of breastfeeding are given in Table 2.

All associations between exclusive breastfeeding and JIA remained statistically significant when factors such as parental smoking, parents′ education, parental country of birth, parental age, heredity for rheumatism, preterm birth and introduction of formula and infections during the first year of life were included in the analysis (aOR 1.30, 95% CI 1.07-1.57; $p = 0.008$).

The group with non-chronic arthritis had the same mean (4.55 months) as the general population and there was no significant association between exclusive breastfeeding and non-chronic arthritis.

Risk factors associated with short-term exclusive breastfeeding

The main logistic regression showed that short-term exclusive breastfeeding was positively associated with older maternal age (aOR 1.42, 95% CI 1.25-1.42), paternal age (over 37 years) (aOR 0.74; 95% CI 0.55–0.99; $p = 0.045$), maternal BMI >30 (aOR 1.07; 95% CI 1.05–1.09; $p < 0.001$) and with maternal smoking (aOR 1.43; 95% CI 1.05–1.95; $p = 0.023$). Short-term exclusive breastfeeding was more often reported by single parents (aOR 2.10; 95% CI 1.43–3.09; $p < 0.001$).

Short-term exclusive breastfeeding was less common if one of the parents had a university degree (Mother: aOR 0.74; 95% CI 0.61–0.90; $p = 0.003$, Father: aOR 0.73; 95% CI 0.58–0.92; $p = 0.008$).

Total duration of breastfeeding

The mean duration of total breastfeeding was 1.5 months less in the affected children than the unaffected children

Table 1 Risk of JIA and non-chronic arthritis according to early feeding and family history. *P*-values from logistic regression. Classification according to ILAR criteria. The number (n) and proportion (%) of patients in each category

	Controls	Non-chronic arthritis			JIA				
		Univariate analysis[a] vs controls			Univariate analysis vs controls			Adjusted for potential confounding factors[b]	
	(*n* = 10,883)	(*n* = 111)	OR (95% CI)	p	(*n* = 32)	OR (95% CI)	p	aOR (95% CI)	p
Duration of exclusive breastfeeding									
Mean (SD) months	4.5 (1.9)	4.6 (1.9)			3.6 (1,6)				
Median (Range) months	4 (1 - 9)	4 (1 - 9)	1.0 (0.9-1.1)	0.879	4 (1 - 7)	1.3 (1.1-1.6)	**0.004**	**1.3 (1.1-1.6)**	**0.008**
Mean (SD) days[c]	126 (60)	135 (61)			109 (55)	1.0 (1.0-1.0)	**0.005**	**1.0 (1.0-1.0)**	**0.009**
Exclusive breastfeeding <4 months (n)	5351 (52.3%)	61 (51%)	1.3 (0.9-2.1)	0.220	22 (73%)	2.5 (1.2-5.6)	**0.026**	**2.5 (1.2-5.6)**	**0.029**
Duration of total breastfeeding									
Mean (SD) months	7.1 (2.4)	7.2 (2.4)			5.7 (2.8)				
Median (Range) months	8 (1 - 9)	8 (1 - 9)	0.99 (0.9-1.1)	0.940	6 (1 - 9)	1.2 (1.1-1.4)	**<0.001**	**1.2 (1.1-1.3)**	**<0.001**
Mean (SD) days[d]	219 (82)	225 (90)	0.97 (0.9-1.1)	0.982	166 (100)	1.0 (1.0-1.0)	**<0.001**	**1.0 (1.0-1.0)**	**<0.001**
Total breastfeeding <4 months (n)	1694(16%)	19 (18%)	1.1 (0.7-1.8)	0.715	11 (36%)	2.8 (1.3-5.8)	**0.006**	**2.8 (1.3-5.7)**	**0.009**
Total breastfeeding <6 months (n)	3166 (31%)	33 (31%)	1.0 (0.7-1.5)	0.981	19 (61%)	3.6 (1.7-7.4)	**<0.001**	**3.5 (1.6-6.2)**	**<0.001**
Introduction of cow's milk formula									
Mean (SD) months	4.8 (2.5)	4.9 (2.7)	1.0 (0.9-1.1)	0.770	3.9 (2.2)	1.2 (1.0-1.3)	0.052	1.0 (1.0-1.3)	0.055
Median (Range) months	5 (1 - 9)	6 (1 - 9)			4 (1 - 9)				
Introduction of gluten									
Mean (SD) months	6.0 (1.39)	5.9 (1.4)	1.0 (0.9-1.2)	0.563	5.8 (1.27)	1.1 (0.9-1.4)	0.483	No analysis performed	
Median (Range) months	6 (1 - 9)	6 (3 - 9)			6 (4 - 8)				
Family history / Heredity for JIA/RA									
Mother with RA (n)	100 (1%)	1 (1%)	0.9 (0.3-6.7)	0.941	1 (3%)	3.5 (0.5-2.6)	0.223	No analysis performed	
Father with RA (n)	31 (0%)	0 (0%)	0	1.000	0 (0%)	0	1.000	No analysis performed	
Siblings with JIA/RA (n)	0 (0%)	0 (0%)	0	1.000	0 (0%)	0	1.000	No analysis performed	
2nd degree family member with RA (n)	940 (9%)	16 (14%)	1.7 (0.98-2.8)	0.06	3 (9%)	1.7 (0.98-2.8)	0.910	No analysis performed	
Category at Onset (ILAR) (n)									
Oligoarticular[a]					14 (44%)				
Polyarticular[e]					4 (13%)				
Enthesitis-related arthritis					2 (6%)				
Psoriatic arthritis					3 (9%)				
Systemic					4 (13%)				
Unclassifiable					5 (16%)				

[a] Patients with oligoarticular disease, not possible to classify as extended or persistent because of missing data

[b] Potential confounding factors were heredity for rheumatism (JIA or RA in first- and second-degree relatives), parity, mode of delivery, preterm birth, infections during the first year of life, introduction of formula, the parents' level of education, smoking and age as well as country of birth

[c] Data from diary: Control (*n* = 8913); Non-chronic arthritis (*n* = 79); JIA (*n* = 29)

[d] Data from diary: Control (*n* = 9732); Non-chronic arthritis (*n* = 105); JIA (*n* = 31)

[e] Patients with polyarticular disease, not possible to classify as RF positive or negative because of missing data

(5.65 v. 7.09 months). The percentages of control infants who were breastfed at 3, 6 and ≥9 months of age were 87.9, 69.1 and 43.6, respectively. The corresponding percentages for any breastfeeding in the JIA-affected group were 73.3, 40.0 and 26.7 (Fig. 1). A short duration of total breastfeeding was associated with an increased risk of JIA in logistic regression with continuous variables.

Total duration of breastfeeding less than 4 months was associated with increased risk of developing JIA (aOR 2.75, 95% CI 1.33-5.71, p = 0.009), with a attributable risk percent at 64,17%.

The adjusted odds ratio for increased risk of JIA was 3.5 (95% CI 1.6-6,2; p = 0.001) if the total duration of breastfeeding stopped at or before 6 months of age, with a attributable risk percent at 71.97%.

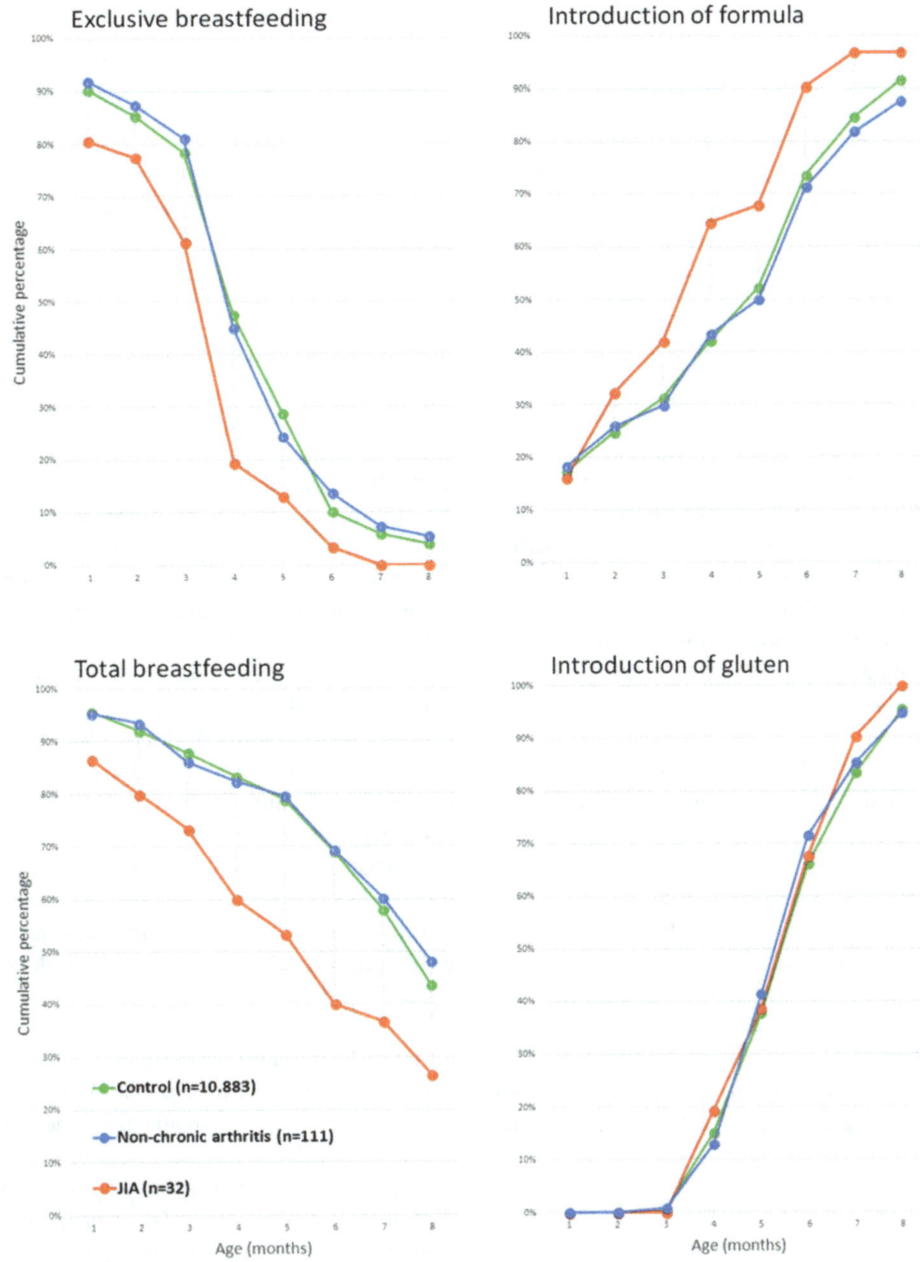

Fig. 1 Cumulative percentages for duration of exclusive and total breastfeeding, as well as cumulative percentages for time of introduction of formula and gluten

Estimates between total duration of breastfeeding and JIA remained significant after adjusting for potential confounders including parental smoking, education, parental country of birth, parental age, heredity, preterm birth, introduction of formula, and infections during the first year of life (aOR 1.20, 95% CI 1.07-1.34 $p < 0.001$).

Non-chronic arthritis had the same mean duration (7.15 months) as the general population and there were no significant associations.

Risk factors associated with total duration of breastfeeding

Both maternal ($P < 0.001$) and paternal age ($P < 0.001$) were positively associated with the total duration of breastfeeding. Short-term exclusive breastfeeding was more often reported by younger mothers.

Introduction of cow's milk formula

According to the questionnaire at 1 year, the mean age of introduction of formulas containing cow's milk was 1

Table 2 End of breastfeeding comparison between JIA and Non-chronic arthritis vs. Controls. OR and *P*-values from logistic regression

	Controls	Non-chronic arthritis			JIA		
	(*n* = 10,189)	(*n* = 105)	OR (95% CI)	p	(*n* = 29)	OR (95% CI)	p
End of exclusive breastfeeding							
Months 1-4 (0-120 days)	3261 (37%)	27 (34%)	1 (ref)	0.700	16 (57%)	1 (ref)	**0.023**
Months 5-8 (121-240 days)	5374 (60%)	48 (61%)	0.9 (0.6-1.3)	0.458	12 (43%)	0.3 (0.1-0.7)	**0.006**
Months 9-12 (241-365 days)	269 (3%)	4 (5%)	1.1 (0.5-2.8)	0.800	0 (0%)	0	0.994
End of total breastfeeding							
Months 1-4 (0-120 days)	1579 (15%)	20 (19%)	1 (ref)	0.558	11 (38%)	1 (ref)	**0.003**
Months 5-8 (121-240 days)	3569 (35%)	34 (32%)	0.8 (0.4-1.3)	0.315	11 (38%)	0.4 (0.2-1.0)	0.056
Months 9-12 (241-365 days)	5041 (50%)	51 (49%)	0.8 (0.5-1.3)	0.397	7 (24%)	0.2 (0.1-0.5)	**0.001**

month less in the JIA affected group than the unaffected (3.94 v. 4.82 months) (Fig. 1). In logistic regression analysis, early introduction of cow's milk formula (before 4 months of age) was associated with an increased risk of developing JIA (OR 2.49, 95% CI 1.19-5.21; p = 0.015). There was only a tendency of association between introduction of cow's milk and JIA (aOR 0.87, 95% CI 0.997-1.32; p = 0.055) in logistic regression with continuous variables.

Non-chronic arthritis had the same mean (4.92 months) as the general population and there were no significant associations.

The age at introduction of formulas containing cow's milk correlated negatively with both duration of exclusive breastfeeding (r 0.6, $p < 0.001$) and total duration of breastfeeding (r 0.575, $p < 0.001$).

Introduction of gluten

We did not observe any significant association between age at introduction of gluten and risk of JIA or non-chronic arthritis (Fig. 1).

Discussion

In the present study, we found that a short total duration of breastfeeding as well as a short duration of exclusive breastfeeding was associated with an increased risk of JIA. An early introduction of formula (<4 months of age) was associated with an increased risk of JIA. All associations remained statistically significant when potential confounders were included in the model.

Children with non-chronic arthritis had the same pattern of breastfeeding and introduction of formula as the general population. This suggests different disease mechanisms for different types of arthritis in children. Breastfeeding appears to be involved in the origin of autoimmunity causing Juvenile idiopathic arthritis.

Breastfeeding data

The average breastfeeding duration in our study was similar to that among infants in Norway [16], Iceland [17] and Denmark [18], showing a relatively high prevalence of breastfeeding in Scandinavia compared with other parts of the Western world [19–21].

The data on total duration of breastfeeding is in good agreement with data from Official Statistics of Sweden [22] for the same area during the study period 1997–1999. Data is also consistent with the breastfeeding prevalence in the entire country during the years 1997–1999 (The National Board of Health and Welfare, 2001, . This indicates that the frequency of breastfeeding in ABIS infants during 1997–1999 was in line with current national recommendations, i.e. almost 85% of infants were breastfed until 4 months of age and more than 90% were introduced to solid food during the recommended 4 to 6 months.

Study strengths and limitations

Earlier studies on the association between breastfeeding and JIA/JCA are all retrospective, and the results may be compromised by recall bias. Mason et al. [6] showed that children with Juvenile Rheumatoid Arthritis were less likely, then their matched controls, to have been breastfed. This could not be confirmed in subsequent studies [8–10]. However, these reports have mainly excluded children with Enthesitis-related arthritis and Psoriatic arthritis. In a relatively large study, Hyrich et al. recently showed that breastfeeding is associated with milder onset of JIA [11]. This, in addition to our results, provides the most reliable evidence so far for an association between breastfeeding and JIA. Breastfeeding may be associated with lesser occurrence, milder or delayed onset of this autoimmune disease.

Our study has several notable strengths. First, our prospective study design avoids the potential recall and selection biases of retrospective, case-control studies which collect data on diet, nutrition, feeding practice and lifestyle after the diagnosis of JIA. Second, all cases of JIA collected through the unique 10-digit PIN with codes from the Swedish National Patient Register have been confirmed via The Swedish pediatric JIA-registry and the medical records, a significant advantage over studies that rely on self-report. Third, the availability of detailed information on parental smoking, socio economic factors, parental age and heredity, and other important early life factors allowed us to control for a number of potential confounding factors that may have influenced our observed associations. Finally, we have detailed information regarding other potential early life factors, including infectious diseases and early exposure to antibiotics, which may also influence risk of JIA.

Even though we find significant correlations one has to be cautious in the conclusions. A limitation of our study is the small patient sample, due to the nature of the study i.e. a birth cohort of a relative rare disease. There are large variations in the clinical severity of the disease between the JIA categories. Therefore, different categories of JIA should be studied as separate groups [23, 24]. The patient sample in this study was too small to allow subgroup analysis.

Another weakness of the current study could be that the nutritional data was collected from the questionnaire at 1 year after birth, and there is a risk of recall bias [25]. However, this risk should not be overestimated as Launer et al. [26] have shown that mothers may well be aware of the breastfeeding duration of their latest child. When we compare breastfeeding data from the 1 year questionnaires and from the diary, the durations were comparable, indicating minimal risk of recall bias.

Although this is a cohort study we have chosen to analyze it with a case-control design since the exposure, duration of breastfeeding, is a continuous variable.

Possible mechanisms underlying the protective effect of breastfeeding

Socioeconomic status affects the duration of breastfeeding, as was shown in our study. However, the relationship between breastfeeding and JIA persisted after adjusting for socioeconomic differences.

In Sweden, most children receive cow's milk formula as their first source of foreign protein. The early introduction of cow's milk formula correlated significantly with both the duration of exclusive breastfeeding and the duration of total breastfeeding, which is a confounding factor in this kind of study [27]. However, the statistical analysis with logistic regression shows that exclusive duration of breastfeeding (OR 1.28) and adjusting for introduction of cow's milk formula (OR 1.32), indicating that breastfeeding has an independent protective effect against JIA.

Introduction of foreign proteins during breastfeeding favors the development of oral tolerance [28, 29]. Breast milk supports the development of tolerance [30–32]. Furthermore, breast milk is a source of other bioactive components such as hormones, immunoglobulins, enzymes and anti-inflammatory agents, which probably stimulates the development of the immune system [31, 32].

Breastfeeding could be linked indirectly to JIA through the gut microbiota of the infant. Gut bacteria play a fundamental role in the human body by promoting intestinal homeostasis [33–36]. The dysbiosis of the gut microbiota has been associated to an increasing number of diseases, including autoimmune diseases such as diabetes and inflammatory bowel disease [35, 37, 38].

Breastfeeding has been reported to influence infant gut microbiota development [39–41]. Breast milk is recognized as one of the most important postpartum elements modulating metabolic and immunologic programming in the child [42]. Formula-fed infants have increased richness of species compared with breastfed infants [43]. However, a fully developed bacterial flora is established within the intestinal tract only with the start of solid food consumption. [44–47].

Conclusions

We cannot point to any specific mechanism effect, and we call for caution as the population-based finding is difficult to transfer to the individual situation. Still, the conclusion of our results is that a short duration of both total and exclusive breastfeeding seems to be associated with an increased risk of JIA in an unselected population of Swedish children. This indicates that breastfeeding might protect against development of JIA. Mothers should be encouraged to exclusively breastfeed their babies, if at all possible, for at least 4 months and continue partial breastfeeding during the time when foreign proteins are introduced via food.

Abbrevations

ABIS: All Babies in Southeast Sweden; aOR: Adjusted odds ratio; CI: Confidence Interval; ICD: International Classification of Diseases; ILAR: International League of Associations for Rheumatology; JCA: Juvenile Chronic Arthritis; JIA: Juvenile Idiopathic Arthritis; JRA: Juvenile Rheumatoid Arthritis; OR: Odds Ratio; PIN: Personal Identification Number; RA: Rheumatoid Arthritis; RR: Relative risk

Acknowledgement

We are very grateful to all children and families participating in the ABIS study, as well as to all staff members of the Child Health Service in the region where questionnaires were collected and biological samples taken. We thank the following colleagues for their participation: Ingela Danielsson (Linköping); Nils-Åke Nilsson (Motala); Per Lewander (Norrköping); Maria Ekelund and Sven Johansson (Jönköping); Johan Jonsson (Växjö); Sofia Hellerfelt (Karlskrona). We are also grateful to Lars Brudin for excellent help with statistics, and to Bo Magnusson and his colleagues at the Board of registry of the Swedish pediatric JIA-registry.

Funding

This study was supported by The Research Unit of Kalmar County Council, Swedish Rheumatism Association and the Jerring Foundation. ABIS has been supported mainly by the Swedish Child Diabetes Foundation (Barndiabetesfonden), the Juvenile Diabetes Research Foundation and the Medical Research Council of Southeast Sweden (FORSS). The funders had no role in study design, data collection and analysis, decision to publish, or preparation of the manuscript.

Authors' contributions

EK was responsible of the collection of JIA-patients, statistical analyses, figures, data interpretation and the writing of the manuscript. MF was responsible for critical review of the statistical analyses and review of the manuscript. JL, founder and project leader of the All Babies In Southeast Sweden study, had the primary responsibility for the study concept and design, collection of materials, and revision of the manuscript.

Competing interests

The authors declare that they have no competing interests.

Author details

[1]Department of Pediatrics, Västervik Hospital, Västervik, Sweden. [2]Division of Pediatrics, Department of Clinical and Experimental Medicine, Linköping University, Linköping, Sweden. [3]Division of Occupational and Environmental Medicine, Department of Clinical and Experimental Medicine, Linköping University, Linköping, Sweden. [4]Forum Östergötland, Faculty of Medicine, Linköping University, Linköping, Sweden.

References

1. Petty RE, Southwood TR, Manners P, Baum J, Glass DN, Goldenberg J, et al. International league of associations for rheumatology classification of juvenile idiopathic arthritis: second revision, Edmonton, 2001. J Rheumatol. 2004;31(2):390–2.
2. Lemke H, Lange H. Is there a maternally induced immunological imprinting phase a la Konrad Lorenz? Scand J Immunol. 1999;50(4):348–54.
3. M'Rabet L, Vos AP, Boehm G, Garssen J. Breast-feeding and its role in early development of the immune system in infants: consequences for health later in life. J Nutr. 2008;138(9):1782S–90S.
4. Bjorksten B. Environmental influences on the development of the immune system: consequences for disease outcome. Nestle Nutr Workshop Ser Pediatr Program. 2008;61:243–54.
5. Bjorksten B. Environment and infant immunity. Proc Nutr Soc. 1999;58(3):729–32.
6. Mason T, Rabinovich CE, Fredrickson DD, Amoroso K, Reed AM, Stein LD, et al. Breast feeding and the development of juvenile rheumatoid arthritis. J Rheumatol. 1995;22(6):1166–70.
7. Kasapcopur O, Tasdan Y, Apelyan M, Akkus S, Caliskan S, Sever L, et al. Does breast feeding prevent the development of juvenile rheumatoid arthritis? J Rheumatol. 1998;25(11):2286–7.
8. Rosenberg AM. Evaluation of associations between breast feeding and subsequent development of juvenile rheumatoid arthritis. J Rheumatol. 1996;23(6):1080–2.
9. Ellis JA, Ponsonby AL, Pezic A, Chavez RA, Allen RC, Akikusa JD, et al. CLARITY - ChiLdhood arthritis risk factor identification sTudY. Pediatric rheumatology online journal. 2012;10(1):37.
10. Shenoi S, Shaffer ML, Wallace CA. Environmental risk factors and early-life exposures in juvenile idiopathic arthritis: a case-control study. Arthritis Care Res. 2016;68(8):1186–94.
11. Hyrich KL, Baildam E, Pickford H, Chieng A, Davidson JE, Foster H, et al. Influence of past breast feeding on pattern and severity of presentation of juvenile idiopathic arthritis. Arch Dis Child. 2016;101(4):348–51.
12. Sverige. Socialstyrelsen: Kvalitet och innehåll i patientregistret : utskrivningar från slutenvård 1964-2006 och besök i öppenvård (exklusive primärvårdsbesök) 1997-2006. Stockholm: Socialstyrelsen; 2008.
13. Lunde AS, Lundeborg S, Lettenstrom GS, Thygesen L, Huebner J. The person-number systems of Sweden, Norway, Denmark, and Israel. Vital and health statistics Series 2, Data evaluation and methods research. 1980;1(84):1–59.
14. Organization WH. Indicators for assessing breastfeeding practices. Geneva: World Health Organization; 1991. In.: WHO/CDD/SER/91.14
15. Rockhill B, Newman B, Weinberg C. Use and misuse of population attributable fractions. Am J Public Health. 1998;88(1):15–9.
16. Lande B, Andersen LF, Baerug A, Trygg KU, Lund-Larsen K, Veierod MB, et al. Infant feeding practices and associated factors in the first six months of life: the Norwegian infant nutrition survey. Acta Paediatr. 2003;92(2):152–61.
17. Atladottir H, Thorsdottir I. Energy intake and growth of infants in Iceland-a population with high frequency of breast-feeding and high birth weight. Eur J Clin Nutr. 2000;54(9):695–701.
18. Michaelsen KF, Larsen PS, Thomsen BL, Samuelson G. The Copenhagen cohort study on infant nutrition and growth: breast-milk intake, human milk macronutrient content, and influencing factors. Am J Clin Nutr. 1994;59(3):600–11.
19. Briefel RR, Reidy K, Karwe V, Devaney B. Feeding infants and toddlers study: improvements needed in meeting infant feeding recommendations. J Am Diet Assoc. 2004;104(1 Suppl 1):s31–7.
20. Freeman V, van't Hof M, Haschke F. Patterns of milk and food intake in infants from birth to age 36 months: the euro-growth study. J Pediatr Gastroenterol Nutr. 2000;31(Suppl 1):S76–85.
21. Giovannini M, Riva E, Banderali G, Scaglioni S, Veehof SH, Sala M, et al. Feeding practices of infants through the first year of life in Italy. Acta Paediatr. 2004;93(4):492–7.
22. The National Board of Health and Welfare CfE. Statistics - health and diseases. Stockholm: Breast-feeding, Children Born 1999. In; 2001.
23. Prakken B, Albani S, Martini A. Juvenile idiopathic arthritis. Lancet. 2011; 377(9783):2138–49.
24. Gowdie PJ, Tse SM. Juvenile idiopathic arthritis. Pediatr Clin N Am. 2012;59(2):301–27.
25. Huttly SR, Barros FC, Victora CG, Beria JU, Vaughan JP. Do mothers overestimate breast feeding duration? An example of recall bias from a study in southern Brazil. Am J Epidemiol. 1990;132(3):572–5.
26. Launer LJ, Forman MR, Hundt GL, Sarov B, Chang D, Berendes HW, et al. Maternal recall of infant feeding events is accurate. J Epidemiol Community Health. 1992;46(3):203–6.
27. Akerblom HK, Knip M. Putative environmental factors in type 1 diabetes. Diabetes Metab Rev. 1998;14(1):31–67.
28. Sansotta N, Piacentini GL, Mazzei F, Minniti F, Boner AL, Peroni DG. Timing of introduction of solid food and risk of allergic disease development: understanding the evidence. Allergol Immunopathol (Madr). 2013;41(5):337–45.
29. Prescott SL, Smith P, Tang M, Palmer DJ, Sinn J, Huntley SJ, et al. The importance of early complementary feeding in the development of oral tolerance: concerns and controversies. Pediatr Allergy Immunol. 2008;19(5):375–80.
30. Garofalo R. Cytokines in human milk. J Pediatr. 2010;156(2 Suppl):S36–40.
31. Lonnerdal B. Bioactive proteins in human milk: mechanisms of action. J Pediatr. 2010;156(2 Suppl):S26–30.
32. Walker A. Breast milk as the gold standard for protective nutrients. J Pediatr. 2010;156(2 Suppl):S3–7.
33. Sjogren YM, Tomicic S, Lundberg A, Bottcher MF, Bjorksten B, Sverremark-Ekstrom E, et al. Influence of early gut microbiota on the maturation of childhood mucosal and systemic immune responses. Clin Exp Allergy. 2009; 39(12):1842–51.
34. Maynard CL, Elson CO, Hatton RD, Weaver CT. Reciprocal interactions of the intestinal microbiota and immune system. Nature. 2012;489(7415):231–41.
35. Young VB. The intestinal microbiota in health and disease. Curr Opin Gastroenterol. 2012;28(1):63–9.
36. El Aidy S, Hooiveld G, Tremaroli V, Backhed F, Kleerebezem M. The gut microbiota and mucosal homeostasis: colonized at birth or at adulthood, does it matter? Gut Microbes. 2013;4(2):118–24.
37. Le Chatelier E, Nielsen T, Qin J, Prifti E, Hildebrand F, Falony G, et al. Richness of human gut microbiome correlates with metabolic markers. Nature. 2013;500(7464):541–6.
38. Soyucen E, Gulcan A, Aktuglu-Zeybek AC, Onal H, Kiykim E, Aydin A. Differences in the gut microbiota of healthy children and those with type 1 diabetes. Pediatrics international : official journal of the Japan Pediatric Society. 2014;56(3):336–43.

39. Gronlund MM, Gueimonde M, Laitinen K, Kociubinski G, Gronroos T, Salminen S, et al. Maternal breast-milk and intestinal bifidobacteria guide the compositional development of the Bifidobacterium microbiota in infants at risk of allergic disease. Clin Exp Allergy. 2007;37(12):1764–72.
40. Martin R, Jimenez E, Heilig H, Fernandez L, Marin ML, Zoetendal EG, et al. Isolation of bifidobacteria from breast milk and assessment of the bifidobacterial population by PCR-denaturing gradient gel electrophoresis and quantitative real-time PCR. Appl Environ Microbiol. 2009;75(4):965–9.
41. Roger LC, Costabile A, Holland DT, Hoyles L, McCartney AL. Examination of faecal Bifidobacterium populations in breast- and formula-fed infants during the first 18 months of life. Microbiology. 2010;156(Pt 11):3329–41.
42. Aaltonen J, Ojala T, Laitinen K, Poussa T, Ozanne S, Isolauri E. Impact of maternal diet during pregnancy and breastfeeding on infant metabolic programming: a prospective randomized controlled study. Eur J Clin Nutr. 2011;65(1):10–9.
43. Azad MB, Becker AB, Guttman DS, Sears MR, Scott JA, Kozyrskyj AL. Canadian healthy infant longitudinal development study I: gut microbiota diversity and atopic disease: does breast-feeding play a role? J Allergy Clin Immunol. 2013;131(1):247–8.
44. Eckburg PB, Bik EM, Bernstein CN, Purdom E, Dethlefsen L, Sargent M, et al. Diversity of the human intestinal microbial flora. Science. 2005;308(5728):1635–8.
45. Lotz M, Gutle D, Walther S, Menard S, Bogdan C, Hornef MW. Postnatal acquisition of endotoxin tolerance in intestinal epithelial cells. J Exp Med. 2006;203(4):973–84.
46. Gill SR, Pop M, Deboy RT, Eckburg PB, Turnbaugh PJ, Samuel BS, et al. Metagenomic analysis of the human distal gut microbiome. Science. 2006; 312(5778):1355–9.
47. Palmer C, Bik EM, DiGiulio DB, Relman DA, Brown PO. Development of the human infant intestinal microbiota. PLoS Biol. 2007;5(7):e177.

23

Design and implementation of a decision aid for juvenile idiopathic arthritis medication choices

William B. Brinkman[1*], Ellen A. Lipstein[1], Janalee Taylor[1], Pamela J. Schoettker[1], Katherine Naylor[2], Karla Jones[3], Sheetal S. Vora[4], Catherine C. Mims[5], Elizabeth Roth-Wojcicki[6], Beth Gottlieb[7], Nancy Griffin[1], Carole Lannon[1] and Esi Morgan[1]

Abstract

Background: Randomized trials have demonstrated the efficacy of patient decision aids to facilitate shared decision making in clinical situations with multiple medically reasonable options for treatment. However, little is known about how best to implement these tools into routine clinical practice. In addition, reliable implementation of decision aids has been elusive and spread within pediatrics has been slow. We sought to develop and reliably implement a decision aid for treatment of children with juvenile idiopathic arthritis.

Methods: To design our decision aid, we partnered with patient, parent, and clinician stakeholders from the Pediatric Rheumatology Care and Outcomes Improvement Network. Six sites volunteered to use quality improvement methods to implement the decision aid. Four of these sites collected parent surveys following visits to assess outcomes. Parents reported on clinician use of the decision aid and the amount of shared decision making and uncertainty they experienced. We used chi-square tests to compare eligible visits with and without use of the decision aid on the experience of shared decision making and uncertainty.

Results: After 18 rounds of testing and revision, stakeholders approved the decision aid design for regular use. Qualitative feedback from end-users was positive. During the implementation project, the decision aid was used in 35% of visits where starting or switching medication was discussed. Clinicians used the decision aid as intended in 68% of these visits. The vast majority of parents reported high levels of shared decision making following visits with (64/76 = 84%) and without (80/95 = 84%) use of the decision aid ($p = 1$). Similarly, the vast majority of parents reported no uncertainty following visits with (74/76 = 97%) and without (91/95 = 96%) use of the decision aid ($p = 0.58$).

Conclusions: Although user acceptability of the decision aid was high, reliable implementation in routine clinical care proved challenging. Our parsimonious approach to outcome assessment failed to detect a difference between visits with and without use of our aid. Innovative approaches are needed to facilitate use of decision aids and the assessment of outcomes.

Keywords: Juvenile idiopathic arthritis, Patient education, Shared decision-making, Decision aids

* Correspondence: Bill.Brinkman@cchmc.org
[1]Department of Pediatrics, Cincinnati Children's Hospital Medical Center, 3333 Burnet Avenue, Cincinnati, OH 45229, USA
Full list of author information is available at the end of the article

Background

Juvenile idiopathic arthritis (JIA) is the most common form of arthritis in children and adolescents, affecting approximately 1 in every 1000 young people. This chronic inflammatory disease is characterized by persistent joint inflammation that results in joint pain and swelling and restricted joint range of motion [1]. Several new, very effective drugs for JIA have been developed in recent years [2]. Because these medications differ in a variety of important attributes, such as mechanism of action, dosing interval, mode of administration, safety profile, and cost, some patients and families struggle to make treatment decisions and seek wide-ranging information from multiple sources [3]. The challenging process of obtaining enough information to make decisions can leave parents with long-lasting questions and concerns [4]. There is a need for improved communication with rheumatology clinicians about treatment decisions.

Decisions with multiple reasonable options that differ in ways that matter to families are conducive to shared decision making (SDM). SDM is a best practice in patient-centered care [5] and a recognized method to translate comparative effectiveness data into practice [6] and decrease unwarranted variation in healthcare [7]. In the SDM process, clinicians share information about treatment options and patients/parents share information about their goals and preferences. Working together, a treatment plan is developed that is the best fit for the individual patient and their family.

Decision aids, such as issue cards [8], are one way to implement SDM in practice by making decisions explicit and providing information about treatment options and their associated outcomes. Issue cards are designed to enable clinicians and patients/parents to efficiently discuss medications when there are multiple reasonable options that differ on a variety of attributes in a given clinical context [8]. Pioneered at the Mayo clinic [8], the issue card format has consistently led to patients/parents that are better informed and more involved in decision making in a variety of clinical contexts, including adults with rheumatoid arthritis [9–13].

However, while randomized trials have demonstrated the efficacy of patient decision aids [9, 14, 15], little is known about how best to implement these tools into routine clinical practice [16]. In addition, reliable implementation of SDM with decision aids has been elusive [17] and spread within pediatrics has been slow [18]. Commonly cited barriers to use of decision aids include time constraints, the absence of a reliable way to identify patients before decisions are made, the perception of too many educational materials, and lack of applicability due to patient characteristics and clinical situations [13, 19, 20].

Learning networks use the creative energies of patients, families, clinicians, and researchers to accelerate innovation, discovery and the application of new knowledge [21]. These learning health systems [22, 23] use continuing education and adult learning principles and an adaptation of the Breakthrough Series model [24] to guide improvement. The Breakthrough Series model promotes collaborative learning methods to understand and evaluate the issues, and begin testing changes that can help an organization make breakthrough improvements in the quality and value of health care [25]. The robust format of learning networks provides the infrastructure needed to understand and address the challenges of implementing SDM.

The Pediatric Rheumatology Care and Outcomes Improvement Network (PR-COIN) is a learning network launched in 2011 to improve outcomes of JIA care using quality improvement approaches [26, 27]. We designed a two-stage quality improvement project within PR-COIN to develop and reliably implement a decision aid to facilitate SDM between clinicians, patients with JIA, and their families around medication choices for treatment of inflammatory arthritis.

Methods

Setting

The project was conducted within PR-COIN during 2012–2014. At that time, the new and growing network consisted of 11 sites in the United States and Canada. Using a modified Breakthrough Series model [28], PR-COIN teams meet monthly via webinar and semi-annually for face-to-face workshops to review data, share best practices, and participate in improvement science training [27]. Teams at each site test innovative ideas and processes to improve care and outcomes for children with JIA. Data collected during clinical care are submitted to a shared registry and analyzed to produce aggregate and site-specific reports to identify patterns of care associated with better outcomes.

Project improvement team

The improvement team was based at Cincinnati Children's Hospital Medical Center and consisted of a quality improvement consultant and clinician researchers with expertise in pediatric rheumatology, SDM and the development of decision aids, family/self-management of chronic disease, and quality improvement methods.

Development of the decision aid

To develop JIA medication choice cards [12], the team partnered with a graphic design graduate student from the University of Cincinnati and patients, parents, and clinicians from PR-COIN. Development steps included review of existing decision aids [10, 12, 29], qualitative interviews with patients [30], parents [3], and clinicians [31] and direct observation of clinical encounters, especially encounters with conversations regarding treatment options, benefits and risks/uncertainties, mode of administration, and need for monitoring. A stakeholder panel of patients, parents, physicians, advanced practice nurses, registered nurses, educational specialists, and project staff discussed and prioritized educational needs from their perspective and contributed suggestions to address these needs via face-to-face meetings, conference calls, and internet communications. This group prioritized a focus on long-term medications that control disease activity (e.g., disease modifying anti-rheumatic drugs and biologics) over medications that are intended for short-term use, or to control pain (e.g., non-steroidal anti-inflammatory medication, joint injections, steroids, etc.) because this conversation is more challenging. Prototype issue cards were critiqued by panel members and tested using plan-do-study-act cycles [25] during outpatient clinical encounters observed by improvement team members. Feedback to guide card revisions was elicited via weekly electronic surveys of teams, discussions during webinars, and following direct observation of encounters using the cards. After 18 revisions, PR-COIN stakeholders found the medication choice cards to be acceptable for use. The improvement team also developed a one-page instruction sheet with pictures depicting the intended use of the cards, a short training video, and a pamphlet containing the content of the cards for families to take home. The cards were also adapted to an interactive electronic portable document format (PDF) to facilitate implementation at PR-COIN sites that employed electronic media for patient education in the clinic setting.

Implementation of the decision aid

The goals of this phase of the project were to (1) identify patients with JIA facing a decision to start or switch medicine, (2) provide SDM support during visits by using the medication choice cards, and (3) measure outcomes.

Four PR-COIN sites volunteered to use quality improvement methods to implement the SDM materials, provide feedback, administer parent surveys, and contribute data to assess SDM outcomes. Participants set a specific, measurable, achievable, realistic and timely aim [32] of increasing the proportion of patients with JIA who received SDM with JIA medication issue cards during visits discussing a medication change from 0 to 65% within three months (March to May 2014). Due to institutional review board delays at some sites, the project period was extended to early August 2014. A key driver diagram (Fig. 1) was

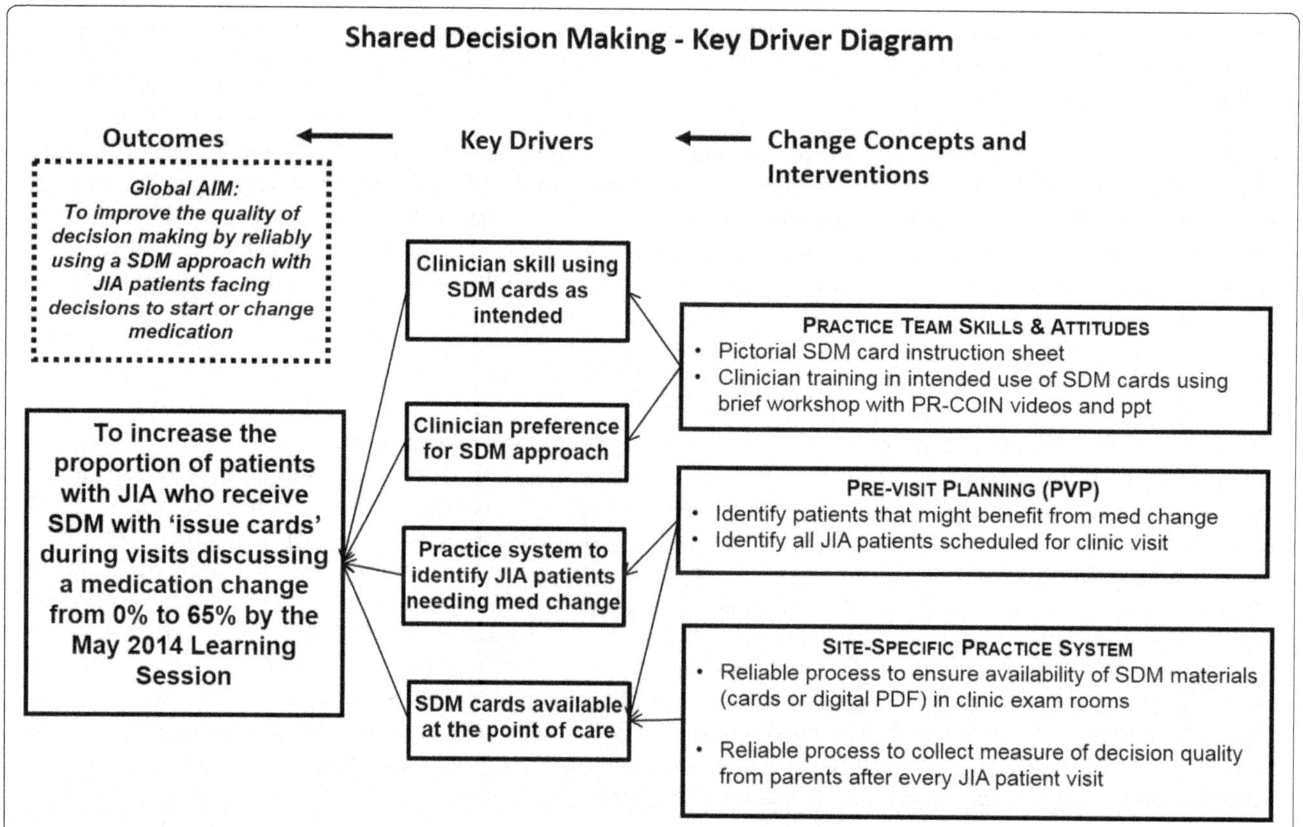

Fig. 1 Key driver diagram

developed to describe the relationship between the outcomes of interest, the desired characteristics of the system (the so-called "drivers"), and the structures, processes and interventions theorized to lead, via the drivers, to the desired outcomes.

A 'train the trainer' workshop was held at a face-to-face PR-COIN Learning Session [28] in November 2013 to enable clinician (i.e., physician and advanced practice nurses) champions from each site to train other clinicians on the intended use of the cards. Clinicians were trained to present the medication choice cards to a patient and/or parent(s) during a clinic visit and ask which of the cards they would like to discuss first. It was explained that, by picking a card, the patient or parent shows the clinician what is most important to her/him and sets the agenda for discussion. For example, parents concerned about the side effects of medications may choose to discuss that first. The cards are meant to be a flexible tool to augment the conversation that clinicians have with families. Clinicians can highlight the options most relevant for the patient given the specifics of their situation. Moreover, the clinician can share their experience and preferences while eliciting what matters most to the family about the relevant options. After reviewing and discussing the cards that the family and clinician choose to discuss, they should be able to decide together which medication best matches the family's circumstances and preferences. A supporting video demonstrating ideal use of the cards was developed and shared with sites.

Process maps produced by each site demonstrated how SDM and the collection of outcome measures could be implemented into clinic flow processes using existing staff. The PR-COIN teams conducted iterative plan-do-study-act cycles to (1) identify all JIA patients scheduled for a clinic visit and those that might benefit from a medication change, (2) establish reliable processes to ensure the availability of SDM materials in exam rooms, (3) collect SDM outcome measures, and (4) increase clinician skill in using medication choice cards as intended.

SDM outcome measures

Outcome measures included the three-item CollaboRATE scale, the 4-item SURE measure (Sure of myself, Understand information, Risk-benefit ratio, Encouragement), and three items developed by the improvement team to assess eligibility for use of the SDM issue cards and, if eligible, fidelity of use. The CollaboRATE scale (0–9 scale on each item, with higher scores indicating more clinician effort to engage and involve the parent) is a validated measure of SDM that is easily understood and accepted by respondents [33] and has good discriminant and concurrent validity, intra-rater reliability, and sensitivity to change [34]. The SURE measure (response options of "yes" and "no") is a validated patient/parent report screening version of the Decisional Conflict Scale [35, 36]. A response of "yes" to all 4 items indicates no uncertainty.

Data collection procedures

Data collection was embedded in the delivery of routine clinical care. A nurse or medical assistant responsible for discharging the patient from the clinic distributed a voluntary, anonymous, paper survey to parents after every encounter with a patient with JIA. The first question on the survey asked parents if starting or switching medication was discussed at the visit. For parents who answered "no" to this question, the survey ended. Parents who answered "yes" to this question were further asked if their child's clinician had shown them the issues cards (pictured below the question) during the visit. If so, the final question assessed fidelity of issue card use by asking the parent if their child's clinician asked her/him to pick the first card to discuss [8]. Each parent who received a survey was asked to place their completed survey in a collection container near the clinic exit. One PR-COIN site also tested electronic distribution of the survey where an administrative assistant for the practice sent a hyperlink for the electronic version of the survey to each parent by email or text message. To enable assessment of the completion rates achieved by the various survey collection methods, two of the four sites that collected data intermittently reviewed the clinic schedule and each patient's medical record to determine a count of JIA patients seen on days surveys were distributed.

Clinician impressions regarding the benefits and barriers to use of the issue cards were documented during the final debriefing call with the lead clinician from each participating site.

Data analysis

Completion rates were calculated by dividing the number of parent-completed surveys by the total number of JIA parents seen that day. The proportion of eligible visits with use of issue cards was calculated by dividing the number of parents who reported "yes" to having a been shown the issue cards by their child's clinician by the total number of parents who reported "yes" to having a discussion about starting or switching medication. Fidelity to intended use of the cards was calculated by dividing the number of parents who reported "yes" to having been asked to pick the first card to discuss by the total number of parents who were shown the cards by their child's doctor.

For the experience of SDM, we calculated the proportion of parents with a top score (9 s on all 3 items) on the CollaboRATE scale. For the experience of uncertainty, we calculated the proportion experiencing no uncertainty ("yes" on all 4 items) on the SURE scale. We used chi-square tests to compare eligible visits with and without use of the cards on the experience of SDM and uncertainty.

Ethics, consent and permissions

We conducted this project in compliance with the research ethics standards of the United States of America. The teams at Cincinnati Children's Hospital Medical Center and the four PR-COIN sites that collected data each received authorization from their local institutional review boards to conduct the study. At each location, the boards determined that the project did not involve the use and/or disclosure of protected health information and waived the requirement to obtain documentation of informed consent.

Results

Six medication choice cards were created to enable clinicians and patients/parents to efficiently discuss medications that are reasonable options in a given clinical context (available at https://www.cincinnatichildrens.org/-/media/cincinnati%20childrens/home/service/j/anderson-center/evidence-based-care/decision-aids/arthritis%20medication%20choice%20cards.pdf?la=en and through the PR-COIN website https://pr-coin.org). Using plain language and pictorial representations, each card covered a key issue on which potential medications differ. The topics addressed by the cards were how often each potential medication must be taken, how soon the medications take effect, side effects, cost, how long each medication must be taken, and other things to consider before starting or while taking each medication.

Following implementation of the medication choice cards by the four PR-COIN sites, we collected 223 parent surveys over 18 weeks of data collection. We assessed completion rates during 7 of the 15 weeks that paper surveys were collected. During these weeks, we collected 103 surveys after 226 visits with patients with JIA, for a completion rate of 45.6%. During the 2 weeks that one site tested electronic administration of surveys by sending a link to the parent's email account, we collected 9 surveys after 64 visits (14% completion rate). During the one week that one site tested electronic administration of surveys by sending a link to the parent by text message, we collected 2 surveys following 29 visits (7% completion rate).

During the study period, the decision aid cards were used in a median of 35% of visits where starting or switching medication was discussed. The cards were used as intended (parent was asked to pick the first card to discuss) in a median of 68% of visits where cards were used.

There were a total of 171 surveys from parents who reported that the visit involved a discussion about starting or switching medicine. The vast majority of these parents reported high levels of SDM on the CollaboRATE scale (i.e., 9 s on all 3 items) following visits with (64/76 = 84%) and without (80/95 = 84%) use of the issue cards (p = 1). Similarly, the vast majority of parents reported no uncertainty on the SURE scale (i.e., "yes" on all 4 items) following visits with (74/76 = 97%) and without (91/95 = 96%) use of the issue cards (p = 0.58).

Comments from clinicians documented during the final debriefing call with the participating PR-COIN sites were generally positive (Table 1). Reflection on facilitators of successful use of issue cards was buy-in from clinicians on the value of SDM, training and familiarity in use of issue cards, and reminders and prompts for card use and ready access at time of discussion of medication choice. Pre-clinic huddles contributed to higher rates of survey distribution and collection.

Discussion

We sought to develop and reliably implement a decision aid to facilitate SDM between clinicians, patients with JIA, and their families concerning medication choices for arthritis. We co-produced a decision aid that met the needs of stakeholders and is publicly available for use [37]. However, in surveyed situations where use of the decision aid might have been appropriate, use occurred only one-third of the time. Efforts to embed decision aid use as part of medication discussions between patients and clinicians in routine clinical care fell short of our a priori goal (65%).

Reliable implementation of decision aids remains elusive. Our rate of 35% is similar to that seen by Group Health in Seattle over the first year during their recent decision aid implementation project for knee and hip surgery among adults [17]. In that study, however, decision aids were mailed to the home, rather than being the subject of an interactive exchange at the point of care. Our rate was less than half that reported by Canadian Cystic Fibrosis Centers that implemented a decision aid for lung transplantation [38]. The differences in the

Table 1 Comments from clinicians

If the goal was to get the patients more engaged and involved then it definitely did that. One family actually said to me, "wow you are actually showing me choices"
We did get a lot of really good feedback. We used the ones on the computer. Because it is a shared clinic space. The families did really like them.
The cards take a little longer as you discuss medications that you are not going to use at that visit. But the thing is that parents want to know, and they ought to know for it to be part of their decision.
This may be a culture change, opening up medication choices for discussion and being less directive.

levels of reliability achieved in these implementation efforts likely reflect differences in clinical contexts, clinician training, capacity for quality improvement, resource allocation, and methods of outcome assessment. For example, this initiative was one of the first attempted interventions in the PR-COIN cohort of centers, which were gaining new experience with quality improvement methods. Therefore, the low rate of implementation may reflect insufficient quality improvement capacity at the time of the study rather than an intrinsic problem with the SDM cards. In regard to methods of outcome assessment, Arterburn et al. [17] relied on documentation that the clinician ordered the decision aid for their patient and Stacey et al. [38] relied on retrospective self-report of clinicians about their own use of the decision aid with patients. Certainly, the latter method has been shown to overestimate performance markedly across a number of settings [39]. It is possible that our measurement, based on patient/parent report, was an underestimate since the result was based on the screening item "did you discuss starting or switching medicine to treat your child's arthritis" and didn't specify the type of medicine. This distinction is important because the issue cards focus on discussion of disease modifying anti-rheumatic drugs and biologics, and don't include other classes of medications, such as NSAIDs, joint injections, or steroids etc., which may have been the focus of their discussion about starting or switching medicine and for which the issue cards would not have been applicable.

Clinicians who chose to use the cards largely used them as intended. Two-thirds of parents reported that their clinician allowed them to pick the first card to discuss. One-third did not. Given the limitations to our measurement strategy, we are unable to comment on how the cards were used during these visits. It is possible that our 'train the trainer' approach was inadequate. We did not track the number of clinicians at each site that were exposed to the training. In hindsight, more rigorous training with knowledge assessment completed by all site clinicians, including fellows in training, may have helped uptake. Alternatively, some clinicians may have been trained but felt uncomfortable relinquishing control over the discussion agenda. Regardless of the reasons that underlie this phenomenon, past studies that video-recorded encounters show that clinician decision aid usage often lacks fidelity to intended use [40].

Embedding outcome assessment in routine clinical care also proved challenging. Completion rates were low by all methods we attempted. Distribution of a paper survey after each clinic visit performed best but yielded a completion rate of only 45%. This approach faced multiple challenges. We do not know if the surveys were distributed as intended; it was an added task competing for staff attention in a busy clinical setting. Even if distributed by staff, patient families may have been eager to leave clinic at the end of their encounter and chose not to complete the survey. Parents who didn't face medication decisions may have been less likely to complete and return the survey. Certainly, surveying only those parents who experience the decision of interest could be more efficient, but this approach creates new challenges related to accurate and reliable case ascertainment.

Our parsimonious approach to measuring the outcomes of SDM and uncertainty failed to detect a difference between visits with and without use of the decision aid. Even though it is possible at participating sites that high levels of SDM and low levels of patient uncertainty happen without decision aids, it would be counter to observational research that has shown limited SDM in JIA visits [41]. Furthermore, systematic reviews have demonstrated low levels of SDM across a range of settings during 'usual care' visits that do not involve a decision aid [42] and efficacy of decision aids to improve outcomes [14]. While ceiling effects may have occurred with the measures, this was not experienced in adult healthcare settings where the measures were validated. Perhaps parents did not feel comfortable providing less than the highest score. We attempted to guard against social desirability response bias and/or concerns about loss of confidentiality by making the survey anonymous, but collecting surveys in the clinic setting may increase this threat. When we attempted to mitigate this possibility by distributing surveys electronically, our completion rate plummeted. Testing additional approaches to assess SDM outcomes is warranted.

Our project was limited by the small number of participating sites, the short 18-week data collection period, the absence of patient characteristics collected on our anonymous survey, and the observational design. Future studies could address these limitations by expanding the number of sites, extending the length of data collection, collecting more information to characterize the sample, and utilizing a randomized controlled design. Future mixed methods studies might lead to a better understanding of the barriers to implementation experienced at each site. Nonetheless, our findings make a meaningful contribution given the paucity of research on implementing decision aids and assessing outcomes related to SDM as part of routine clinical care [16].

Conclusions

Although user acceptability of the decision aid was high, reliable implementation in routine clinical care proved challenging. Clinician leaders at each site expressed enthusiasm for using the decision aid, but it is unclear how broadly this enthusiasm was shared by their colleagues. We further reason that what appears to be a shortcoming of implementation may not reflect an intrinsic problem with the SDM cards, but rather it may be attributed to the quality improvement inexperience of the network at time of the study. Our parsimonious approach to outcome assessment failed to detect a difference between visits with and without use of our decision aid.

Our next steps include revising the JIA medication choice issue cards based on ongoing stakeholder feedback and to reflect medication changes (e.g., new modes of administration, new products). Periodic training of new clinicians and centers entering the network and sharing of best practices on implementation will continue in the context of PR-COIN to promote spread of SDM. Our findings raise interesting questions for future research. Might an electronic format that is enabled by decision support from the electronic health record engender more reliable use? If SDM represents a culture change in the practice of rheumatology, are additional tools needed to facilitate this process with a broader range of decisions faced by children with JIA (e.g., pain relief, etc.)? Could the burden of outcome measurement be lessened by leveraging the infrastructure that is used to collect patient reported outcomes and satisfaction? Indeed, it appears there are miles to go before reliable implementation of decision aids becomes a reality in routine clinical practice [16, 33]. Innovative approaches are needed to facilitate use of decision aids and assessment of outcomes.

Abbreviations

JIA: Juvenile idiopathic arthritis; PDF: Portable document format; PR-COIN: Pediatric rheumatology care and outcomes improvement network; SDM: Shared decision making; SURE: Sure of myself, understand information, risk-benefit ratio, encouragement

Acknowledgements

This project was conducted with the cooperation and assistance of the Pediatric Rheumatology Care and Outcome Improvement Network (PR-COIN) and the physicians, clinicians and families participating in this multicenter Quality Improvement Collaborative, https://pr-coin.org.

The authors are grateful for the participation of clinicians, patients and staff from the Pediatric Rheumatology units of the following institutions for participating in the reliability of implementation project: Cincinnati Children's Hospital, Levine Children's Hospital, Medical University of South Carolina, Nationwide Children's Hospital, Children's Hospital of Wisconsin, and Cohen Children's Medical Center of New York. We thank Jesse Pratt for assistance with data analysis.

Additionally, we acknowledge participation of all active PR-COIN centers during the period of development and piloting of the JIA Medication Choice Cards, as well as the parents and patients who provided valued input into their formation: Cincinnati Children's Hospital Medical Center (PI Esi Morgan), Hackensack University Medical Center (PI Yukiko Kimura, Jennifer Weiss); The Hospital for Sick Children, Toronto (PI Ronald Laxer), Medical College Wisconsin (PI Judyann Olson), Medical University of South Carolina (PI Murray Passo), Nationwide Children's Hospital (PI Stacy Ardoin, Cagri Toruner), Penn State Hershey Children's Hospital (PI C. April Bingham), and Stanford Children's Hospital (PI Tzielan C. Lee).

Funding

This project was funded by a grant from the Agency for Healthcare Research and Quality U19HS021114 to PI Carole Lannon for "Pursuing Perfection in Pediatric Therapeutics." Dr. Brinkman was supported by Award Number K23MH083027 from the National Institute of Mental Health. Dr. Lipstein was supported by award number K23HD073149 from the Eunice Kennedy Shriver National Institute of Child Health and Human Development. The funding sources had no role in study design; in the collection, analysis and interpretation of data; in the writing of the report; and in the decision to submit the article for publication.

Authors' contributions

WBB, EAL, and EM conceived of the study. WBB, EAL, JT, KN, KJ, SV, CCM, ERW, BG, NG, CL, and EM participated in the design and coordination of the study. WBB, EAL, JT, PJS, KN, KJ, SV, CCM, ERW, BG, NG, CL, and EM helped to interpret the data, draft and critically revise the manuscript. All authors read and approved the final manuscript.

Competing interests

The authors declare that they have no competing interests.

Consent for publication

Not applicable.

Ethics approval and consent to participate

We conducted this research in compliance with the research ethics standards of the United States of America. The teams at Cincinnati Children's Hospital Medical Center and the four PR-COIN sites that collected data each received authorization from their local institutional review boards to conduct the study. At each location, the boards determined that the project did not involve the use and/or disclosure of protected health information and waived the requirement to obtain documentation of informed consent. This study was reviewed by the following Institutional Review Boards: Cincinnati Children's Hospital Medical Center: Study number #2014–0555; Levine Children's Hospital: Study number #061508E; Medical University of South Carolina: Study number Pro00035057; Nationwide Children's Hospital: Study IRB11–00032.

Author details

[1]Department of Pediatrics, Cincinnati Children's Hospital Medical Center, 3333 Burnet Avenue, Cincinnati, OH 45229, USA. [2]University of Cincinnati College of Design, Architecture, Art and Planning, 5470 Aronoff, Cincinnati, OH 45221, USA. [3]Nationwide Children's Hospital, 700 Children's Drive, Columbus, OH 43205, USA. [4]Levine Children's Hospital, 1000 Blythe Blvd, Charlotte, NC 28203, USA. [5]Medical University of South Carolina, 171 Ashley Ave, Charleston, SC 29425, USA. [6]Medical College of Wisconsin, 8701 W Watertown Plank Rd, Milwaukee, WI 53226, USA. [7]Cohen Children's Medical Center of New York, 269-1 76th Ave, Queens, NY 11040, USA.

References

1. Rochette E, Duche P, Merlin E. Juvenile idiopathic arthritis and physical activity: possible inflammatory and immune modulation and tracks for interventions in young populations. Autoimmun Rev. 2015;14(8):726–34.
2. Tugwell P, Singh J, Wells G. Biologics for rheumatoid arthritis. BMJ. 2011;343:d4027.
3. Lipstein E, Lovell D, Denson L, Moser D, Saeed S, Dodds C, et al. Parents' information needs in tumor necrosis factor-α inhibitor treatment decisions. J Pediatr Gastroenterol Nutr. 2013;56(3):244–50.
4. Lipstein E, Britto M. Evolution of pediatric chronic disease treatment decisions: a qualitative, longitudinal view of parents' decision-making process. Med Decis Mak. 2015;35(6):703–13.
5. Barry M, Edgman-Levitan S. Shared decision making - pinnacle of patient-centered care. N Engl J Med. 2012;366(9):780–1.

6. Shah N, Mullan R, Breslin M, Yawn B, Ting H, Montori V. Translating comparative effectiveness into practice: the case of diabetes medications. Med Care. 2010;48(6 Suppl):S153–S8.
7. O'Connor A, Llewwllyn-Thomas H, Flood A. Modifying unwarranted variations in health care: shared decision making using patient decision aids. Health Aff (Millwood). 2004;Suppl Variation:VAR63-VAR72. https://www.ncbi.nlm.nih.gov/pubmed/15471770?dopt=Citation.
8. Breslin M, Mullan R, Montori V. The design of a decision aid about diabetes medications for use during the consultation with patients with type 2 diabetes. Patient Educ Couns. 2008;73(3):465–72.
9. Barton J, Trupin L, Schillinger D, Evans-Young G, Imboden J, Montori V, et al. Use of a low-literacy decision aid to enhance knowledge and reduce decisional conflict among a diverse population of adults with rheumatoid arthritis: results of a pilot study. Arthritis Care Res. 2016; 68(7):889–98.
10. Brinkman W, Hartl Majcher J, Poling L, Shi G, Zender M, Sucharew H, et al. Shared decision-making to improve attention-deficit hyperactivity disorder care. Patient Educ Couns. 2013;93(1):95–101.
11. LeBlanc A, Bodde A, Branda M, Yost K, Herrin J, Williams M, et al. Translating comparative effectiveness of depression medications into practice by comparing the depression medication choice decision aid to usual care: study protocol for a randomized controlled trial. Trials. 2013;14:127.
12. Mullan R, Montori V, Shah N, Christianson T, Bryant S, Guyatt G, et al. The diabetes mellitus medication choice decision aid: a randomized trial. Arch Intern Med. 2009;169(17):1560–8.
13. Tugwell P, Shea B, Boers M, Brooks P, Simon L, Strand V, et al., editors. Evidence-Based Rheumatology. London: BMJ Books; 2004.
14. Stacey D, Legare F, Col N, Bennett C, Barry M, Eden K, et al. Decision aids for people facing health treatment or screening decisions. Cochrane Database Syst Rev. 2014;1:CD001431.
15. Fraenkel L, Matzko C, Webb D, Oppermann B, Charpentier P, Peters E, et al. Use of decision support for improved knowledge, values clarification, and informed choice in patients with rheumatoid arthritis. Arthritis Care Res. 2015;67(11):1496–505.
16. Elwyn G, Scholl I, Tietbohl C, Mann M, Edwards A, Clay C, et al. "Many miles to go ...": a systematic review of the implementation of patient decision support interventions into routine clinical practice. BMC Med Inform Decis Mak. 2013;13(Suppl 2):S14.
17. Arterburn D, Wellman R, Westbrook E, Rutter C, Ross T, McCulloch D, et al. Introducing decision aids at Group Health was linked to sharply lower hip and knee surgery rates and costs. Health Aff (Millwood). 2012;31(9):2094–104.
18. Wyatt K, List B, Brinkman W, Prutsky Lopez G, Asi N, Erwin P, et al. Shared decision making in pediatrics: a systematic review and meta-analysis. Acad Pediatr. 2015;15(6):573–83.
19. Feibelmann S, Yang T, Uzogara E, Sepucha K. What does it take to have sustained use of decision aids? A programme evaluation for the Breast Cancer Initiative. Health Expect. 2011;14(Suppl 1):85–95.
20. Legare F, Ratte S, Gravel K, Graham I. Barriers and facilitators to implementing shared decision making in clinical practice: update of a systematic review of health professionals' perceptions. Patient Educ Couns. 2008;73(3):526–35.
21. Crandall W, Margolis P, Kappelman M, King E, Pratt J, Boyle B, et al. Improved outcomes in a quality improvement collaborative for pediatric inflammatory bowel disease. Pediatrics. 2012;129(4):e1030–e41.
22. Olsen L, Aisner D, McGinnis J. The Learning Healthcare System. Washington: National Academy Press; 2007.
23. Smith M, Saunders R, Stuckhardt L, McGinnis J. Committee on the Learning Health Care System in America. Best Care at Lower Cost: The Path to Continuously Learning Health Care In America. Washington: National Academies Press; 2013.
24. Kilo C. A framework for collaborative improvement: lessons from the Institute for Healthcare Improvement's Breakthrough Series. Qual Manag Health Care. 1998;6(4):1–13.
25. Langley G, Nolan K, Nolan T, Norman C, Provost L. The Improvement Guide. A Practical Approach to Enhancing Organizational Performance. San Francisco: Jossey-Bass; 1996.
26. Harris J, Bingham C, Morgan E. Improving care delivery and outcomes in pediatric rheumatic diseases. Curr Opin Rheumatol. 2016;28(2):110–6.
27. Pediatric Rheumatology Care & Outcomes Improvement Network (PR-COIN). About the PR-COIN Collaborative. [cited March 28, 2017]; Available from: https://pr-coin.org/about.
28. Institute for Healthcare Improvement. The Breakthrough Series: IHI's Collaborative Model for Achieving Breakthrough Improvement. Cambridge, MA: Institute for Healthcare Improvement; 2003 (Available on www.IHI.org).
29. Barton J, Koenig C, Evans-Young G, Trupin L, Anderson J, Ragouzeos D, et al. The design of a low literacy decision aid about rheumatoid arthritis medications developed in three languages for use during the clinical encounter. BMC Med Inform Decis Mak. 2014;14:104.
30. Lipstein E, Muething K, Dodds C, Britto M. "I'm the one taking it": adolescent participation in chronic disease treatment decisions. J Adolesc Health. 2013; 53(2):253–9.
31. Lipstein E, Brinkman W, Sage J, Lannon C, Morgan DE. Understanding treatment decision making in juvenile idiopathic arthritis: a qualitative assessment. Pediatr Rheumatol Online J. 2013;11(1):34.
32. Doran G. There's a S.M.A.R.T. way to write management's goals and objectives. Manag Rev. 1981;70(11):35–8.
33. Elwyn G, Barr P, Grande S, Thompson R, Walsh T, Ozanne E. Developing CollaboRATE: a fast and frugal patient-reported measure of shared decision making in clinical encounters. Patient Educ Couns. 2013;93(1):102–7.
34. Barr P, Thompson R, Walsh T, Grande S, Ozanne E, Elwyn G. The psychometric properties of CollaboRATE: a fast and frugal patient-reported measure of the shared decision-making process. J Med Internet Res. 2014;16(1):e2.
35. Legare F, Kearing S, Clay K, Gagnon S, D'Amours M, Rousseau M, et al. Are you SURE?: assessing patient decisional conflict with a 4-item screening test. Can Fam Physician. 2010;56(8):e308–e14.
36. O'Connor A. Validation of a decisional conflict scale. Med Decis Mak. 1995; 15(1):25–30.
37. Pediatric Rheumatology Care & Outcomes Improvement Network (PR-COIN). Arthritis Medication Choice Cards readily available. [cited March 28, 2017]; Available from: https://pr-coin.org/announcements/05-05-15.
38. Stacey D, Vandemheen K, Hennessey R, Gooyers T, Gaudet E, Mallick R, et al. Implementation of a cystic fibrosis lung transplant referral patient decision aid in routine clinical practice: an observational study. Implement Sci. 2015; 10:17.
39. Davis D, Mazmanian P, Fordis M, Van Harrison R, Thorpe K, Perrier L. Accuracy of physician self-assessment compared with observed measures of competence: a systematic review. JAMA. 2006;296(9):1094–102.
40. Wyatt K, Branda M, Anderson R, Pencille L, Montori V, Hess E, et al. Peering into the black box: a meta-analysis of how clinicians use decision aids during clinical encounters. Implement Sci. 2014;9:26.
41. Lipstein E, Dodds C, Britto M. Real life clinic visits do not match the ideals of shared decision making. J Pediatr. 2014;165(1):178–83. e1
42. Couet N, Desroches S, Robitaille H, Vaillancourt H, Leblanc A, Turcotte S, et al. Assessments of the extent to which health-care providers involve patients in decision making: a systematic review of studies using the OPTION instrument. Health Expect. 2015;18(4):542–61.

Education and employment in patients with juvenile idiopathic arthritis – a standardized comparison to the German general population

Jenny Schlichtiger[1*], Johannes-Peter Haas[2], Swaantje Barth[1], Betty Bisdorff[1], Lisa Hager[1], Hartmut Michels[2], Boris Hügle[2] and Katja Radon[1]

Abstract

Background: Although several studies show that JIA-patients have significantly lower employment rates than the general population, the research on educational and occupational attainments in patients with juvenile idiopathic arthritis (JIA) remain conflicting most likely due to small sample sizes. Therefore, aim of this study is to compare the educational achievements and employment status of 3698 JIA-patients with the German general population (GGP).

Methods: "SEPIA" was a large cross-sectional study on the current status of a historic cohort of JIA-patients treated in a single center between 1952 and 2010. For the analyses of education and employment a sub-cohort was extracted, including only adult cases with a confirmed diagnosis of JIA ($N = 2696$). Participants were asked to fill out a standardized written questionnaire on education and employment. Outcome measures (education/unemployment) were directly standardized to the GGP using data obtained from the National Educational Panel Study 2013 ($N = 11{,}728$) and the German Unemployment Statistics 2012 of the Federal Statistical Office ($N = 42{,}791{,}000$).

Results: After age- and sex-standardization, 3% (95% Confidence Interval 1.9 to 4.1%) more of the JIA-patients (26%) than of the GGP (23%) had only reached primary education. In contrast, parents of JIA-patients had similar levels of education as parents in the GGP. With a standardized difference of 0.2% (95% CI: 0.16 to 0.19%), the unemployment rate in JIA-patients was slightly, but not significantly higher than in the GGP. Stratifying for disease duration and the current treatment status, differences were confirmed for persons diagnosed before 2001, whilst for patients diagnosed after 2000, differences were found only in JIA-patients with ongoing disease. Medium and high educational achievements did not differ statistically significant between JIA patients and the GPP.

Conclusion: Educational achievements in German JIA-patients are significantly lower than in the GGP. Furthermore we were able to identify a slightly higher level of unemployment, especially in those with still under treatment and longer disease duration. Better treatment options as well as further development of social support programs might help to overcome this lifelong secondary effect of JIA.

Keywords: Juvenile idiopathic arthritis, Jia, Education, Chronic disease, Direct standardization, German general population

* Correspondence: Jenny.Schlichtiger@gmail.com
[1]Unit of Occupational and Environmental Epidemiology and NetTeaching, Institute and Outpatient Clinic for Occupational, Social and Environmental Medicine, University Hospital of Munich (LMU), Ziemssenstrasse 1, D-80336 Munich, Germany
Full list of author information is available at the end of the article

Background

Juvenile idiopathic arthritis (JIA) is a heterogeneous multifactorial autoimmune disease [1–3], characterized by persistent joint inflammation causing severe swellings, pain and limitation of movement [3]. The current definition of JIA unifies the previous classifications juvenile chronic arthritis (JCA) and juvenile rheumatic arthritis (JRA) [2, 4]. Incidence of JIA in Germany is estimated with 35 per 100,000/year, whereas in the Unites States the incidence rate is lower with 12 per 100,000/year [5]. Despite these comparatively low incidence rates, JIA is the most common rheumatic disease in children and adolescents and one of the most important causes of disability in this age group [1, 6, 7].

Although JIA-patients are frequently affected by severe functional impairment caused by inflammation and inflammation-related complications, some studies suggest that JIA-patients have a higher school graduation and postgraduate degrees compared to the general population [7–9]. Nevertheless, research on the educational attainments in patients with JIA remains conflicting [4, 10–12]. Concerning the employment status several studies have shown that adult JIA-patients have significantly lower employment rates than their healthy counterparts [1, 7, 8, 13–15]. Other research were able to show an association between arthritis and increased employment rates [15–17]. However, for the general description of the transition process into adulthood, the results of several studies suggest, that there is no significant difference between patients with rheumatic disease and their healthy peers [18].

Inconsistent findings across studies might mainly be caused by a variable age range of the participants or limited power due to the mostly low number of JIA-patients included [7]. Therefore the different results of recent studies make further research indispensable.

Considering previous contradictions the presented cross-sectional study compares the age- and sex-standardized educational achievements and the employment status of a large sample, including 3698 JIA-patients, to the German general population (GGP).

Since, in Germany parental level of education is still a major predictor of one's educational achievement [19], the age- and sex-standardized parental level of education of the patients and the German population was also compared.

Methods

Study population and study design

JIA patients

The SEPIA study (**S**tudie zu malignen **E**rkrankungen bei **P**atienten mit juveniler **i**diopathischer **A**rthritis) is a single-center hospital-based study. 10,580 patients who were hospitalized in the German Center for Pediatric and Adolescent Rheumatology (GCPAR) in Garmisch-Partenkirchen (GCPAR) between 1952 and 2010 were contacted. The GCPAR is the largest clinic for pediatric rheumatology in Europe with 60 years of experience it treats approximately 2500 inpatients and 900 outpatient patients a year. The clinic is focused on the treatment of children with inflammatory rheumatic diseases and chronic pain.

For our study patients were eligible if they had been diagnosed with JIA, JCA or JRA. Furthermore, they had to live in Germany and to be fluent in German. All participants had to sign an informed consent form; if they were under the age of 18 a parent/legal guardian had to give his/her permission for their participation. The Medical Ethical Committee of the University Hospital of Munich (LMU) approved the study. (Project- Nr.: 226-11).

General population

Data on the education of the German general population was extracted from the National Educational Panel Study (NEPS). In addition, the German Employment Statistics 2012 including the German population aged between 20 and 64 years were obtained from the Federal Statistical Office.

Recruitment

After a pilot test for comprehensibility and feasibility, the main study started in 2012 when 10,580 postal questionnaires were sent out. In the following 5970 residential addresses had to be searched via local registration offices.

Disease status

Two of the authors extracted the diagnosis made at the first admission and the date of the first admission to the GCPAR from the medical records. As information on the onset of disease was not available in one third of the patients, the date of the first admission to the GCPAR was calculated as a proxy for disease duration.

As the definition of childhood chronic arthritis was changed several times since 1952 [20, 21] we had to re-diagnose patients treated before 1997, the year when the current definition of JIA was put into place. This procedure has formerly been performed in order to evaluate the ILAR criteria for JIA [22].

Therefore the definition of JIA followed established criteria:

- Patients diagnosed before 1978 were re-classified according to the ILAR-classification based on their medical recordings [N = 433 (11.7%)] [23] This included patients diagnosed with Spondylarthitis, Psoriatic Arthritis, Rheumatoid Arthritis or Still's disease (with an onset before the age of 16 years, disease duration of at least 6 weeks and no other cause of symptoms)
- JCA-patients diagnosed between 1978 and 1996 according the classification criteria of the European League Against Rheumatism [N = 1290 (34.9%)] [24]

- JIA-patients diagnosed after 1996 had been classified based on the classification criteria of the International League of Associations for Rheumatology [N = 1975 (53.4%)] [20, 25]

Questionnaire

In 2012, data was collected via a self-administered standardized questionnaire, containing validated questions of the ISAAC [26] and the ECRHS [27] study on the following aspects:

- Socio-demographics: sex; age; participants' and parental education; employment status

Disease related questions were newly designed and face-validated by two experts:

Disease related data: holding a disability card (yes/no - For the determination of the requirement of a disability card, there are nationwide guidelines, which contain general assessment rules on the disease specific determination of the degree of disability [28]; current intake of anti-rheumatic drugs (yes/no - the medication classified as anti-rheumatic drugs included cytostatics, glucocorticoids, immunosuppressives, DMARDs, biologic agents); current treatment (yes/no).

Variable definition

Participants' educational level

The highest school degree of the participants was available from the questionnaire in the following categories: Primary School ("Hauptschule/Volksschule"), Secondary School ("Mittlere Reife/Realschule"), College ("Abitur/Fachabitur"), University ("Hochschule/Fachhochschule/Universität"), other degree.

In Germany the average age for the attendance of Primary School ranges from 5 to 18 years, for Secondary School and Collage from 8 to 18 years and for University the average entrance date is 21 years [29, 30].

Parental education

Highest level of schooling achieved by the parents was used to define parental level of education applying the same coding scheme as for the participants' educational level. Information on the parents' highest educational degree was available for 1801 participants [Missing values: n = 382 (21%)].

For both groups we categorized the educational achievements into *"Primary School Degree"*, *"Secondary School Degree"* and *"College or University Degree"*, in order to differentiate between low, medium and high level of education [31]. Participants that indicated "Other degree" were excluded as no definite level of schooling can be determined.

Employment

All participants indicating full- or at least part-time employment were categorized as being employed. Participants who indicated to carry out a profession less than 8 h per day or less than 40 h a week were categorized as being part-time employed.

Data management and statistical analyses

Eligible study population

Statistical analyses using level of education as outcome needed to be restricted to JIA-patients older than 19 years (n = 2696) due to the restrictions of the National Educational Panel Study (NEPS). Therefore, JIA-patients were excluded (Fig. 1) if:

- aged under 20 years [32],
- not graduate from school (pupils) yet
- no clear assignment was possible to the group of pupils or already graduated persons (students, trainees, working population, homemakers, retired) due to contradictory information within the questionnaire. (e.g. participants indicated a highest school degree but mentioned in the questionnaire that they were currently attending further education and that they worked part-time)
- missing information on educational degree

For the analyses of unemployment participants were excluded (Fig. 1) if:

- younger than 20 years or older than 64 years. As the national data on the employment status of the German general population [33] only considers the working population between 20 and 64;
- data classify them to be a pupil, student, trainee, homemaker or retired subject as profession
- no clear classification was possible to the group of pupils or already graduated persons (students, trainees, working population, homemakers, retired) due to contradictory information within the questionnaire. (e.g. participants indicated a school degree, but noted within the questionnaire that they were currently doing further education and that they worked part-time)
- employment status was missing.

Data entry

Double-entry of data and congruence checking was performed using Surveymonkey database (Surveymonkey Inc., USA) and Synkronizer Version 10.0 (©2000-2014, XL Consulting GmbH, Schweiz).

Statistical analyses

SPSS program version 22.0 (IBM Corporation, USA) was used for the statistical analyses.

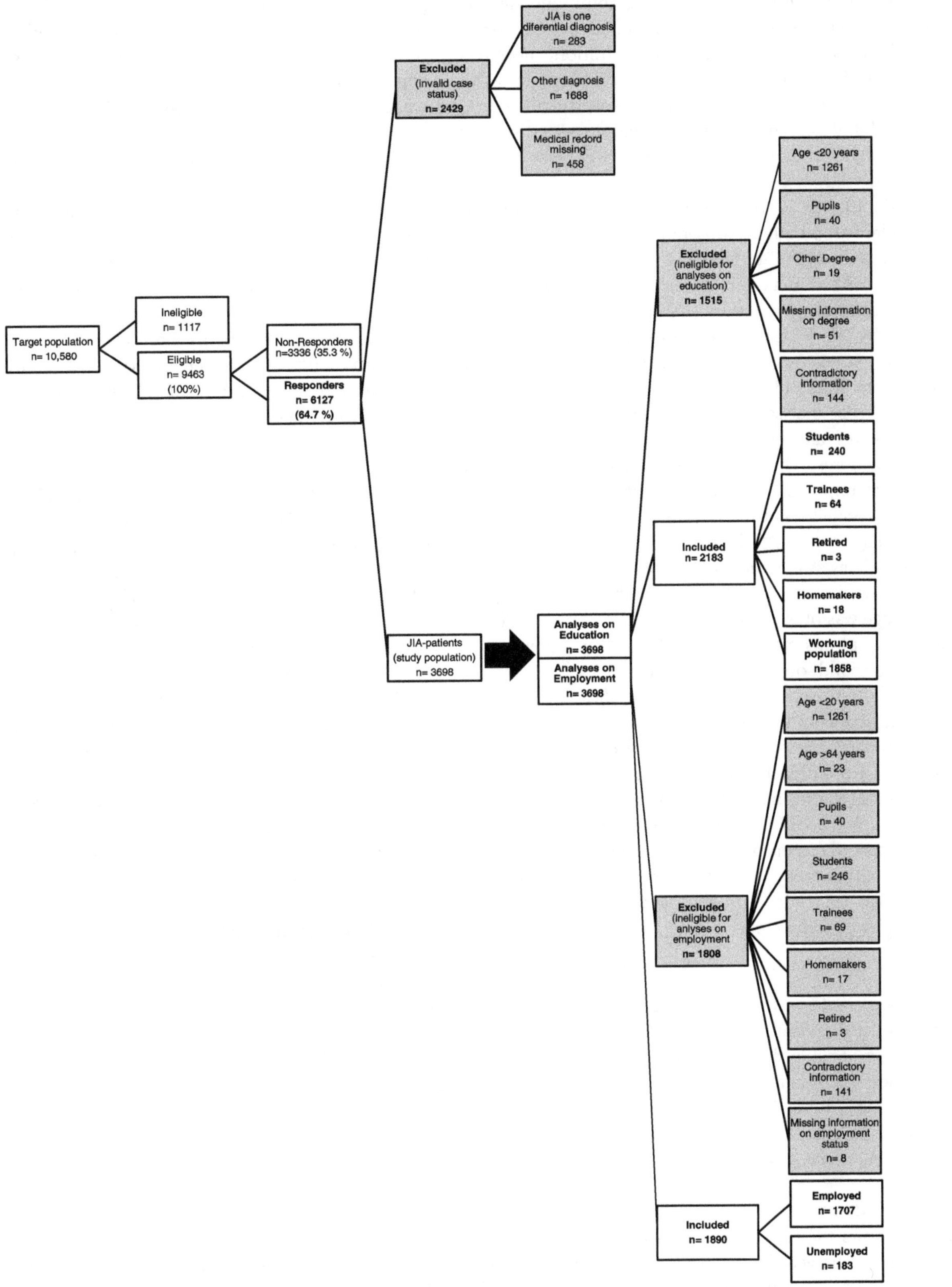

Fig. 1 Response and inclusion criteria of the study population. Eligibility criteria for the analyses on educational achievement and employment

For the description of socio-demographic and disease related characteristics absolute and relative frequencies were calculated. For age and disease duration, measures of the central tendency (mean, median) and measures of dispersion (range, standard deviation) were calculated.

Patients' and parental level of education were directly sex- and age-standardized to the NEPS-dataset for the general population [32]. For this, we stratified age (20–29; 30-39; 40–49; 50–59; ≥60 yrs) and sex according to the standard population. Subsequently the age- and sex-standardized relative differences were calculated with 95% confidence interval between the study population and the general population. Using the age categories provided by the Federal Statistical Office Germany (20–34; 35–49; 50–64 yrs) the same method was applied for employment status [34].

For sensitivity analyses the age- and sex-standardized educational degree and employment status were stratified by year of diagnoses. This was done as changes in treatment might have improved educational achievements and employment possibilities of JIA-patients [34]. For this two time periods, diagnoses made before 2001 or after 2000 were compared. This was done as biologics were approved for treatment of JIA in Germany around the year 2000 [35]. This change was of great clinical significance, since biologics alleviate symptoms rapidly and can be used in patients who did not respond on conventional therapies [36, 37]. In addition, within both time periods, stratification was performed for patients that were still under treatment due to their rheumatic disease and those who were not. Small age strata (n < 10) within the study population were excluded from analyses as they may produce invalid results [38].

As 31% of the SEPIA study population was from the Bavarian part of Germany, which has the lowest unemployment rate in Germany [39], a separate standardization of the Bavarian JIA-patients to the Bavarian general population (BGP) was conducted.

Results

The response rate was 66% with 6127 filled out questionnaires returned and of these, 3698 (60%) were identified as JIA-patients. The excluded patients (n = 2429) suffered from other (rheumatic) diseases. A total of 2183 fulfilled the inclusion criteria for the analyses about their own as well as the parental level of education. For the analyses on employment status, 1890 JIA-patients were eligible (Fig. 1).

Descriptive data

Table 1 shows the non-standardized distribution of socio-demographic characteristics of the SEPIA study population and the GGP. A significantly higher proportion of JIA-patients were female in comparison to the general population. In addition, JIA-patients were on average more than 10 years younger than the GGP. About half of the JIA-patients reported taking anti-rheumatic drugs at the time of the survey (Table 1). Over one third of the study population were disability cardholders. The median disease duration approximated by the date of first admission to the hospital was 20 years with a wide range (1 to 60 years).

Educational degree of the JIA-patients and the German general population

The non-standardized distribution of the educational degree of the JIA-patients indicated a higher level of schooling than in GGP with 51% of the JIA-patients having achieved a high educational degree as compared to 44% in GGP (Table 2). However, after age- and sex-standardization, 3% more of the JIA-patients had only achieved the lowest level of education (95% Confidence Interval: 1.91 to 4.12%) while medium and high educational achievements did not differ statistically significant.

Sensitivity analyses

JIA-patients admitted to the GCPAR before 2001

Stratifying for the date of admission (treated **before the year 2001** (n = 1887)) a 3% (95% CI: 1.94 to 4.15%) higher proportion of patients were shown to have a lower level of education as compared to the GGP. The differences in medium and high education remained non-significant. In patients still **under treatment** (n = 922) no statistically significant difference in the education was found as compared to the general population. Among patients who indicated **not being under treatment** at time of the survey (n = 962) 5% more than in GGP achieved only a primary school degree (3.34 to 5.57%) and 4% less than the general population reached a secondary school degree (−5.18 to −2.18%). There was no statistically significant difference between the proportions of highly educated persons in both groups. (Additional file 1).

JIA-patients admitted to the GCPAR after 2000

Comparing JIA-patients admitted **after 2000** (n = 288) to the German general population revealed no significant differences. When stratifying for current treatment status 5% (2.09 to 8.11%) more of participants that indicated to be still **in need of treatment** were less educated than the general population. Furthermore, there was no statistical significant difference in the educational achievements of JIA-patients and the German general population for those admitted after the year 2000 and **not receiving treatment** at the time of the survey (Additional file 1).

Standardized comparison of the parental education of the SEPIA study population and the German general population

Educational level of participants' parents was almost equally distributed between low, medium and high level of education (Table 3). Comparing the standardized educational

Table 1 Comparison of socio-demographic and disease related characteristics of the SEPIA study population and the GGP

	SEPIA study population		German general population[a]	
Total	N = 2183	$n_{missing}$	N = 11,799	$n_{missing}$
Sex				
Female	60.8% (n = 1327)	0	50.8% (n = 6065)	0
Age (years)				
Mean (± SD[b])	34.4 (± 10.8)	0	46.9 (± 11.2)	10
Median (Range)	32.0 (20.0 – 73.0)		47.9 (20.3 – 67.5)	
Current intake of anti-rheumatic drugs	49.0% (n = 1068)	0	N.a.[c]	
Disability cardholder	37.3% (n = 815)	0	N.a.[c]	
Disease duration[d]				
Mean (± SD[b]) Median (Range)	22.8 (± 11.6) 20.0 (1.0 - 60.0)	0	N.a.[c]	

[a]NEPS Data
[b]SD = Standard Deviation
[c]N.a. = Not available
[d]Disease duration approximated by the date of the 1st admission to the GCPAR

achievement to the general population, JIA-patients' parents were equally likely to have only reached primary education, while they were more likely to hold a *"Secondary School Degree"* (difference 3%; 95% CI: 2.31 to 4.37%) and less frequently held *"College or University Degree"* (–3%; –4.21 to –2.03%).

Unemployment among the SEPIA study population and the German general population.

For JIA-patients, a non-standardized unemployment of 9.7% was observed which went up to 12.9% after direct age- and sex-standardization to GGP. The 0.2% difference compared to the GGP was statistically significant (95% CI 0.16 to 0.19%) (Table 4).

Sensitivity analyses

JIA-patients admitted to the GCPAR before 2001

In sensitivity analyses a standardized difference of 0.1% (95% CI: 0.07 to 0.10%) indicated that the proportion of unemployed JIA-patients **admitted before 2001** (n = 1691) was almost equal to that of the general population. However, those still **receiving treatment** due to JIA were more likely to be unemployed (6%; 6.27 to 6.30%) while those **not requiring treatment** were statistically significantly less likely to be unemployed (–4%; –4.23 to –4.21%). (Additional file 2).

JIA-patients admitted to the GCPAR after 2000

Comparing JIA-patients admitted after 2000 to the general population, a 0.5% (–0.45 to –0.49%) lower standardized proportion of unemployment was observed (n = 195). Again, this differed by treatment status: Of the patients still **reliant on treatment** (n = 126) the proportion of unemployment was 1.5% (1.47 to 1.51%) higher, among those **not requiring treatment** it was 2% (–2.29 to –2.25%) lower than in the general population. (Additional file 2).

Subgroup of Bavarian JIA-patients

The Bavarian study population had in total a 3% higher proportion of unemployment (95% CI: 3.27 to 3.34%) than the Bavarian general population.

Patients admitted to the GCPAR before 2001 were significantly more likely to be unemployed (3%; 3.12 to 3.28%) when restricting the analyses to the Bavarian sub-cohort. In patients still **reliant on treatment** the unemployment was 8% (7.42 to 7.49%) above that of the BGP. However, in those who did **not require treatment** at the time of the survey, the unemployment was almost equal (–0.1%; –0.17 to –0.11%) to that of the BGP.

The standardized difference in Bavarian JIA-patients **admitted to the GCPAR after 2000** remained comparable to that of the total study population (–0.5%; –0.53 to –0.42%). Patients' still **receiving treatment** at the time of the survey had a 4% (4.04 to 4.16%) higher unemployment rate than in the BGP. Patients that were **not reliant on treatment** any more were statistically significantly less likely (–4%; –4.29 to –4.20%) to be unemployed than the general population. (Additional file 3).

Discussion

In the present study, JIA-patients had on average achieved a lower level of education and were slightly but statistically significantly more likely to be unemployed than the GGP. Distinctions in parental level of education could not explain this difference indicating that this might be a consequence of their disease.

Our findings are in line with some but not all previous studies. E.g., Packham et al. reported that JIA-patients from the UK were better educated while their unemployment rate was twice as high compared to the control population. They investigated 246 JIA-patients of which 72% were female, the mean age was 35 years, the patients

Table 2 Age- and sex-standardized comparison of the educational degree of the study population and the GGP

				Primary School Degree			Secondary School Degree			College or University Degree		
	Age groups[a] [years]	N GGP[b]	N Sepia	GGP[b] n (%)	SEPIA n (%)	Standardized SEPIA n (%) [c]	GGP[b] n (%)	SEPIA n (%)	Standardized SEPIA n (%)[c]	GGP[b] n (%)	SEPIA n (%)	Standardized SEPIA n (%)[c]
Men	20–29	624	306	99 (15.87)	55 (17.97)	112 (17.97)	170 (27.24)	95 (31.05)	194 (31.05)	355 (56.89)	156 (50.98)	318 (50.98)
	30–39	772	230	157 (20.34)	50 (21.74)	168 (21.74)	209 (27.07)	69 (30.00)	232 (30.00)	406 (52.59)	111 (48.26)	373 (48.26)
	40–49	1542	231	348 (22.57)	52 (22.51)	347 (22.51)	501 (32.49)	69 (29.87)	461 (29.87)	693 (44.94)	110 (47.62)	734 (47.62)
	50–59	2052	59	553 (26.95)	14 (23.73)	487 (23.73)	555 (27.05)	19 (32.20)	661 (32.20)	944 (46.00)	26 (44.07)	904 (44.07)
	≥60	812	30	359 (44.21)	13 (43.33)	352 (43.33)	177 (21.80)	8 (26.67)	217 (26.67)	276 (33.99)	9 (30.00)	244 (30.00)
Women	20–29	482	618	35 (7.26)	61 (9.87)	48 (9.87)	136 (28.22)	201 (32.52)	157 (32.52)	311 (64.52)	356 (57.61)	278 (57.61)
	30–39	820	344	118 (14.39)	36 (10.47)	86 (10.47)	285 (34.76)	110 (31.98)	262 (31.98)	417 (50.85)	198 (57.56)	472 (57.56)
	40–49	1753	242	227 (12.95)	37 (15.29)	268 (15.29)	786 (44.84)	97 (40.08)	703 (40.08)	740 (42.21)	108 (44.63)	782 (44.63)
	50–59	2182	97	538 (24.66)	40 (41.24)	900 (41.24)	847 (38.82)	28 (28.87)	630 (28.87)	797 (36.53)	29 (29.90)	652 (29.90)
	≥60	740	26	290 (39.19)	11 (42.31)	313 (42.31)	240 (32.43)	8 (30.77)	228 (30.77)	210 (28.38)	7 (26.92)	199 (26.92)
Total		11,789	2183	2724 (23.11)	369 (16.90)	3080 (26.13)	3906 (33.13)	704 (32.25)	3742 (31.75)	5149 (43.68)	1110 (50.85)	4956 (42.04)
Standardized Difference %[d] (95% CI)[e]						3.02 (1.91; 4.12)			−1.39 (−2.59; −0.19)			−1.63 (−2.91; −0.37)

[a]Categorization of age groups was set by NEPS dataset of the German general population
[b]GGP = German general population [Ref.]
[c]Standardized proportion of the SEPIA study population
[d]Standardized Difference (%) = Standardized Proportion of SEPIA (%) − Proportion of GGP (%)
[e]95% CI = 95% Confidence Interval

Table 3 Age- and sex-standardized comparison of the parental education within the study population and the GGP

	Age groups[a] [years]	N GGP[b]	N Sepia	Primary School Degree			Secondary School Degree			College or University Degree		
				GGP[b] n (%)	SEPIA n (%)	Standardized SEPIA n (%)[c]	GGP[b] n (%)	SEPIA n (%)	Standardized SEPIA n (%)[c]	GGP[b] n (%)	SEPIA n (%)	Standardized SEPIA n (%)[c]
Men	20–29	618	257	153 (24.76)	52 (20.23)	125 (20.23)	179 (28.96)	93 (36.19)	224 (36.19)	286 (46.28)	112 (43.58)	269 (43.58)
	30–39	767	192	303 (39.50)	77 (40.10)	308 (40.10)	197 (25.68)	58 (30.21)	232 (30.21)	267 (34.81)	57 (29.69)	228 (29.69)
	40–49	1527	180	907 (59.40)	113 (62.78)	959 (62.78)	240 (15.72)	47 (26.11)	399 (26.11)	380 (24.89)	20 (11.11)	170 (11.11)
	50–59	2053	50	1336 (65.08)	33 (66.00)	1355 (66.00)	301 (14.66)	11 (22.00)	452 (22.00)	416 (20.26)	6 (12.00)	246 (12.00)
	> = 60	809	22	592 (73.18)	16 (72.73)	588 (72.73)	98 (12.11)	3 (13.64)	110 (13.64)	119 (14.71)	3 (13.64)	110 (13.64)
Women	20–29	481	532	117 (24.32)	105 (19.74)	95 (19.74)	158 (32.85)	190 (35.71)	172 (35.71)	206 (42.83)	237 (44.55)	214 (44.55)
	30–39	818	277	331 (40.46)	100 (36.10)	295 (36.10)	219 (26.77)	68 (24.55)	201 (24.55)	268 (32.76)	109 (39.35)	322 (39.35)
	40–49	1729	195	981 (56.74)	109 (55.90)	967 (55.90)	333 (19.26)	37 (18.97)	328 (18.97)	415 (24.00)	49 (25.13)	435 (25.13)
	50–59	2179	79	1399 (64.20)	52 (65.82)	1434 (65.82)	323 (14.82)	12 (15.19)	331 (15.19)	457 (20.97)	15 (18.99)	414 (18.99)
	> = 60	747	17	515 (68.94)	11 (64.71)	483 (64.71)	96 (12.85)	2 (11.76)	88 (11.76)	136 (18.21)	4 (23.53)	176 (23.53)
Total		11,728	1801	6634 (56.57)	668 (37.09)	6609 (56.35)	2144 (18.28)	521 (28.93)	2536 (21.62)	2950 (25.15)	612 (33.98)	2584 (22.03)
Standardized Difference %[d] (95% CI)[e]						−0.21 (−1.49; 1.06)			3.34 (2.31; 4.37)			−3.12 (−4.21; −2.03)

[a]Categorization of age groups was set by NEPS dataset of the German general population
[b]GGP = German general population [Ref.]
[c]Standardized proportion of the SEPIA study population
[d]Standardized Difference (%) = Standardized Proportion of SEPIA (%) – Proportion of GGP (%)
[e]95% CI = 95% Confidence Interval

Table 4 Age- and sex-standardized comparison of the unemployment rate of the study population and the GGP

	Age groups[a] [years]	N GGP[b]	N Sepia	Unemployment GGP[b] n (%)	SEPIA n (%)	Standardized SEPIA n (%)[c]
Men	20–34	6,135,000	342	427,000 (6.96)	13 (3.80)	233,202 (3.80)
	35–49	8,431,000	355	381,000 (4.52)	20 (5.63)	474,986 (5.63)
	50–64	9,904,000	74	3,680,000 (37.16)	11 (14.86)	1,472,216 (14.86)
Women	20–34	5,335,000	616	312,000 (5.85)	36 (5.84)	311,786 (5.84)
	35–49	7,336,000	391	336,000 (4.58)	69 (17.65)	1,294,588 (17.65)
	50–64	5,650,000	112	291,000 (5.13)	34 (30.36)	1,715,178 (30.36)
Total		42,791,000	1890	5,427,000 (12.68)	183 (9.68)	5,501,956 (12.86)
Standardized Difference %[d] (95% CI)[e]						0.18 (0.16; 0.19)

[a]Categorization of age groups was set by the data on employment of the German General population of the Federal Statistical Office Germany
[b]GGP = German general population [Ref.]
[c]Standardized proportion of the SEPIA study population
[d]Standardized Difference (%) = Standardized Proportion of SEPIA (%) − Proportion of GGP (%)
[e]95% CI = 95% Confidence Interval

siblings served as controls [8]. Foster and colleagues, however, did not observe a difference in the educational attainment of JIA-patients compared to local controls in the UK. They included 82 patients of which 83% were female, the median age was 30 years and the local population severed as controls [4]. In line with our results Bouaddi et al. found that the schooling of Moroccan children with JIA was negatively impacted by their chronic illness. They included 33 JIA-patients and 74 healthy controls, 46% of the observed patients were female with a median age of 11 years [3]. Within the SEPIA study we investigated the educational achievements of 2183 JIA-patients of which 61% were female; the median age was 32 years. The age- and sex-standardized comparison to the GGP showed that JIA-patients received statistical significantly lower educational degrees. Although within Germany the number of young people entering university is constantly increasing [40], the proportion of students suffering from health restrictions remained around 7% (n = 137,000) within the time range from 2000 to 2012 [41]. One explanation for poor educational performance might be increased absenteeism-rates within pupils that suffer from chronic diseases [3, 42–44]. Bouaddi et al. observed that JIA-patients were 3-times more often absent then the healthy controls and 33% were not even able to attend school [3]. Moreover, patients with chronic conditions were found to have more days of absences than could be attributed to their chronic disease [43]. Confirming these findings a study by Moonie et al. reported a negative impact of absenteeism on the test performance for all participants comparing the educational achievements of asthma patients to their non-asthmatic peers [44]. In accordance with these findings adolescents with chronic conditions were found to have higher school dropout rates [43].

Interpreting these inconsistencies between studies, differences in health- [45] and education systems as well as the social insurance systems have to be taken into account. In Germany, 90% of the pupils attend public schools, [46] and 93% of all students are enrolled at a public university [47]. In addition, about 86% of the German population are members of public health insurances [48], which covers e.g. the JIA treatment costs. Therefore, the disease might not have a large impact on families' income as it could be the case in other countries where families have to cover costs for treatment and education.

In Germany, since 2002, programs supporting employers to hire persons with disability which offer an extended protection from termination, contribute a part of the salary and offer financial support for better accessibility are in place [49]. Additionally entrepreneurs with more than 20 employers are legally obligated to employ at least 5% disabled persons [50]. Despite disability legislations we showed a higher overall rate of unemployment in JIA-patients compared to the GGP. These differences were mainly due to higher likelihood of unemployment in patients with active disease. Sensitivity analyses further showed that the unemployment in participants admitted to the GCPAR after the year 2000 was 0.5% lower than in the GGP. This circumstance could on one hand be due to the already mentioned disability legislations; on the other hand they might be a result of better treatment options. Due to progress in early detection and holistic treatment options better patient outcomes could be achieved [36, 37, 51]. The increased unemployment rates within the Bavarian subset are due to Bavaria being a rather prosperous region of Germany where the unemployment is on average lower [39, 52].

The recruitment of a large sample of JIA-patients followed from childhood until adulthood is the main strength of the study. Furthermore, data was collected via a detailed questionnaire containing validated standardized questions. As only questionnaire data on the highest school degree, sex (categorical items) and age (calculated via date of birth) was considered, we do not assume major reporting bias. Additionally, direct standardization enabled an unbiased comparison to the GGP.

Some limitations of our study have to be taken into account as well. As the National Disability Program and the use of biologic drugs were introduced in early 2000, young patients might be more likely to have experienced the beneficial effects of the improved access to employment and new treatment possibilities. However, future studies might be more likely to show the beneficial effects of these measures as many of the participants admitted after 2000 were still under the age of 20 years and had therefore been excluded from our analyses. Furthermore, we were not able to conduct analyses on the non-responders, as no data was available. This group of patients might contain more severe cases, which were not able to answer the questionnaire because of their health condition. In addition, on the basis of the available data we were not able to consider the impact of the disease on delaying the graduation or the entry into the work force. No further analyses on patients classified as students, trainees, homeworkers or retired persons were conducted because no data on the background of their employment status was available, although it might be associated to disease related factors. It is also due to a lack of data, that we had to approximate the disease duration by the date of the first admission to the GCPAR. This might lead to biased results since the delay between the onset of symptoms and the first admission could be highly variable. However, we choose this approach as it rather underestimates the effect of disease duration.

Although a response of 66% can be considered as reasonably high in an epidemiological study of this kind, one still has to take selection bias into account. In general, persons with a higher level of education are more likely to participate in studies [53–55]. This would have led to an underestimation of effect, i.e., the true level of education among JIA-patients would even be lower than in our study. Generalizability of our results to all JIA-patients might be limited by the fact that we recruited JIA-patients from a specialized hospital where more severe cases are likely to be treated.

Conclusion

In conclusion, our findings indicate that especially JIA-patients with longer disease duration or active disease still have a lower educational attainment and higher unemployment rate than the general population. This calls for further improvement of treatment options in order to minimize the permanent impact of JIA on patients' life. Further progress in maintaining mobility and effective pain management could facilitate the access to higher educational degrees and a successful profession. Furthermore, more supporting programs within the education system are necessary to increase the chance on higher educational qualifications. Occupational therapy interventions could improve the entry into the working environment.

Acknowledgements

The authors would like to thank the "Verein Hilfe für das rheumakranke Kind e.V." for funding this study. Furthermore, they would like to thank all the study participants as well as Birgit Huber and colleagues from the GCPAR in Garmisch-Partenkirchen for their invaluable support during fieldwork.

Funding

The "Verein Hilfe für das rheumakranke Kind" has provided financial support for this study. The funders had no role in study design, data collection and analysis, decision to publish, or preparation of the manuscript.

Authors' contributions

JS conducted the fieldwork, performed the statistical analysis and drafted the manuscript. JPH designed the study, supported fieldwork and interpretation of data and helped draft the manuscript. SB coordinated the fieldwork, was involved in interpretation of the data and helped draft the manuscript. BB designed the study, coordinated the fieldwork, contributed to the interpretation of the data and helped draft the manuscript. LH participated in the fieldwork and interpretation of the data and helped to draft the manuscript. HM and BH participated in the design of the study, interpretation of data and helped draft the manuscript. KR designed the study, supported fieldwork, statistical analysis and interpretation of data and helped draft the manuscript. All authors read and approved the final manuscript.

Competing interests

The authors declare that they have no competing interests.

Consent for publication

Not applicable.

Financial support

"Verein Hilfe für das Rheumakranke Kind e.V."

Author details

[1]Unit of Occupational and Environmental Epidemiology and NetTeaching, Institute and Outpatient Clinic for Occupational, Social and Environmental Medicine, University Hospital of Munich (LMU), Ziemssenstrasse 1, D-80336 Munich, Germany. [2]German Center for Pediatric and Adolescent Rheumatology, Garmisch-Partenkirchen, Germany.

References

1. Malviya A, Rushton SP, Foster HE, Ferris CM, Hanson H, Muthumayandi K, et al. The relationships between adult juvenile idiopathic Arthritis and employment. Arthritis Rheum. 2012;64(9):3016–24.
2. Ravelli A, Martini A. Juvenile idiopathic arthritis. Lancet. 2007;369(9563):767–78.
3. Bouaddi I, Rostom S, El Badri D, Hassani A, Chkirate B, Amine B, et al. Impact of juvenile idiopathic arthritis on schooling. BMC Pediatr. 2013;13:2.
4. Foster HE, Marshall N, Myers A, Dunkley P, Griffiths ID. Outcome in adults with juvenile idiopathic arthritis: a quality of life study. Arthritis Rheum. 2003;48(3):767–75.
5. Eisenstein EM, Berkun Y. Diagnosis and classification of juvenile idiopathic arthritis. J Autoimmun. 2014;(48-49):31–3.
6. Minden K, Niewerth M, Listing J, Mobius D, Thon A, Ganser G, et al. The economic burden of juvenile idiopathic arthritis-results from the German paediatric rheumatologic database. Clin Exp Rheumatol. 2009;27(5):863–9.
7. Gerhardt CA, McGoron KD, Vannatta K, McNamara KA, Taylor J, Passo M, et al. Educational and occupational outcomes among young adults with juvenile idiopathic Arthritis. Arthritis Rheumatism Arthritis Care Res. 2008;59(10):1385–91.
8. Packham JC, Hall MA. Long-term follow-up of 246 adults with juvenile idiopathic arthritis: social function, relationships and sexual activity. Rheumatology. 2002;41(12):1440–3.
9. Minden K, Niewerth M, Listing J, Biedermann T, Bollow M, Schontube M, et al. Long-term outcome in patients with juvenile idiopathic arthritis. Arthritis Rheum. 2002;46(9):2392–401.
10. Miller JJ 3rd. Psychosocial factors related to rheumatic diseases in childhood. J Rheumatol Suppl. 1993;38:1–11.
11. White PH, Shear ES. Transition/job readiness for adolescents with juvenile arthritis and other chronic illness. J Rheumatol Suppl. 1992;33:23–7.
12. Archenholtz B, Nordborg E, Bremell T. Lower level of education in young adults with arthritis starting in the early adulthood. Scand J Rheumatol. 2001;30(6):353–5.
13. Peterson LS, Mason T, Nelson AM, O'Fallon WM, Gabriel SE. Psychosocial outcomes and health status of adults who have had juvenile rheumatoid arthritis - a controlled, population-based study. Arthritis Rheum. 1997;40(12): 2235–40.
14. Flato B, Lien GH, Smerdel A, Vinje O, Dale K, Johnston V, et al. Prognostic factors in juvenile rheumatoid arthritis: a case-control study revealing early predictors and outcome after 14.9 years. J Rheumatol. 2003;30(2):386–93.
15. Diaz-Mendoza AC, Modesto Caballero C, Navarro-Cendejas J. Analysis of employment rate and social status in young adults with childhood-onset rheumatic disease in Catalonia. Pediatr Rheumatol Online J. 2015;13:29.
16. Jetha A. The impact of arthritis on the early employment experiences of young adults: a literature review. Disabil Health J. 2015;8(3):317–24.
17. Gerhardt CA, McGoron KD, Vannatta K, McNamara KA, Taylor J, Passo M, et al. Educational and occupational outcomes among young adults with juvenile idiopathic arthritis. Arthritis Rheum. 2008;59(10):1385–91.
18. Jetha A, Badley E, Beaton D, Fortin PR, Shiff NJ, Gignac MA. Unpacking early work experiences of young adults with rheumatic disease: an examination of absenteeism, job disruptions, and productivity loss. Arthritis Care Res (Hoboken). 2015;67(9):1246–54.
19. Fischer M, Geis W. Bestimmungsgrößen der Bildungsmobilität in Deutschland. IW-Trends : Vierteljahresschrift zur empirischen Wirtschaftsforschung aus dem Institut der Deutschen Wirtschaft Köln. 2013;40(1):3–17.
20. Duffy CM, Colbert RA, Laxer RM, Schanberg LE, Bowyer SL. Nomenclature and classification in chronic childhood arthritis - time for a change? Arthritis Rheum. 2005;52(2):382–5.
21. Petty RE, Southwood TR, Manners P, Baum J, Glass DN, Goldenberg J, et al. International league of associations for rheumatology classification of juvenile idiopathic arthritis: second revision, Edmonton, 2001. J Rheumatol. 2004;31(2):390–2.
22. Krumrey-Langkammerer M, Hafner R. Evaluation of the ILAR criteria for juvenile idiopathic arthritis. J Rheumatol. 2001;28(11):2544–7.
23. Brewer EJ Jr, Bass J, Baum J, Cassidy JT, Fink C, Jacobs J, et al. Current proposed revision of JRA criteria. JRA criteria Subcommittee of the Diagnostic and Therapeutic Criteria Committee of the American rheumatism section of the Arthritis Foundation. Arthritis Rheum. 1977;20(2 Suppl):195–9.
24. Wood P. Special meeting on nomenclature and classification of arthritis in children. In: The care of rheumatic children [internet]. Basel: EULAR Publisher; 1978. p. 47–50.
25. Petty RE. Classification of childhood arthritis: a work in progress. Bailliere Clin Rheum. 1998;12(2):181–90.
26. Weiland SK, Bjorksten B, Brunekreef B, Cookson WO, von Mutius E, Strachan DP. Phase II of the international study of asthma and allergies in childhood (ISAAC II): rationale and methods. Eur Respir J. 2004;24(3):406–12.
27. European Community Respiratory Health survey. Available from: http://www.ecrhs.org/Quests/ECRHSIImainquestionnaire.pdf. Accessed 15 May 2017.
28. Verbraucherschutz BfJu. Verordnung zur Durchführung des § 1 Abs. 1 und 3, des § 30 Abs. 1 und des § 35 Abs. 1 des Bundesversorgungsgesetzes (Versorgungsmedizin-Verordnung - VersMedV) Anlage zu § 2 der Versorgungsmedizin-Verordnung vom 10. Dezember 2008 2008. Available from: http://www.gesetze-im-internet.de/versmedv/anlage.html. Accessed 15 May 2017.
29. Entwicklung des Durchschnittsalters von Studierenden und Absolventen an deutschen Hochschulen seit 2000. 2008. https://www.destatis.de/DE/Publikationen/WirtschaftStatistik/BildungForschungKultur/DurchschnittsalterStudierende.pdf?__blob=publicationFile. Accessed 15 May 2017.
30. Bildung und Kultur. Allgemeinbildende Schulen. Schuljahr 2014/2015. 2015.
31. Jöckel K-H, Babitsch B, Bellach B-M, Bloomfield K, Hoffmeyer-Zlotnik J, Winkler J, et al. Messung und Quantifizierung soziodemographischer Merkmale in epidemiologischen Studien. Messung Soziodemographischer Merkmale Epidemiologie RKI-Schriften. 1998;1(1998):7–38.
32. Blossfeld H-P, von Maurice J. Education as a lifelong process. Z Erziehungswiss. 2011;14(2):19–34.
33. Mikrozensus Bevölkerung und Erwerbstätigkeit: Stand und Entwicklung der Erwerbstätigkeit in Deutschland. https://www.destatis.de/DE/Publikationen/Thematisch/Arbeitsmarkt/Erwerbstaetige/StandEntwicklungErwerbstaetigkeit2010411127004.pdf?__blob=publicationFile. Accessed 15 May 2017
34. Minden K, Niewerth M, Zink A, Seipelt E, Foeldvari I, Girschick H, et al. Long-term outcome of patients with JIA treated with etanercept, results of the biologic register JuMBO. Rheumatology. 2012;51(8):1407–15.
35. Horneff G, Forster J, Seyberth HW, Michels H, Arbeitgemeinschaft Kinder- und J. Recommendations by the pediatric and adolescent rheumatology study committee on therapy with Etanercept (p75 TNF-alpha receptor immunoglobulin fusion protein. Pharmacotherapy committee Z Rheumatol 2000;59(6):365-9.
36. Hashkes PJ, Uziel Y, Laxer RM. The safety profile of biologic therapies for juvenile idiopathic arthritis. Nat Rev Rheumatol. 2010;6(10):561–71.
37. Klein A, Horneff G. Treatment strategies for juvenile idiopathic arthritis. Expert Opin Pharmacother. 2009;10(18):3049–60.
38. Curtin LR, Klein RJ, Statistics NCfH. Direct standardization (age-adjusted death rates). Hyattsville: U.S. Department of Health and Human Services, Public Health Service, Centers for Disease Control and Prevention, National Center for Health Statistics; 1995.
39. Durchschnittliche Arbeitslosenquote nach Bundesländern im Jahr 2014: statista; 2014. Available from: http://de.statista.com/statistik/daten/studie/2192/umfrage/durchschnittliche-arbeitslosenquote-nach-bundeslaendern/. Accessed 15 May 2017.
40. Wachsender Studentenberg – Entwicklung der Studierendenzahlen in Deutschland: Bundeszentrale für Politische Bildung; 2014. Available from: http://www.bpb.de/gesellschaft/kultur/zukunft-bildung/190350/wachsender-studentenberg-entwicklung-der-studierendenzahlen-in-deutschland. Accessed 15 May 2017.
41. Middendorff EABPJKMNN. Die wirtschaftliche und soziale Lage der Studierenden in Deutschland 2012 - 20. Sozialerhebung des Deutschen Studentenwerks durchgeführt durch das HIS-Institut für Hochschulforschung: Bundesministerium für Bildung und Forschung; 2012. Available from: https://www.studentenwerke.de/sites/default/files/01_20-SE-Hauptbericht.pdf. Accessed 15 May 2017.
42. Sturge C, Garralda M, Boissin M, Dore C, Woo P. School attendance and juvenile chronic arthritis. Br J Rheumatol. 1997;36(11):1218–23.
43. Suris JC, Michaud PA, Viner R. The adolescent with a chronic condition. Part I: developmental issues. Arch Dis Child. 2004;89(10):938–42.
44. Moonie S, Sterling D, Figgs L, Castro M. The relationship between school absence, academic performance, and asthma status. J Sch Health. 2008;78(3):140–8.
45. Hugle B, Haas JP, Benseler SM. Treatment preferences in juvenile idiopathic arthritis - a comparative analysis in two health care systems. Pediatr Rheumatol Online J. 2013;11(1):3.
46. Statistisches Bundesamt W. Schulen auf einen Blick 2012. Available from: https://www.destatis.de/DE/Publikationen/Thematisch/BildungForschungKultur/Schulen/BroschuereSchulenBlick0110018129004.pdf?__blob=publicationFile.

47. Statistisches Bundesamt W. Bildung und Kultur 2014. Available from: https://www.destatis.de/DE/Publikationen/Thematisch/BildungForschungKultur/Hochschulen/PrivateHochschulen5213105127004.pdf?__blob=publicationFile.
48. Statistisches Bundesamt W. Angaben zur Krankenversicherung - (Ergebnisse der Mikrozensus 2011) 2012. Available from: https://www.destatis.de/DE/Publikationen/Thematisch/Bevoelkerung/HaushalteMikrozensus/KrankenversicherungMikrozensus2130110119004.pdf?__blob=publicationFile.
49. Behindertengleichstellungsgesetze. Available from: http://www.behindertenbeauftragte.de/DE/Themen/RechtlicheGrundlagen/Behindertengleichstellungsgesetz/Behindertengleichstellungsgesetz_node.html. Accessed 15 May 2017.
50. Allgemeines Gleichbehandlungsgesetz (AGG): Bundesministerium der Justiz und Verbraucherschutz; 2006. Available from: https://www.gesetze-im-internet.de/agg/BJNR189710006.html.
51. Davies R, Gaynor D, Hyrich KL, Pain CE. Efficacy of biologic therapy across individual juvenile idiopathic arthritis subtypes: a systematic review. Semin Arthritis Rheum. 2016;
52. Nettoeinkommen und verfügbares Nettoeinkommen pivater Haushalte im Monat nach Bundesländern Essen: statista; 2015. Available from: http://de.statista.com/statistik/daten/studie/5758/umfrage/verfuegbares-nettoeinkommen-nach-bundeslaendern/. Accessed 15 May 2017.
53. Sonne-Holm S, Sorensen TI, Jensen G, Schnohr P. Influence of fatness, intelligence, education and sociodemographic factors on response rate in a health survey. J Epidemiol Community Health. 1989;43(4):369–74.
54. Korkeila K, Suominen S, Ahvenainen J, Ojanlatva A, Rautava P, Helenius H, et al. Non-response and related factors in a nation-wide health survey. Eur J Epidemiol. 2001;17(11):991–9.
55. Langhammer A, Krokstad S, Romundstad P, Heggland J, Holmen J. The HUNT study: participation is associated with survival and depends on socioeconomic status, diseases and symptoms. BMC Med Res Methodol. 2012;12:143.

Permissions

All chapters in this book were first published in PR, by BioMed Central; hereby published with permission under the Creative Commons Attribution License or equivalent. Every chapter published in this book has been scrutinized by our experts. Their significance has been extensively debated. The topics covered herein carry significant findings which will fuel the growth of the discipline. They may even be implemented as practical applications or may be referred to as a beginning point for another development.

The contributors of this book come from diverse backgrounds, making this book a truly international effort. This book will bring forth new frontiers with its revolutionizing research information and detailed analysis of the nascent developments around the world.

We would like to thank all the contributing authors for lending their expertise to make the book truly unique. They have played a crucial role in the development of this book. Without their invaluable contributions this book wouldn't have been possible. They have made vital efforts to compile up to date information on the varied aspects of this subject to make this book a valuable addition to the collection of many professionals and students.

This book was conceptualized with the vision of imparting up-to-date information and advanced data in this field. To ensure the same, a matchless editorial board was set up. Every individual on the board went through rigorous rounds of assessment to prove their worth. After which they invested a large part of their time researching and compiling the most relevant data for our readers.

The editorial board has been involved in producing this book since its inception. They have spent rigorous hours researching and exploring the diverse topics which have resulted in the successful publishing of this book. They have passed on their knowledge of decades through this book. To expedite this challenging task, the publisher supported the team at every step. A small team of assistant editors was also appointed to further simplify the editing procedure and attain best results for the readers.

Apart from the editorial board, the designing team has also invested a significant amount of their time in understanding the subject and creating the most relevant covers. They scrutinized every image to scout for the most suitable representation of the subject and create an appropriate cover for the book.

The publishing team has been an ardent support to the editorial, designing and production team. Their endless efforts to recruit the best for this project, has resulted in the accomplishment of this book. They are a veteran in the field of academics and their pool of knowledge is as vast as their experience in printing. Their expertise and guidance has proved useful at every step. Their uncompromising quality standards have made this book an exceptional effort. Their encouragement from time to time has been an inspiration for everyone.

The publisher and the editorial board hope that this book will prove to be a valuable piece of knowledge for researchers, students, practitioners and scholars across the globe.

List of Contributors

Anne M. Selvaag and Vibke Lilleby
Department of Rheumatology, Oslo University Hospital, Rikshospitalet, Nydalen, 0424 Oslo, Norway

Eva Kirkhus
Department of Radiology and Nuclear Medicine, Oslo University Hospital, Rikshospitalet, Oslo, Norway
Institute of Clinical Medicine, Faculty of Medicine, University of Oslo, Oslo, Norway

Berit Flatø
Department of Rheumatology, Oslo University Hospital, Rikshospitalet, Nydalen, 0424 Oslo, Norway
Institute of Clinical Medicine, Faculty of Medicine, University of Oslo, Oslo, Norway

Lena Törnqvist
Department of Radiology and Nuclear Medicine, Oslo University Hospital, Rikshospitalet, Oslo, Norway
Department of Radiology, Linköping University, Linköping, Sweden

Hanne A. Aulie
Department of Rheumatology, Oslo University Hospital, Rikshospitalet, Nydalen, 0424 Oslo, Norway
Department of Internal Medicine, Diakonhjemmet Hospital, Oslo, Norway

Leyla S. Namazova-Baranova, Saniya I. Valieva, Rina V. Denisova, Tatyana V. Sleptsova, Kseniya B. Isaeva, Alexandra M. Chomahidze, Nikolay I. Taibulatov, Anna N. Fetisova, Anna V. Karaseva and Alexandr A. Baranov
Federal State Autonomous Institution "National Scientific and Practical Center of Children's Health" Of the Ministry of Health of the Russian Federation, Moscow, Russia

Tatyana M. Bzarova
Federal State Autonomous Institution "National Scientific and Practical Center of Children's Health" Of the Ministry of Health of the Russian Federation, Moscow, Russia
Federal State Autonomous Educational Institution of Higher Education I.M. Sechenov First Moscow State Medical University of the Ministry of Health of the Russian Federation, Moscow, Russia

Ekaterina I. Alexeeva
Federal State Autonomous Institution "National Scientific and Practical Center of Children's Health" Of the Ministry of Health of the Russian Federation, Moscow, Russia
Federal State Autonomous Educational Institution of Higher Education I.M. Sechenov First Moscow State Medical University of the Ministry of Health of the Russian Federation, Moscow, Russia
Rheumatology Department, Federal State Autonomous Institution "National Scientific and Practical Center of Children's Health" Of the Ministry of Health of the Russian Federation, Moscow, Russia

Sonja Falvey
University of Mississippi School of Pharmacy, Oxford, USA

Lauren Shipman and Timothy Beukelman
Division of Pediatric Rheumatology, University of Alabama Birmingham, Birmingham, USA

Norman Ilowite
Children's Hospital at Montefiore, Albert Einstein College of Medicine, Bronx, USA

Helen Strike
Department of Paediatric Rheumatology, Bristol Royal Hospital for Children, Upper Maudlin Street, Bristol BS2 8BJ, UK

Ethan S. Sen and Athimalaipet V. Ramanan
Department of Paediatric Rheumatology, Bristol Royal Hospital for Children, Upper Maudlin Street, Bristol BS2 8BJ, UK
School of Clinical Sciences, University of Bristol, Bristol, UK

Michelle J. Morgan
Sirona Care & Health, Community Children's Health Partnership, Bristol, UK

Rachael MacLeod
Department of Paediatrics, Bristol Royal Hospital for Children, Bristol, UK

Ann Hinchcliffe
Retinal Treatment and Research Unit, Bristol Eye Hospital, Bristol, UK

Andrew D. Dick
School of Clinical Sciences, University of Bristol, Bristol, UK
Retinal Treatment and Research Unit, Bristol Eye Hospital, Bristol, UK
National Institute for Health Research Biomedical Research Centre at Moorfields Eye Hospital NHS Foundation Trust and UCL Institute of Ophthalmology, London, UK

Brinda Muthusamy
Department of Ophthalmology, Cambridge University Hospitals NHS Foundation Trust, Cambridge, UK

M. S. Camacho-Lovillo, W. Goycochea-Valdivia, L. Fernández-Silveira and O. Neth
Unidad de Enfermedades Infecciosas e Inmunopatologías Pediátrica, Hospital Universitario Virgen del Rocío/Instituto de Biomedicina de Sevilla (IBIS), Sevilla, Spain

A. Bulnes-Ramos and P. Pérez-Romero
Instituto de Biomedicina de Sevilla (IBIS), University Hospital Virgen del Rocío/CSIC/University of Sevilla, Unidad Clínica de Enfermedades Infecciosas, Microbiología y Medicina Preventiva, Sevilla, Spain

E. Núñez-Cuadros
Unidad de Reumatología Pediátrica, Hospital Materno Infantil, Hospital Regional Universitario de Málaga, Málaga, Spain

Marinka Twilt
Department of Paediatrics, Section of Rheumatology, Alberta Children's Hospital, University of Calgary, Calgary, AB, Canada
Department of Paediatrics, Division of Rheumatology, Aarhus University Hospital, Aarhus, Denmark

Dan Pradsgaard, Anne Helene Spannow and Carsten Heuck
Department of Paediatrics, Division of Rheum-atology, Aarhus University Hospital, Aarhus, Denmark

Arne Horlyck
Department of Radiology, Aarhus University Hospital, Aarhus, Denmark

Troels Herlin
Department of Paediatrics, Division of Rheumatology, Aarhus University Hospital, Aarhus, Denmark
Pediatric Rheumatology Clinic, Department of Pediatrics, Aarhus University Hospital, Palle Juul-Jensens Boulevard 99, DK-8200 Århus N, Denmark

Ellen Nordal and Veronika Rypdal
Department of Pediatrics, University Hospital of North Norway, and Department of Clinical Medicine, UiT the Arctic University of Norway, Tromsø, Norway

Terje Christoffersen
Department of Ophtalmology, University Hospital of North Norway, and Department of Clinical Medicine, UiT the Arctic University of Norway, Tromsø, Norway

Kristiina Aalto and Suvi Peltoniemi
Pediatric Rheumatology Clinic, Hospital for Children and Adolescents, University of Helsinki, Helsinki, Finland

Lillemor Berntson
Department of Women's and Children's Health, Uppsala University, Uppsala, Sweden

Anders Fasth
Department of Pediatrics, Institute of Clinical Sciences, Sahlgrenska Academy, University of Gothenburg, Gothenburg, Sweden

Troels Herlin
Department of Pediatrics, Aarhus University Hospital, Aarhus, Denmark

Susan Nielsen and Marek Zak
Pediatric Rheumatology Clinic, Rigshospitalet Copenhagen University Hospital, Copenhagen, Denmark

Bjørn Straume
Department of Community Medicine, UiT the Arctic University of Norway, Tromsø, Norway

Marite Rygg
Department of Clinical and Molecular Medicine, NTNU - Norwegian University of Science and Technology, and Department of Pediatrics, St. Olavs Hospital, Trondheim, Norway

Kristin Houghton, Kimberly Morishita, David A. Cabral, Ross E. Petty, Stuart E. Turvey and Lori B. Tucker
From British Columbia Children's Hospital and University of British Columbia, Vancouver, Canada

Jaime Guzman
From British Columbia Children's Hospital and University of British Columbia, Vancouver, Canada
Division of Pediatric Rheumatology, BC Children's Hospital, 4500 Oak St, Suite K4-122, Vancouver, BC V6H 3N1, Canada

Roxana Bolaria and Katherine Gross
Department of Pediatrics University of British Columbia, Vancouver, Canada

Janet Ellsworth
Stollery Children's Hospital and University of Alberta, Edmonton, Canada

Nicole Johnson, Paivi Miettunen, Heinrike Schmeling and Susanne Benseler
Alberta Children's Hospital and University of Calgary, Calgary, Canada

Alan M. Rosenberg
Royal University Hospital and University of Saskatchewan, Saskatoon, Canada

Kiem Oen
Department of Pediatrics and Child Health, University of Manitoba, Winnipeg, Canada

Roberta A. Berard
London Health Sciences Centre and Western University, London, Canada

Maggie Larché
McMaster University, Hamilton, Canada

Brian M. Feldman, Deborah M. Levy, Ronald M. Laxer, Earl Silverman, Lynn Spiegel, Rayfel Schneider, Shirley M. L. Tse, Bonnie Cameron and Rae S. M. Yeung
Hospital for Sick Children and University of Toronto, Toronto, Canada

Leanne M. Ward, Jinhui Ma, Karen Watanabe Duffy, Johannes Roth, Roman Jurencak, Michele Gibbon and Ciarán M. Duffy
Children's Hospital of Eastern Ontario and University of Ottawa, Ottawa, Canada

Rosie Scuccimarri, Sarah Campillo, Gaëlle Chédeville and Claire LeBlanc
McGill University Health Centre and McGill University, Montreal, Canada

Elie Haddad and Claire St. Cyr
Centre Hospitalier Universitaire Ste. Justine and Université de Montréal, Montréal, Canada

Debbie Feldman
Université de Montréal, Montréal, Canada

Gilles Boire and Alessandra Bruns
Centre Hospitalier Universitaire de Sherbrooke and Université de Sherbrooke, Sherbrooke, Canada

Anne-Laure Chetaille and Jean Dorval
Centre Hospitalier Universitaire de Laval and Université Laval, Quebec, Canada

Adam M. Huber, Elizabeth Stringer, Bianca Lang and Suzanne E. Ramsey
IWK Health Centre and Dalhousie University, Halifax, Canada

Paul Dancey
Janeway Children's Health and Rehabilitation Centre and Memorial University, Saint John's, Canada

Natalie J. Shiff
Shands Children's Hospital and University of Florida, Gainesville, USA

Tristan Kerr
Division of Pediatric Rheumatology, BC Children's Hospital, 4500 Oak St, Suite K4-122, Vancouver, BC V6H 3N1, Canada

Alexander Sauer and Thomas Pabst
Department of Diagnostic and Interventional Radiology, University Hospital Wuerzburg, 97080 Wuerzburg, Germany

Mengxia Li
Department of Radiation Oncology, University Hospital Wuerzburg, 97080 Wuerzburg, Germany

Annette Holl-Wieden
Department of Paediatrics, University Hospital Wuerzburg, 97080 Wuerzburg, Germany

Henning Neubauer
Department of Diagnostic and Interventional Radiology, University Hospital Wuerzburg, 97080 Wuerzburg, Germany

Department of Diagnostic and Interventional Radiology, University Hospital Ulm, Albert-Einstein-Allee 23, Ulm 89081, Germany
SRH Clinic of Radiology, 98527 Suhl, Germany

Anjali Sura, Christopher Failing, Julie Sturza and Meredith Riebschleger
University of Michigan, 1500 E Medical Center Dr, Ann Arbor, MI 48109, USA

Jasmine Stannard
IHA Rheumatology Consultants, 4990 W Clark Rd, Suite 300, Ypsilanti, MI 48197, USA

Boris Hügle
German Center for Pediatric and Adolescent Rheumatology (DZKJR), Gehfeldstrasse 24, 82467 Garmisch-Partenkirchen, Germany

Lea Höfel, Bruno Eppler, Magdalena Storf and Johannes-Peter Haas
German Center for Pediatric and Adolescent Rheumatology (DZKJR), Gehfeldstrasse 24, 82467 Garmisch-Partenkirchen, Germany
Center for Pain Treatment in Young People, Garmisch-Partenkirchen, Germany

Elizabeth Schnöbel-Müller
Center for Pain Treatment in Young People, Garmisch-Partenkirchen, Germany

Sarah L. Finch
College of Pharmacy and Nutrition, University of Saskatchewan, Saskatoon, Canada

Alan M. Rosenberg
Department of Pediatrics, University of Saskatchewan, Saskatoon, Canada

Hassan Vatanparast
College of Pharmacy & Nutrition and School of Public Health, University of Saskatchewan, 104 Clinic Place, Saskatoon, SK S7N 2Z4, Canada

Liane D. Heale, Victoria A. Maksymiuk and Greg D. Wells
Division of Rheumatology, The Hospital for Sick Children, 555 University Ave, Toronto, ON M5G 1X8, Canada

Y. Ingrid Goh
Division of Rheumatology, The Hospital for Sick Children, 555 University Ave, Toronto, ON M5G 1X8, Canada
Child Health Evaluative Sciences, The Hospital for Sick Children Research Institute, 686 Bay St, Toronto, ON M5G 0A4, Canada

Saunya Dover
Child Health Evaluative Sciences, The Hospital for Sick Children Research Institute, 686 Bay St, Toronto, ON M5G 0A4, Canada

Brian M. Feldman
Division of Rheumatology, The Hospital for Sick Children, 555 University Ave, Toronto, ON M5G 1X8, Canada
Department of Pediatrics and the Dalla Lana School of Public Health, University of Toronto, 155 College St., Toronto, ON M5T 3M7, Canada

Kristin M. Houghton, Jaime Guzman and Lori Tucker
Division of Rheumatology, K4-123 ACB, British Columbia Children's Hospital, 4480 Oak Street, Vancouver, BC V6H 3V4, Canada
Department of Pediatrics, University of British Columbia, Vancouver, BC, Canada

Heather M. Macdonald
Department of Family Practice, University of British Columbia, Vancouver, BC, Canada
Centre for Hip Health and Mobility, Vancouver Coastal Health Research Institute, Vancouver, BC, Canada

Heather A. McKay
Department of Family Practice, University of British Columbia, Vancouver, BC, Canada
Centre for Hip Health and Mobility, Vancouver Coastal Health Research Institute, Vancouver, BC, Canada
Department of Orthopaedics, University of British Columbia, Vancouver, BC, Canada

Ciarán Duffy
Division of Rheumatology, Department of Pediatrics, Children's Hospital of Eastern Ontario and University of Ottawa, Ottawa, Canada

Grace O'Sullivan, Siobhán O'Higgins, Sophia Saetes and Brian E. McGuire
Centre for Pain Research; School of Psychology, College of Arts, Social Sciences & Celtic Studies, Galway, NUI, Ireland

Line Caes
Division of Psychology; Faculty of Natural Sciences, University of Stirling, Stirling, Scotland, UK

Jennifer Stinson
The Hospital for Sick Children, Toronto, Canada
Child Health Evaluative Sciences, The Hospital for Sick Children, Toronto, Canada
Lawrence S. Bloomberg Faculty of Nursing, University of Toronto, Toronto, Canada

Georgina Tiller, Roger Allen, Peter Gowdie and Angela Cox
Department of Rheumatology, The Royal Children's Hospital, 50 Flemington Rd, Parkville, Melbourne, VIC 3052, Australia

Joanne Buckle, Jane Munro and Jonathan Akikusa
Department of Rheumatology, The Royal Children's Hospital, 50 Flemington Rd, Parkville, Melbourne, VIC 3052, Australia
Murdoch Childrens Research Institute, Melbourne, Australia

Tracy V. Ting
Cincinnati Children's Hospital Medical Center, Department of Pediatric Rheumatology, 3333 Burnet Ave, MLC 4010, Cincinnati, OH 45229, USA

Leslie A. Favier
Cincinnati Children's Hospital Medical Center, Department of Pediatric Rheumatology, 3333 Burnet Ave, MLC 4010, Cincinnati, OH 45229, USA
Cincinnati Children's Hospital Medical Center, Behavioral Medicine and Clinical Psychology, Center for Adherence and Self-Management, 3333 Burnet Ave, MLC 7039, Cincinnati, OH 45229, USA

Avani C. Modi
Cincinnati Children's Hospital Medical Center, Behavioral Medicine and Clinical Psychology, Center for Adherence and Self-Management, 3333 Burnet Ave, MLC 7039, Cincinnati, OH 45229, USA

Frances C. Sherratt, Louise Roper and Bridget Young
Department of Psychological Sciences, University of Liverpool, Whelan Building, Brownlow Hill, Liverpool L69 3GB, UK

Simon R. Stones
School of Healthcare, University of Leeds, Leeds, UK

Flora McErlane and Helen Foster
Great North Children's Hospital, Newcastle upon Tyne, UK
Institute Cellular Medicine, Newcastle University, Newcastle upon Tyne, UK

Matthew Peak
Clinical Research Division, Alder Hey Children's NHS Foundation Trust, Liverpool, UK

Eileen Baildam
Department of Paediatric Rheumatology, Alder Hey Children's NHS Foundation Trust, Liverpool, UK

Michael W. Beresford
Department of Paediatric Rheumatology, Alder Hey Children's NHS Foundation Trust, Liverpool, UK
Department of Women's and Children's Health, Institute of Translational Medicine, University of Liverpool, Liverpool, UK

Athimalaipet V. Ramanan
University Hospitals Bristol NHS Foundation Trust & Bristol Medical School, University of Bristol, Bristol, UK

Madeleine Rooney
School of Medicine, Dentistry and Biomedical Sciences, Queens University of Belfast, Belfast, UK

Paweł Więch, Izabela Sałacińska and Dariusz Bazaliński
Institute of Nursing and Health Sciences, Faculty of Medicine, University of Rzeszów, Al. mjr. W. Kopisto 2 a, 35-310 Rzeszów, Poland

Mariusz Dąbrowski
Institute of Nursing and Health Sciences, Faculty of Medicine, University of Rzeszów, Al. mjr. W. Kopisto 2 a, 35-310 Rzeszów, Poland
Diabetic Outpatient Clinic, Medical Center "Beta Med", Pl. Wolności 17, 35-073 Rzeszów, Poland

Anne Marit Selvaag and Vibke Lilleby
Department of Rheumatology, Oslo University Hospital, Rikshospitalet, Oslo, Norway

Hanne Aaserud Aulie
Department of Rheumatology, Oslo University Hospital, Rikshospitalet, Oslo, Norway

Department of Internal Medicine, Diakonhjemmet Hospital, Oslo, Norway

Mette-Elise Estensen
Department of Cardiology, Oslo University Hospital, Rikshospitalet, Oslo, Norway

Berit Flatø
Department of Rheumatology, Oslo University Hospital, Rikshospitalet, Oslo, Norway
Institute for Clinical Medicine, Medical Faculty, University of Oslo, Oslo, Norway

Svend Aakhus
Department of Circulation and Imaging, Faculty of Medicine and Health Science, Norwegian University of Science and Technology, NTNU, Trondheim, Norway
Clinic of Cardiology, St. Olavs Hospital, Trondheim, Norway

Damjana Ključevšek
Radiology Unit, University Children's Hospital Ljubljana, Ljubljana, Slovenia

Nina Emeršič
Department of Allergology, Rheumatology and Clinical Immunology, University Children's Hospital Ljubljana, Ljubljana, Slovenia

Nataša Toplak and Tadej Avčin
Department of Allergology, Rheumatology and Clinical Immunology, University Children's Hospital Ljubljana, Ljubljana, Slovenia
Department of Pediatrics, Medical Faculty, University of Ljubljana, Ljubljana, Slovenia

Erik Kindgren
Department of Pediatrics, Västervik Hospital, Västervik, Sweden
Division of Pediatrics, Department of Clinical and Experimental Medicine, Linköping University, Linköping, Sweden

Johnny Ludvigsson
Division of Pediatrics, Department of Clinical and Experimental Medicine, Linköping University, Linköping, Sweden

Mats Fredrikson
Division of Occupational and Environmental Medicine, Department of Clinical and Experimental Medicine, Linköping University, Linköping, Sweden
Forum Östergötland, Faculty of Medicine, Linköping University, Linköping, Sweden

William B. Brinkman, Ellen A. Lipstein, Janalee Taylor, Pamela J. Schoettker, Nancy Griffin, Carole Lannon and Esi Morgan
Department of Pediatrics, Cincinnati Children's Hospital Medical Center, 3333 Burnet Avenue, Cincinnati, OH 45229, USA

Katherine Naylor
University of Cincinnati College of Design, Architecture, Art and Planning, 5470 Aronoff, Cincinnati, OH 45221, USA

Karla Jones
Nationwide Children's Hospital, 700 Children's Drive, Columbus, OH 43205, USA

Sheetal S. Vora
Levine Children's Hospital, 1000 Blythe Blvd, Charlotte, NC 28203, USA

Catherine C. Mims
Medical University of South Carolina, 171 Ashley Ave, Charleston, SC 29425, USA

Elizabeth Roth-Wojcicki
Medical College of Wisconsin, 8701 W Watertown Plank Rd, Milwaukee, WI 53226, USA

Beth Gottlieb
Cohen Children's Medical Center of New York, 269-1 76th Ave, Queens, NY 11040, USA

Jenny Schlichtiger, Swaantje Barth, Betty Bisdorff, Lisa Hager and Katja Radon
Unit of Occupational and Environmental Epidemiology and Net Teaching, Institute and Outpatient Clinic for Occupational, Social and Environmental Medicine, University Hospital of Munich (LMU), Ziemssenstrasse 1, D-80336 Munich, Germany

Johannes-Peter Haas, Hartmut Michels and Boris Hügle
German Center for Pediatric and Adolescent Rheumatology, Garmisch-Partenkirchen, Germany

Index

www.ingramcontent.com/pod-product-compliance
Lightning Source LLC
LaVergne TN
LVHW080705210926
848485LV00003B/423
* 9 7 8 1 6 3 9 2 7 4 2 1 5 *